P9-DTK-022

HEALTH CARE IN AMERICA

HEALTH CARE IN AMERICA

The Political Economy of Hospitals and Health Insurance

Edited by
H.E. Frech III

Foreword by
Richard Zeckhauser

PACIFIC RESEARCH INSTITUTE FOR PUBLIC POLICY
San Francisco, California

Cloth ISBN 0–936488–18–2
Paperback ISBN 0–936488–19–0

Library of Congress Catalog Card Number 87–63451

Printed in the United States of America

Pacific Research Institute for Public Policy
177 Post Street
San Francisco, CA 94108
(415) 989-0833

Library of Congress Cataloging-in-Publication Data

Health Care in America.

Bibliography: p.
Includes indexes.
1. Medical economics—United States.   2. Hospitals—Economic aspects—United States.   3. Insurance, Health—United States.   4. Medical care—United States—Cost effectiveness.   I. Frech, H. E.
RA410.53.H417   1988   338.4'73621'0973   87–63451
ISBN 0–936488–18–2
ISBN 0–936488–19–0 (pbk.)

CONTENTS

PART I   HEALTH CARE COMPETITION

1

A Primer on Competition in Medical Markets
—*Mark V. Pauly*   27

PART II THE HOSPITAL INDUSTRY

2

An Economic History of American Hospitals
—Peter Temin   75

3

Property Rights in the Hospital Industry
—Frank A. Sloan   103

PART IV   PRIVATE HEALTH INSURANCE

LIST OF FIGURES

LIST OF TABLES

FOREWORD

Health economics is no longer a neglected child. One parent, the economics profession, once slighted the field as insufficiently rigorous. The other, the health care profession, rejected it on the grounds that it failed to understand the basic medical and institutional issues that underlie the structure of the health care industry. Moreover, the profession criticized economics, with its reliance on prices and incentives, as insensitive to values issues, in particular the special nature of medical care.

ENHANCED STATUS

Trends over the past couple of decades have enhanced the status of health economics with both parents. Economists welcome the fact that the original pioneers in the health economics field—mostly broad-ranging thinkers more concerned with exploring policy than with impressing their disciplinary colleagues—have been joined by a younger generation. That generation, though still interested in policy, is equipped with the latest economic tools and econometric techniques, the keys to many of their colleagues' hearts. The best of the second and third generations of health economists are represented in this volume.

In the industry, moreover, executives and policy-makers have embraced and implemented a range of proposals originally set forth by

xvii

economists. The messages of economists have been simple: try to give decision-makers the right incentives; promote competition; get prices right; where possible, let the market work; where that is impossible, promote market-like instruments.

It is interesting that such simple messages have been systematically neglected in other policy areas. The economist's standard suggestion that we employ effluent charges, for example, has been effectively ignored in the environmental area. When political necessity dictates that the nation limit imports of cars or textiles, it has typically used quotas despite the economists' consensus that tariffs could produce the same import levels while yielding revenues to the United States instead of monopoly profits to exporting nations. Proposals to substitute cash for in-kind transfers have also been ignored. A few policy innovations have pursued the economist's goal of promoting competition; airline deregulation is an example. For the most part, however, the ideas of economics have been kibitzing around the edges, influencing policy proposals but not policy.

One might have expected the health care field in particular to shun the message of economics. Its output, improved survival and life quality, is not sold on markets. Delicate values and ethical issues, rarely the chosen domain of economics, abound. Physicians have a strong professional interest in keeping economists out. And if health planners tend to have values and mind-sets somewhat inimical to economic approaches, health activists can be positively hostile. The substantial roles of third-party payers, nonprofit institutions, and governments suggest that standard economic models do not apply. And the politics of health care, which often focus on redistribution of services and health care as a right, are quite contrary to the economic frame of mind.

One might also have expected that economics would have had difficulties in the health field; health care is not a highly market-oriented industry. Nonprofit organizations still dominate in the hospital sector. Competition among doctors hardly conforms to the market norm, given their ability to influence demand for their own services, the difficulties patients encounter switching among providers, the effective absence of advertising, and the salient role assigned to ethics in guiding physician behavior. The product cannot be standardized and put on a shelf. Finally, the customer is rarely the prime decision-maker on major medical purchases, and the payer is usually a third party. In sum, the lessons of economics textbooks are not easily translated to the health care sector.

Why, then, has economics been successful in this domain? Three factors, I would argue, account for its success. First, there was a strong need. The sector was so poorly organized from the standpoint of incentives and appropriate pricing that even a little attention to resource costs and the effective arrangement of rewards and penalties would yield substantial gains. Second, costs were escalating out of sight, so that policy proposals oriented toward efficiency and cost control found a receptive ear. Physicians, often hostile to such proposals, found their control over health care and health policy ebbing. Indeed, efforts to make physicians behave more appropriately became a major consideration in the design of policies to constrain expenditures. Third, the health care field was ripe for entrepreneurs using economic concepts for their own purposes, for example exploiting economics of scale in providing medical supplies, or using expenditure control methods of modern for-profit management in building hospital chains. Moreover, the political climate was becoming more receptive to business and to market-oriented approaches to policy issues.

CONTRIBUTIONS OF ECONOMICS

To what extent were economists themselves responsible for the extensive introduction of economic concepts? Economists in general believe that markets induce participants—even those unfamiliar with econometric models of production functions—to come up with beneficial innovations. (See, for example, the discussion in this volume of preferred provider organizations, an entrepreneurial response to the need for both greater consumer choice and cost control.) However, many decisions in health care are public and political. For such decisions, public, political persuasion is required to bring about innovations. Thus economists, as analysts and policy intellectuals, have a role to play.

Surely the notion that competition fosters efficiency, perhaps the central lesson of microeconomics, was well understood by policymakers and health-sector participants long before the authors of this volume made their contributions. But there was always the nagging question of whether competition was appropriate to this sector. Economists helped create a climate in which the belief that competition makes sense for health care could gain support and credence. (Contrast, for example, the position of that beleaguered industry, primary and secondary education, which has received very limited attention from economists. The idea of competition for the public schools has had minimal political support.)

Where has economics played a direct role? Economists can take credit for drawing increased attention to the demand-limiting role of deductibles and coinsurance payments. The Rand Health Insurance Experiment significantly changed the policy debate in this area, as have numerous subsequent studies—some reported here—of the incentive effects of even small charges borne by the patient.

Economists were also instrumental in promoting the HMO concept as part of the broader recognition that prepaid arrangements will encourage care deliverers to economize on resources. For a variety of reasons, the HMO movement would not have developed so swiftly without government action. First, many regulatory hurdles had to be removed. Second, start-up funding was needed in many instances. Third, as predominantly nonprofit institutions, HMOs did not have the profit motive as an incentive for expansion. Fourth, they had to gain legitimacy among prospective subscribers and their employers (who paid most of the bill for HMO services). Economists wrote widely and testified frequently, helping to sway political opinion.

Economists also brought substantial intellectual capital to the health policy debate. They fostered a clear recognition of the inevitable trade-off between risk spreading and the provision of appropriate incentives. They set forth the concept of contingent claims, on which diagnosis-related groups (DRGs) are clearly based. These are new ideas. Though they may lack novelty for individuals brought up with the economics of uncertainty, that subject itself is predominantly a phenomenon of the past three decades.

Economists have also had a great deal to say on the merits of for-profit as opposed to nonprofit or publicly owned hospitals. They have joined both sides of the debate and have employed great ingenuity to test for differences in quality and price performance. That economists are found on both sides of this question reflects not only differences in values within the profession, but the inability of analytic models, by themselves, to give an unambiguous answer. Essays in this volume provide some further evidence on the subject.

More generally, these essays, bristling with discussions of incentives, cost-control mechanisms, and the potential for market-related policy proposals, capitalize on the dramatically improved environment for economic approaches to health policy. A critical question for those who study the history of policy development is how and to what extent such analyses by social scientists help shape our society's approaches to policy. Is their primary role to legitimize and give standing to arguments by government officials or policy activists? Or do they create fundamental preconditions and understanding for new policy directions? Whatever the answer, are their central lessons well understood, or so oversimplified in policy debate as to lose their relevance? For example, in assessing the effects of coinsurance on reducing the demand for services, will attention be paid to whether the curtailed services are those with low marginal benefits? The field having come of age, health economists should perhaps now examine the ways in which their profession has contributed to health policy.

HEALTH CARE AND VALUES

The health care system presents a challenge to the usual values assumptions of economists. Its practitioners, in theory, answer to an ethical code that subordinates revenues to patient care. In an individualistic, materialistic society, this creates a continuing tension, not unlike the one confronted by organized religion. Whether economists like it or not, society sees health care as different from other commodities. That is why most advanced nations have national health insurance. That is why the U.S. government plays such a significant role in financing health care, particularly for the elderly and the poor. That is why many citizens perceive health care to be a right, not a commodity to be purchased. If economists, perhaps emboldened by some recent successes in the health arena, condemn these beliefs too loudly, they may breed antagonisms that lead to the summary dismissal of their ideas. Ordinarily, economists believe that peoples' preferences and values are to be accepted as given. Can we legitimately make an exception when those values conflict with the economist's perspective? On the other hand, does respect for such preferences necessarily bar us, through some philosophical Hatch Act, from participating in values battles?

Values issues surrounding economic concepts foster fierce battles in the health care sector. Many critics sharply criticize the expansion of for-profit hospitals, arguing more from principle than from empirical evidence on performance, which turns out to be ambiguous. Despite clear documentation that they restrain utilization, economic incentives, such as deductibles and copayments, are often denounced. And government has acted to prohibit many instruments developed by those providing health coverage (for example, provisions limiting the coverage for certain conditions or treatments). This last issue will be brought to the fore by the AIDS epidemic and, in the longer term, by various genetic-screening techniques. Yet health care expenditures as a fraction of GNP continue to grow. At the same time, plans that limit reimbursement, such as DRGs, threaten to bankrupt some major health care institutions.

THE AGENDA FOR HEALTH ECONOMICS

Health care is a muddled sector: The visible hand of government, substantially influenced by politics, directs the flow of resources alongside the invisible hand of the market. The result is not close to anyone's ideal. Although private for-profit enterprises will expand or contract with their economic fortunes, and market forces will exert at least some discipline over nonprofits, there is less assurance that government activities will be substantially guided by a performance criterion relating to a cost-benefit or social welfare test. Once government activities (e.g., support for renal dialysis) are established, they are almost impossible to curtail. The argument that we could get more "bang"—progress against morbidity and mortality—"for our buck" elsewhere is unlikely to carry the day.

When matters are muddled in this fashion, the clear logic of careful economic thinking can be helpful. Indeed, economics can probably make a much greater contribution in health than in, say, the restaurant or vegetable-growing sectors of our economy, which have already been well and competitively organized by self-interested actors. But if clear logic were the sole contribution of this volume, it would be of only marginal interest. It also provides substantial evidence on a range of issues that cannot be settled with logic alone. These are questions that must be addressed in a second-best world; clear prescriptions based solely on first principles of economic theory may not apply. What is the evidence on provider-induced demand? Is adverse selection, a *bête noire* for economists, a serious problem in practice?

Given regulatory restrictions on expansion and the tax, fund-raising, and supposed agency advantages of non-profit hospitals, how might we expect the hospital sector to evolve? Are informational imperfections such that for-profit institutions can skim off the most desirable cases and deliver lower-quality care? For whose benefit does the non-profit hospital actually operate, the patients, the physicians, the trustees? When hospitals use DRGs as a cost-control mechanism, do they dismiss patients prematurely, or does the Hippocratic ethic, combined with the fact that a single doctor's contribution to total costs is trivial, provide sufficient protection?

Recognizing that any insurance plan warps incentives, how should plans be designed? What can we expect from private insurers? To whom should they be responsive? Why haven't they been effective in carrying out their insuring duties, controlling costs, prices, and quality? What are the consequences of supplementary insurance programs that pay deductibles in government programs; should they be taxed or regulated? How have cost-control experiments, such as second opinions for surgery and rebates for individuals not incurring any health costs in a year, performed? And perhaps most important, what does the record tell us about the performance of market discipline— for example, competition versus regulation as mechanisms to promote quality, or the extent of monopoly power within various realms of the health care system?

These questions and many more are addressed in this volume. Some essays draw on specific experiences or case studies, others on broadly based empirical studies. Although these analyses employ up-to-date economic techniques, some of the best aspects of early work in health economics are preserved: a strong attention to institutional detail, a clear recognition that history influences present circumstances, and a helpful blend of fact finding and policy insight.

Richard Zeckhauser
Harvard University

INTRODUCTION

H. E. Frech III

The health care industry is going through exciting changes. Competition is increasing. Preferred provider organizations (PPOs) are proliferating. In Europe, some insurers are giving rebates in the form of a prepaid deductible to policyholders who have not filed claims during a given period. Any kind of insurance scheme seems possible now. Profit-seeking hospitals are growing and even invading the world of high-tech academic medicine, such as heart transplants. Humana, a profit-seeking hospital chain, has offered to build and operate an academic hospital for the University of Southern California. Medicare is now using the diagnosis-related group (DRG) fixed reimbursement for each hospital admission to improve hospital incentives to cut costs. In southern California, health maintenance organizations (HMOs) are advertising for Medicare enrollees. The future seems to hold the promise—or threat—of greater changes. While some of these changes have helped to slow the explosion of health care expenditures, these expenditures are still very large (much larger than the nation's defense budget) and are still growing faster than the American economy. Furthermore, the federal deficit puts continuing pressure on the government to reduce its health care expenditures.

This collection of papers is designed to shed light on the issues underlying these developments. The papers vary a great deal. Some focus on little-known but important problems or facts about health

1

care. Some provide state-of-the-art surveys of important topics. Some interpret recent or historical developments and trends in the rapidly changing health care environment.

All the essays are original and at the frontiers of our knowledge. Thus, they should be of interest to specialized professional researchers or policy analysts. On the other hand, we have striven to make the presentation of the papers as nontechnical as possible. The material is accessible to the nonspecialist, even though some of it is inherently difficult. Where an algebraic, geometric, or statistical argument seemed helpful, we have provided a parallel verbal analysis. Thus a lack of mathematical, economic, or statistical background should be no obstacle to understanding the essays.

With a single exception all the essays are written by economists and thus take a definitely economic viewpoint. They reflect the authors' shared belief that economic and political forces are intertwined and, together with technology, determine the evolution of the health care industry.

This economic viewpoint is especially helpful now because the two major developments, Medicare's DRG system and the growth of PPOs, represent a new public and private adoption of economic ideas. The DRG system is the first national attempt to harness profit and loss incentives to induce hospitals to control costs efficiently and appropriately. This system views the hospital as primarily a business operation, whether it is legally organized as a profit-seeking firm, a private nonprofit firm, or a government firm. PPOs view physicians and hospitals similarly. The idea is to offer them additional customers if they are willing to accept lower prices and aggressive utilization controls. PPOs provide a mechanism whereby providers can choose to compete more aggressively in ways that are beneficial to the insurer and the consumer.

The order of presentation of the papers is purposeful. Mark Pauly's paper on competition in health care, which constitutes Part I of the volume, is the most general of the papers. It captures the dynamism of the growing competition in the health care market and thus provides a background for the remaining essays. It places some of the blame for current health care problems on well-intentioned but misguided government health insurance programs and regulations, which have undermined the efficiency and competitiveness of health care markets. Two contributions on the hospital industry (Part II) follow.

The first details its surprising historical evolution; the second examines the issues surrounding the growth of profit-seeking hospitals. The next section (Part III) contains two papers on government health insurance. The first is a sharply focused essay on a little-known but serious flaw in the design of Medicare health insurance for the elderly. The second is a broad and knowledgeable survey of the economic problems created by the large government health insurance plans, coupled with excellent suggestions for reform.

The last section (Part IV) is the largest because it deals with the area of the most profound and most hopeful change. It covers private health insurance, which in recent years has awakened from its much criticized slumber and is now the driving force behind some vital changes. The first paper in this section examines the possible explanations for the past stagnation of the private insurance industry. Specifically, it asks why private insurance companies passively paid huge and rising claims for years with little effort to control costs. The second paper zeroes in on a little-known fact of the recent history of private health insurance: its rapidly declining price. The third paper looks at a continuing problem in health insurance—the monopoly buying power of some health insurers, in particular that of the powerful Massachusetts Blue Shield. This is followed by a paper that reports on an exciting new development in German private health insurance, whereby consumers are choosing policies that give them large premium rebates in the form of prepaid deductibles if no claims have been made in a given year. Because it does not demand cash out of pocket at the time of illness, this form of deductible may be preferred by some customers or groups.

The last paper ends the book on an upbeat note. It provides an economic rationale for the phenomenal growth of PPOs. In response to wasteful health insurance, the market is creating a new economic institution. Following is a more detailed discussion of the individual papers.

COMPETITION

Mark Pauly takes a broad approach, defining competition as voluntary market response and interaction. He contrasts competition with regulation designed to supplant the market. This approach captures the most important issue in health policy, the power of consumers in the market versus that of governments, bureaucracies, and the medical profession.

Pauly stresses that in making policy comparisons, one must be careful to be realistic. One must compare actual, attainable regulations to market competition. Pauly lives up to this ideal in his essay. He considers six interrelated ways in which the market is conventionally said to have failed. These supposed failures have been used to justify various kinds of regulation and other government and professional interventions. The six failures are

1. Moral hazard and flat-of-the-curve medicine
2. Private supply of cost-containment devices
3. Consumer information imperfections and demand creation
4. Redistribution of income from the sick to the well
5. Excess capacity and the technological imperative
6. Squeezing the poor

These analyses are often iconoclastic. Pauly focuses the most attention on item 6, squeezing the poor.

Alleged market failures 1, 2, and 5 all deal with moral hazard— the idea that insuring against some undesirable event makes such an event more likely because people know they are insured. These criticisms have been historically important in the health planning movement that gave us local and regional health planning, certificate-of-need (CON) laws, and in some states hospital rate regulation. The once-dominant idea behind health planning can be summarized as follows: Health insurance leads consumers to demand, and providers to supply, too much medical care that is too high in quality and therefore wasteful. Private health insurers, employers, and consumers are unable or unwilling to curb this excess. Thus planning should be used directly to reduce the supply of services. Initially this reduction occurred through voluntary planning, which was simply a local cartel or conspiracy among hospitals designed to reduce entry and investment. In the 1970s, after recognizing that private hospital cartels could not completely suppress competition, planners got government backing in the form of the CON laws. Hospital rate regulation was also advocated to reduce the competition in quality and other nonprice aspects of hospital care.

Pauly shows that the planning movement's fall from grace is due not to mere fad, but to the discovery that its central argument is in many ways flawed. Research has shown that regulation has been largely ineffective in controlling costs. But regulation has an additional disadvantage: It treats all consumers as though they were the same. The recent spectacular growth of PPOs and other private insurer cost-control measures has shown that the private market can and now does supply cost control that allows for choice and diversity. Pauly states that there is no longer market failure in cost containment.

Health maintenance organizations (HMOs) control utilization directly by the internal management of the plan and by limiting the number of physicians and hospital beds available. PPOs, as I mention in my essay in this volume, often control utilization by such previously rare devices as mandatory second opinions for surgery and requiring insurer authorization for initial and continued hospitalization. PPOs also control the cost per unit of care by building in incentives to use preferred (lower-cost) providers. Much like indemnity insurance, the PPO does allow consumers to use more costly providers, but they must pay the additional cost per unit out of their pockets. Furthermore, after twenty years of declining consumer copayment and declining popularity of indemnity insurance, the past few years has witnessed a sharp turnaround.

Deductibles are rapidly becoming larger and more common, as is coinsurance. Pauly reports that traditional indemnity insurance (which pays a set dollar amount per unit of service) is undergoing a renaissance. Indemnity insurance has long been praised by economists such as Pauly, Ginsburg, Newhouse, Taylor, and me for its superior incentives. The increasing copayment is important for a couple of reasons. First, it preserves the maximum consumer choice. Second, it is the one cost-control scheme that always works. It is not dependent on the continuing resolve and managerial ability of the insurance company, PPO, or HMO, as are administrative cost controls. Why private insurance has not supplied much administrative or copayment cost control has until recently remained a mystery. Clark Havighurst's essay in this volume is the best effort yet at an explanation.

Pauly also discusses the concern that poorly informed consumers will be induced to consume too much care through dishonest advice from providers. This is called demand creation, or provider-induced demand. In the past, large variations in the intensity of treatment of apparently similar groups of people have been presented as evidence for the demand-creation hypothesis. However, Pauly reports that the huge cross-sectional variation cannot be explained by provider-induced demand. Unfortunately, no one knows which of the observed patterns of cost is appropriate, because no one knows how much and which medical care is really worth the cost. Pauly does see some role for government in helping to provide this information to consumers. Once this information was provided, however, consumers would make their own decisions with respect to the health care they wanted to buy. The choice of the best medical care is often intimately bound up with the values and attitudes of the patient. No objective hard-and-fast rule is possible.

In discussing redistribution from the sick to the well, Pauly directly attacks community rating. Something of a sacred cow, community rating is simply charging the same premium to individuals with different known risks. It is enshrined in the federal HMO act and it is preached and practiced by some Blue Cross and Blue Shield plans. Nonetheless, Pauly says that it is simply a bad idea, based on a misunderstanding of how insurance works. Not only is it unfair, forcing the low risks to pay too much to subsidize insurance for the high risks, but it leads the low risks to purchase too little insurance and the high risks too much. A superior and more honest way to redistribute from the known well to the known sick is through an explicit tax and subsidy. Moreover, this redistribution can prevent redistribution from the poor well to the wealthy sick, while community rating cannot. Indeed, Lien fu Huang and Richard Rosett showed that Blue Cross/Blue Shield community rating transfers wealth from the poor to the rich and from blacks to whites.[1]

Pauly's discussion of adverse selection suggests that (1) the problem is probably not very serious, and (2) the worst of it is that the good risks get priced out of the insurance market by being inadvertently or purposely lumped in with the bad risks. The second of these contradicts the conventional view.

Squeezing the Poor

The possibility that competition will reduce the well-being of the poor is currently considered the major defect of competition. Pauly shows

---

1. See Lien fu Huang and Ricard N. Rosett, "Redistribution of Income through Blue Cross Community-Rated Premiums." (Discussion Paper No. 72–9, Department of Economics, University of Rochester, June 1972).

that this argument is, at its heart, not only economically inefficient but is based on a fundamentally dishonest approach to politics and policy.

The argument against competition runs like this: Monopoly power for hospitals allows them to earn monopoly rents or profits when treating middle- and upper-class consumers. The hospitals then use these monopoly returns to cross-subsidize the other activities the hospital decision-makers favor, including providing uncompensated hospital care to the poor. Protection of this monopoly power is then used as an excuse for regulation. Monopoly and regulation are wrapped in the mantle of charity. An especially clear example is Maryland's hospital rate regulation, where rates are explicitly set high enough to cover uncompensated hospital care.

But caring for the uninsured poor may be very low on hospital's list of preferred activities, especially a research or teaching hospital. One might also note that this argument makes little sense for profit-seeking hospitals.

There is little evidence that increasing hospital competition has, in fact, reduced uncompensated care. There is little evidence that the non-Medicaid poor are missing hospital care of real value to them. It is sobering to note that the uninsured poor are hospitalized at about the same rate as are middle-class consumers who are enrolled in HMOs.

Throughout this discussion, Pauly has noted a confusion between uncompensated hospital care and care for the poor. It is likely that most uncompensated care is provided to those who are not poor. And most of the poor receive compensated care under Medicaid, Medicare, and/or private insurance. There is an efficient, direct, and honest approach to the real problem of underconsumption by the poor—a broadly based tax to support an explicit subsidy. This is not a new idea, of course; it is a description of Medicaid. Medicaid was designed to replace private and public charity and hospital monopoly cross-subsidization with a government insurance program empowering the poor to enter the ordinary private market. For political reasons, Medicaid has not completely achieved its promise, but it has made an enormous difference.

Pauly describes as bizarre and baroque the roundabout and wasteful ways of subsidizing the poor advocated by the defenders of regulation and monopoly. An outright tax on hospitals to pay for uncompensated care would be wasteful and regressive, and would fall particularly hard on the sick. A tax on health insurance might be slightly better.

But both of these are somewhat self-defeating, since they discourage consumers from purchasing health insurance, thus increasing the size of the problem. Monopoly, whatever its source, adds additional inefficiencies to a tax.

Some defenders of monopoly and regulation recognize the waste inherent in these indirect financing schemes. Nonetheless, they argue that these methods must be pursued because direct financing is not politically feasible. Pauly exposes this as a plan to deceive the electorate by "political flim-flam, hiding the costs off-budget, disguising taxation as regulation, and insulating the choice by moving the locus fact that although he might personally prefer more government subsidy of the poor's medical consumption, this does not give him the right to engage in dishonest political maneuvering to force the rest of the country to go along with him. Thus the major remaining objection to growing competition fades away on both efficiency and moral grounds.

The other papers are less sweeping and easier to describe, but not less interesting. For example, Peter Temin's essay on the history of American hospitals paints a fascinating and little-known picture that is relevant to some policy discussions today. In particular, he explains why it is that nonprofit hospitals have come to dominate, in spite of the fact that Robert Clark in his article in *Harvard Law Review,* as well as many others, claim that they are not appropriate for the modern hospital industry.

THE HOSPITAL INDUSTRY

Temin tells us that hospitals were originally wholly charitable institutions, devoted to the care of the poor and supported by public and/ or private contributions, often from churches. They did not charge for services. These early hospitals did not furnish much medical care. And that was probably good, since historians believe that medical care was, on balance, dangerous to one's health. Since it was considered (and was) safer and more comfortable to receive medical treatment at home, the middle class did so. Given their charitable role, it was natural for nineteenth-century hospitals to be organized under the nonprofit form.

This form is superior to the profit-seeking form for receiving contributions and grants. In a profit-seeking firm, the donor would expect his contribution simply to be passed along to the stockholders. Only a large donor, who could execute, monitor, and enforce a contract with a profit-seeking firm, could expect to use such a firm for charitable purposes. For smaller donors and donors with poor ability to monitor contracts, the nonprofit form at least guarantees that the donation will be spent on expanding the work of the firm rather than being transferred to stockholders. It is telling that U.S. government grants, with little monitoring, can be given only to nonprofit firms, while contracts with more monitoring built in can be entered into with profit-seeking organizations. The guarantee that funds will be spent on the work of the firm is not free, however. The cost is that the nonprofit firm is managed and monitored less intensely by its own top decision-makers, so it operates less efficiently.

Since the mid-nineteenth century, the nature of the hospital has been almost totally transformed. Medical care became helpful as effective antitoxins and the radical idea of cleanliness in surgery spread. Moreover, urbanization and the decline of the extended family made home treatment more difficult. Hospitals became superior to home care, especially for surgery. By the turn of the century, the middle class had started to use hospitals. Hospitals began charging patients, philanthropy declined, and hospitals started changing from charities into businesses, a process that continues to this day. By the Great Depression, charity provided less than half of hospital income. Frank Sloan calculates that today private contributions provide less than 10 percent of hospitals' construction funds and less than 2 percent of operating funds. And most of that is for research, not patient care. Of course, this has been partly a result of the purposeful socialization of charity through Medicare and Medicaid.

Temin also provides some insight into the mystery of why health insurers until recently had so little interest in cost control. By founding Blue Cross during the Depression, the hospitals themselves began modern health insurance. From the beginning it was designed to provide revenue for the hospitals and to restrict competition among them. No wonder a commitment to complete coverage and little cost control became traditional. The now-standard explanation for the rise in hospital costs since World War II, associated with Martin Feldstein, is based on a large expansion of private and public insurance.

Surprisingly, Temin expresses some skepticism about two key elements in the Feldstein analysis: the price sensitivity of the demand for health care and the price sensitivity of demand for health insurance. I believe that Temin's skepticism on the price sensitivity of hospital demand comes from a misinterpretation of the Rand Corporation's health insurance experiment. Joseph Newhouse and the other Rand economists found that randomly assigned copayment greatly reduced ambulatory and hospital use. For example, 25 percent coinsurance reduced hospital expenditures by about the same percentage. Length of stay of those who were admitted was little affected. Temin takes this to mean that hospital demand is insensitive to price once one has made the decision to be hospitalized.

But the selection of who goes to the hospital under coinsurance is not random. Only the relatively sicker people are willing to make the financial sacrifice. Thus, based on selection, one would expect longer stays of the sicker people who are hospitalized under coinsurance. That the data show no difference indicates that coinsurance does indeed reduce length of stay. Furthermore, the experimental coinsurance went to zero by the time the patient had been hospitalized for a day or two, so it could not have affected length of stay for many patients. And regardless of whether the main impact of coinsurance is on admission rates or demand for additional days and services for those who are admitted, the Rand study shows the effect to be large.

On the issue of the price sensitivity of the demand for health insurance as distinct from the demand for health care, Temin relies on Martin Feldstein's early work, using state aggregates as observations and gets substantially different results than more recent work. Charles Phelps's work on cross-sectional micro data clearly shows that the demand for insurance is quite price sensitive, substantially more so than the demand for health care. More recently, Phelps has estimated the price elasticity of demand for health insurance, using time-series data, with similar results.

Frank Sloan's paper is a masterful survey of the large but difficult-to-digest literature on hospital property rights and performance. He considers in depth, but finally rejects, the benign public interest arguments for the existence of nonprofit hospitals. He finds Robert Clark's analysis of the tax benefits of nonprofit status and the relative ease of physician dominance most plausible, and notes that if physicians do dominate, then the nonprofit hospital is really a profit-seeking firm in disguise; it's just that the profits go to the physicians who use the hospital rather than to stockholders. To this I would add the historical accident that hospitals started out as charities, even though they have by now changed into businesses.

The standard property rights and public choice theories would predict that nonprofit hospitals would be less efficient than profit-seeking ones. Results from other industries suggest that the differences may be large. After an exhaustive analysis of the literature, however, Sloan finds the efficiency advantage to be quite small—at most a few percentage points, and perhaps zero. Future research may allow more exact measurement, but we know enough now to say that the differences are not large. He finds profit-seeking and private nonprofit hospitals to be surprisingly similar in other ways as well. For example, the amount of free care (charity plus bad debts) provided by profit-seeking hospitals was almost the same as that provided by nonprofit ones. In cities, the profit-seeking free care was slightly less common (3.0 versus 3.7 percent), while outside the cities the profit-seeking hospitals were more generous (4.2 versus 4.0 percent). The fact that both percentages are so low underscores the modern transformation of hospitals from charities to businesses.

Sloan's argument is convincing. First, because of doctor control, nonprofit hospitals' incentives are more like those of profit-seeking ones than meets the eye. Second, owing to incentives for overinsurance that arose in the 1960s and 1970s, no hospital has had a very strong incentive to control costs. I might add that competition, as imperfect as it has been, has prevented the worst of nonprofit waste.

GOVERNMENT HEALTH INSURANCE

Amy Taylor, Pamela Farley, and Constance Horgan analyze a serious weakness in Medicare health insurance for the aged. The system unexpectedly created an incentive for private insurers and enrollees to undermine Medicare's cost control. The problem, first analyzed theoretically by Mark Pauly, is this: Medicare requires cost-sharing on physician and hospital care. However, 66 percent of Medicare enrollees negate this cost-control device by purchasing private supplemental (Medigap) insurance that fills in all or most of the Medicare copayment. Another 11 percent have Medicaid insurance that performs the same function. So the cost controls designed into the system affect only 23 percent of the Medicare population.

An immediate prediction problem is created by the supplemental insurance. If Medicare were to raise copayments to improve cost control, how much of the additional cost containment would be negated by supplemental insurance? Also, would more cost-sharing induce more or less purchase of Medigap insurance? Taylor, Farley, and Horgan quantitatively analyze these difficult issues.

Medigap insurance has an enormous impact on utilization, estimated in their paper to be 27 percent for hospital costs and 23 percent for physician expenditures for those with group supplemental insurance. The authors argue that this difference is not due to selection, because group insurance holders have little choice. I believe that the result does reflect some selection, since groups choose in the interests of their members. However, since these results are close to those found in the Rand experiment, I suspect that the overstatement of the effect due to selection bias is probably small. Since the bulk of this cost increase is picked up by Medicare, Medigap insurance shifts a large burden to the Medicare budget and the taxpayer. Why, it may be asked, is Medigap insurance so popular when Medicare's cost-sharing is modest by modern standards? One answer is that this insurance allows the enrollee and the insurer to exploit Medicare and the taxpayer. In effect, Medicare provides an unwitting subsidy to the very Medigap insurance that is destructive of its own cost controls. The magnitude of the subsidy is surprisingly large.

In 1977, Medicare enrollees with group insurance paid an average of $142 per year for Medigap insurance that reduced their expected out-of-pocket total payment by $11. Thus, the net expected increase in annual out-of-pocket payment, including insurance premiums, was $131. However, Taylor, Farley, and Horgan found that this Medigap insurance raised total expected expenditures by $204. Of this, about 90 percent was paid by Social Security; thus the subsidy from Medicare to those who purchase group Medigap insurance was about $180. Applying these figures to the full 66 percent of the population with private Medigap insurance, we find that about 14 percent of Medicare hospital expenditures and about 12 percent of physicians' services expenditures go for these unintended subsidies of wasteful private supplemental insurance. What's more, the subsidies redistribute income in a way that charitably minded taxpayers are unlikely to approve, favoring the relatively wealthy Medicare enrollees since they are much more likely to purchase supplemental insurance.

Economic efficiency does not require the complete elimination of this private Medigap insurance. But it does require that a tax be placed on it equal to the Medicare subsidy so that Medicare is not harmed by an individual's purchase of the insurance. In this volume, Paul Ginsburg suggests such a tax. In the case of the average 1977 group policy, the tax would be $180 per year, or 127 percent of premiums by my calculation. (Ginsburg suggests a smaller tax of about 35 percent of premiums.) Clearly, such a tax would greatly reduce the popularity of private supplemental insurance, perhaps to the point of virtual disappearance. This in turn would substantially improve Medicare cost containment.

Taylor, Farley, and Horgan also try to estimate the price elasticity of demand for private supplemental insurance, but data limitations force them to use total premiums as a measure of the price of insurance. As Jody Sindelar explains in her essay, the ratio of benefits to premiums is the ideal measure.

The other paper on public insurance, by Paul Ginsburg, provides a general treatment of the problems caused by Medicare and Medicaid and possible policy changes to reform the systems. Ginsburg begins with an excellent, concise history of the federal government's involvement in health care, starting well before the 1965 enactment of Medicare and Medicaid. He demonstrates the rapid rise in costs of both systems, caused by the moral hazard effect of more complete insurance for the aged and the poor. He then traces the series of reforms that have characterized the programs since the very beginning, when, to the apparent surprise of the founders of the programs, costs soared.

But Ginsburg emphasizes the major reforms of the past few years. The most important are the Medicare DRG payment system for hospitals, more freedom and smaller subsidies for state Medicaid programs, Medicare enrollment in private HMOs, and the physicians' fee freeze and participating physician program. Ginsburg reports that the DRG system already appears to have dramatically slowed rises in hospital costs. The physician fee freeze, on the other hand, appears to me to have increased expenditures on physicians' services. Early data from the Congressional Budget Office indicate that the freeze reduced prices and thus increased utilization. It will not be surprising if fuller analysis supports this conclusion, given the work of John

Holahan and others at the Urban Institute. They found that a similar fee freeze during the Nixon price controls in the early 1970s had increased physician expenditures.

Ginsburg predicts that the new and little-known HMO option, in effect a voucher program, will be very popular. Indeed, in California HMOs have begun television advertising for Medicare enrollees.

The paper concludes with an excellent discussion of future policy options, more use of DRG-type prospective payment, more copayments, use of capitation for individual physicians, and use of PPOs. Ginsburg is somewhat less optimistic than I am about increased use of cost-sharing, though he favors a substantial tax on Medigap insurance and at least experimentation with a premium-rebate scheme, such as is described by Peter Zweifel in the section on private insurance.

PRIVATE HEALTH INSURANCE

Clark Havighurst starts off this section by trying to solve a riddle that was noted by Mark Pauly. Why have private health insurers been so reluctant, until recently, to use cost controls? The most important of the missed opportunities for cost control have been cost-sharing, contracting with providers selectively over utilization and price, and prior authorization for hospitalization or costly elective procedures. Of these, only cost-sharing was used, and not nearly enough, until recently. Havighurst contrasts the insurance industry's excellent record of being tough with auto body shops and dentists to its passive payment of any medical claim that was not outrageous. The possible explanations range from the purely psychological and ideological to the purely legal.

One hypothesis explored by Havighurst is that reforms of traditional insurance were hampered by the belief prevailing in the 1970s that only HMOs would work or be acceptable to the government in the long run. Some varieties of HMOs, of course, represent a very high degree of insurer interference in medical care. The belief that HMOs, as defined by the government, were the only practical or acceptable alternative may have prevented smaller movements in the direction of reform of traditional insurance, particularly PPO development. This would not be the first case of the best obstructing the good, or of government's narrow vision precluding desirable change.

A second argument is that there was no demand for cost containment—that insurance customers, particularly large employers, did not favor it. One can find some support for this view in surveys of employee benefit administrators. However, it is hard to believe that companies that expend a great deal of effort to save a small amount of money in production would be happy to waste millions on inefficient insurance. The survey results may simply reflect the fact that middle managers who deal with employee benefit issues adopt the viewpoint of the employees and unions and/or realize that active cost containment would make their jobs more difficult. Havighurst notes the highly political nature of employee benefits and suggests, convincingly, that this climate makes symbolism important and interferes with rational behavior.

The commercial insurers themselves claim that they hold market shares that are too small to make them effective cost controllers— that is, that they do not have the clout to bargain with providers. For years they have tried to get an antitrust exemption to allow them to deal with physicians and hospitals collectively. Havighurst easily dismisses their claim by noting that recently HMOs and PPOs that could steer patients to a price-cutting provider have been able to negotiate substantial price discounts and utilization controls with minuscule market shares. A related argument has been put forward by Mark Pauly and others.

If cost containment were to benefit other consumers and other insurers, there might be little incentive for any one insurer to provide it. Cost control would be, as Havighurst notes, what economists call a public good. This may be true of some cost-containment initiatives, but the growth of PPOs shows that it is far from general. Also, empirical research has shown that, where the Blue Cross/Blue Shield plans have large market shares, health care costs are higher, not lower. At least for the Blues, a large market share is not conducive to good cost control.

Another interesting possibility raised by Havighurst is that the insurers have colluded to prevent cost containment. The incentive for such collusion is there. It is also clear that the industry favors cooperation and the presentation of a united front, partly through the Health Insurance Association of America. But although the industry might like to collude, it is so unconcentrated that any attempt to do so would be likely to fail. There are hundreds of commercial insurers, and Havighurst reports that the top five have less than one-sixth of the group market. While it is probable that no actual conspiracy ever existed, Havighurst notes that the industry is characterized by weak entrepreneurship and aversion to innovation.

In this connection, Havighurst calls attention to two final and related causes for the lack of active cost control by commercial insurers. One is the opposition of providers, especially physicians, to insurer initiatives. The second is the market power and behavior of the Blue Cross/Blue Shield plans, which were founded by, and originally controlled by, the hospitals and physicians. In recent years, the degree of provider control has declined in some of the Blue plans, but this has not made much difference, because the basic philosophy or ideology of the plans has not changed. Havighurst also suggests, as noted below, that the Blues' policies reflect a rational strategy for a nonprofit firm and that their corporate interests were well served by maintaining their close alliances with provider cartels.

Physician opposition to HMOs and to active insurer cost control is not dead. Recently the Medical Society of Michigan organized a boycott of Blue Shield. Indiana dentists organized a similar boycott. Both groups of practitioners were sued successfully by the Federal Trade Commission. Why the insurance industry was, until recently, so easily intimidated by the providers is still puzzling, though Havighurst's hypothesis helps to clarify the matter. Limiting the ability of providers to threaten insurers is a positive role for antitrust enforcement—perhaps the most successful government activity in health care. Although Havighurst stops short of that conclusion, I believe that the most important single cause of health insurers' poor historical record has been their fear of boycott by physicians and/or hospitals. Partly because of more active antitrust enforcement in health care, and partly because the internal discipline of the organized providers appears to be breaking down, this threat is clearly waning.

Because of their origin and early leadership, the Blues offered health insurance that served the interests of hospitals and doctors. That is, they offered overly complete insurance with little cost-sharing. Further, their rules required that they contract with all or most providers, preserve the consumer's free choice of provider, and reimburse in ways that minimized the subscriber's incentive to patronize a low-cost provider. These features of Blue Cross/Blue Shield coverage combined to discourage competition among hospitals or physicians.

Although this pro-provider bias would seem to create a market opportunity for the commercial insurers, the Blue plans have many cost advantages, including favorable tax and regulatory treatment. In many states, the Blues pay no premium tax, while the commercial firms pay 2 percent of gross premiums. More important are provider discounts. In many states, the Blue Cross plans receive a discount from the hospitals of as much as 10 percent, while the Blue Shield plans get a discount from the physicians of as much as 30 percent. These discounts give the Blues a cost advantage that increases their share of the insurance market.

Using Blue Cross and hospitals as his example—though the argument seems applicable to Blue Shield and physicians as well—Havighurst argues that providers as a group may be better off granting discounts to an insurer with policies and practices that are to their benefit. By collectively granting such discounts to a friendly Blue plan, providers could ensure that the plan would continue such policies and would not exert its buying power against them individually, extracting even bigger discounts. With their biggest customer thus converted into an ally, providers could have greater confidence that, as interdependent oligopolists, they would each recognize the long-term harm to them all if any one of them should grant competitive discounts to other payers, such as HMOs, to gain a short-term advantage. According to Havighurst's hypothesis, as long as the provider cartel or oligopoly holds together, a Blue plan is better off not using its power to the fullest extent, because the cartel, by fending off competitors' efforts at cost control, ensures the Blue plan the maximum *net* cost advantage over its competitors. According to Havighurst's theory, it would seem to pay for the Blues to use their monopsony power fully only in markets where provider cartels have become ineffective. Thus Havighurst's hypothesis would probably be far more likely to hold for Blue Cross and hospitals than for Blue Shield and physicians. It would also be less likely to hold in larger urban areas, where oligopolistic interactions are weaker.

My own article on the Kartell case discusses the use of monopsony power by the Blue plans. The paper finds that high Blue Shield market share and high physician discounts are positively associated. Other research indicates that the same is true for Blue Cross market share and Blue Cross hospital discount.

Contrary to Judge Frank Easterbrook's claim in the 1986 Ball Memorial case, the Blues *are* special.[2] It is clear that they have unique advantages, giving them real market power, even though the commercial health insurance sector is quite competitive. As Havighurst suggests, the Blues' close alliance with provider cartels is a way of preserving their cost advantage over payers that might use selective purchasing to control costs. It appears, however, that another important source of the Blues' strength is their monopsony power in health care markets. Providers are increasingly faced with Blue plans willing to exercise monopsony power that they previously had used less aggressively. Some might see poetic justice in the Blues' turning on their one-time masters. Of course, poetic justice and efficiency are not the same. Blue plan monopsony can easily go so far as to cause waste, especially if it serves the traditional Blue plan preference for overly complete insurance, as was the case in *Kartell*.

Fortunately, it seems that, as provider cartels are weakening and HMOs and PPOs are gaining strength, the Blue plans are generally either declining and/or adopting cost-sharing and PPO strategies similar to those of the commercial insurers.

In an essay with a narrower focus, Jody Sindelar brings to light a surprising fact. While medical prices and costs have been soaring, medical insurance prices have been declining. From 1959 to 1981, the average price declined from $1.35 to $1.12, measured by the ratio of total benefits paid to total premiums for all consumers. If the insurance were actuarially fair, with no profits, taxes, or administrative costs, the price measured in this way would be $1. In this very limited sense, private health insurance is already close to perfect. Since we know from Charles Phelps's work that the demand for health insurance is relatively price elastic, the price decline exacerbated the decrease in insurance copayment features that was occurring until about 1975. The most important consequence of these developments has been an increasingly severe moral hazard problem; the presence of cheaper insurance has led to a large increase in the number of claims filed.

Commercial insurance has always been more expensive, owing largely to greater marketing effort and costs, particularly for individual and small group insurance. However, the difference has narrowed

2. *Ball Memorial Hospital, Inc. v. Mutual Hospital Insurance, Inc.*, 584 F.2d 1325 (7th Cir. 1986).

considerably over time. Sindelar finds that the commercial insurers' price declined from $1.55 to $1.26 during the period 1959 to 1979, while the Blues' price fell only slightly, from $1.10 to $1.09. She tries to explain the decline in prices with an econometric model estimated across states and over time. While the results are reasonable and interesting, they do not explain why the price has declined so much for the commercial insurers and so little for the Blues.

My essay, which follows, investigates the ill effect—mentioned by Pauly and Havighurst—of the large market power held by the Blue Cross/Blue Shield plans. It analyzes one of the most powerful of the Blues, Massachusetts Blue Shield. The Kartell antitrust case brought against them provided a uniquely rich source of information. I was in a good position to use this information because I was a consultant and expert witness for the plaintiff-intervenor, the Massachusetts Medical Society.

Conceptually, the Massachusetts situation is typical. The Blues use their large market share to extract large discounts, about 30 percent from physicians and several percentage points from hospitals. This gives them a competitive advantage, allowing them to maintain their large share and giving them the ability to promote overly complete insurance, with little cost-sharing. As in most states, competition with the commercial insurers cannot overcome the Blues' special advantages. Although the essential analysis is the same for most Blue plans, there are some unique twists in the Bay State.

First, the market share, and thus market power over providers of the Massachusetts Blues, is unusually high. The Blues insure about 74 percent of those with private health insurance, while the national average is close to 40 percent. Furthermore, the extent of the exploitation of physicians is much greater than in other states, because physicians must accept the below-market Blue Shield allowance as full payment or receive nothing at all. In virtually every other Blue Shield plan, physicians and consumers can agree on a fee that exceeds the Blue Shield allowance. In Massachusetts this option is not available. The discounts have gotten so high, and are so inescapable, that they are no longer favored by most Massachusetts physicians. Obviously, the Medical Society no longer controls this Blue Shield.

Second, the results are uniquely unfortunate. Massachusetts has the worst cost-control record in the country. This is an excellent example of Havighurst's warning that severing the Blue Cross/Blue Shield plans from provider control may not solve the problem. Havighurst is concerned that independent Blue plans might still favor the type of overly complete insurance that is so destructive of medical markets. Massachusetts Blue Shield is a clear example of his fears come to life. One objection to consumer copayments has always been the consumer's problem of financing them if he has little in liquid savings. The next essay investigates a possible solution to the problem.

Peter Zweifel introduces us to an innovative method of cost-sharing that is in common and growing use in German private health insurance: rebates (in the form of prepaid deductibles) to insureds who present no claims. The insurers offered rebates of two or three months' worth of premiums to enrollees who make no claims in a particular year. In the United States, this would amount to about $600 to $1,000 for a family. (Another innovation that has received some attention is experience-rated rebates. Under this scheme, also in current use, the size of the rebate in any one year depends on the insured's claims experience in past years.) Zweifel cleverly and carefully analyzes the data from two German insurers and finds that rebates to insureds have a large effect in reducing utilization and costs, roughly comparable to that of the deductibles studied in the Rand Corporation's U.S. health insurance experiment. Further research would be very interesting. One might expect that rebates would be less powerful than the cash out-of-pocket requirement, because rebates are less obvious to the consumer. Also, some consumers may be short-sighted and illiquid, so that paying cash becomes a bigger strain than foregoing a future rebate.

In a simple standard economic model, the rebate is identical to the combination of a regular deductible plus having the consumer bank the money saved by the lower premiums. After all, there is no free lunch. In a richer model, however, there are some important advantages to the rebate that account for its popularity in Germany. According to Zweifel, the main advantage is that consumers have the choice of full insurance or a deductible when they become ill.

Another interpretation of Zweifel's results is that the rebate system is a form of forced savings to finance the deductible. Some consumers approve of it because the rebate system aids their own budgeting. They are prevented from spending the money that they may need if they become ill. The rebate plan also appeals to employers or policymakers who take a very paternalistic view of consumers. If one believes that consumers will simply spend all the money available in a

short-sighted way, then conventional cost-sharing may be too oner-
ous. Here the nature of the insurance requires them to save. This is
analogous to the paternalistic argument for Social Security.

Perhaps even more important, the rebate makes it crystal clear that
a deductible is efficient and is in the interests of consumers—not merely
the insurance company or the employer. Starting from 100 percent
coverage with zero cost-sharing, one could introduce a rebate. Since
research has shown that the utilization-reducing effect of deductibles
is quite powerful, this would produce net savings that could be shared
among the employer, the consumer, and possibly the insurer. The size
of the rebate could be chosen so that the cost of the policy to the
consumer and/or the employer would be reduced. Yet the value of
the benefits to the consumer is higher, not lower, than it was before
the rebate was introduced. If the consumer were to become ill, he
could simply ignore the rebate scheme and remain exactly as well off
as he was with complete insurance. Alternatively, if he were not to
become ill, he would be eligible for a substantial rebate. Thus the
rebate can be a way of introducing cost-sharing without making any
consumers worse off or even making them appear to be worse off,
no matter how risk averse they may be.

As far as I know, there has been little or no use of this form of
copayment in the United States. However, similar ideas for health
insurance and other employee benefits have been proposed and successfully put into use. For example, some have suggested the creation
of an employee wellness fund that is credited with a sum of dollars
every year that the employee does not make any health insurance claims.
Some firms and school districts have reduced absenteeism by rebating
all or some of the dollar value of unused sick leave. In any case, this
is an idea that seems worthy of experimentation, particularly for groups
such as labor unions that have historically resisted copayment as a
form of cost control.

The last chapter, which is mine, presents the best news yet on the
health care sector. It reports on and analyzes the appeal of the PPOs,
an exciting new development in health insurance. Interestingly, the
modern PPO was introduced by two small, Los Angeles–based consulting and claims administration firms, Dual-Plus and AdMar, not
the major health insurance firms. This is consistent with Havighurst's
view that the major private health insurers were sluggish and content
with the status quo. It is also consistent with recent developments in

electronics, where it seems that small firms have been the major source of innovation and invention.

PPOs provide a particular type of health insurance. From the consumer's viewpoint, they are similar to an HMO, except that (1) the choice of preferred providers is typically much larger than the choice within the HMO, and (2) coverage for using providers outside the PPO, though less than coverage for using PPO providers, is still substantial. The overall range of choice is substantially larger and thus more attractive. In particular, the consumer who has an established relationship with a particular physician can continue to use him, albeit with lower benefits. Though PPOs offer fuller coverage for using PPO physicians or hospitals, they often maintain some degree of consumer copayment as a further cost control. Moreover, though generalization is difficult, PPOs tend to be less expensive than HMOs.

From the viewpoint of the participating provider, PPOs are much like the independent-practice type of HMO. Typically the provider must agree to grant price discounts and to submit to utilization controls of varying intensity. Some PPOs, at least initially, require price discounts or utilization controls, but not both. One difference between PPOs and HMOs is that PPOs use fee-for-service medicine and often employ cost-sharing. Therefore, the price of care is revealed to the consumer and enters into his decision-making.

Aside from their obviously useful controls on utilization (discussed by both Pauly and Havighurst), PPOs make the health care market more price competitive. By offering providers the opportunity to grant selective price discounts without reducing price to all comers, PPOs encourage price competition. By publishing lists of preferred providers, they efficiently inform consumers about which physicians and hospitals are the low-priced ones. And by reducing benefits for using nonpreferred providers, they sharpen consumer incentives to patronize the price-competitive providers. In so doing, PPOs improve the traditionally poor information and resultant imperfect competition in health care.

One might suspect that PPOs use monopsony power to drive down prices, like the Blue Shield plans discussed in my earlier essay. This hypothesis is easy to disprove. Many of the PPOs that have easily obtained substantial price discounts from all kinds of providers have been very small, with little or even zero market share. This cannot be monopsony power at work. However, there is a danger of monopsony power here, particularly if the larger Blue Cross/Blue Shield plans get involved with PPOs. There is also a danger of provider monopoly if provider-dominated PPOs are used as a disguise and enforcement mechanism for a provider cartel. Physicians in Modesto, California, attempted this, but were thwarted by the Antitrust Division of the U.S. Justice Department.

In spite of these dangers, the PPO movement is the most promising development on the health care scene. It promises improvements in efficiency and competition with a minimal reduction in consumer choice.

PART I

HEALTH CARE COMPETITION

1

A PRIMER ON COMPETITION IN MEDICAL MARKETS

Mark V. Pauly

INTRODUCTION

The purpose of this chapter is to discuss the role that competition does or can play in medical markets. *Competition* will be defined broadly to include the whole panoply of market responses, and it will be contrasted with the alternative of public regulation as a way of controlling the medical care sector. It is interesting that competition and some types of regulation both seem to be on the increase in this sector, sometimes in the same locations. Indeed, some states, notably Wisconsin, have styled their regulatory apparatus as procompetitive, taking the position that competition ought to be given an opportunity to work, but if it does not, regulation should be in place as a backup. The label "competition" has been applied to many arrangements, often for public relations purposes (after all, the opposite of competition is monopoly, and no one—explicitly—favors that). It often happens, however, that the label is misapplied and is used to argue for a truly noncompetitive advantage for a particular set of firms. (The key here is usually some value-laden word like *fair*.) It also happens that state regulation, in bestowing on government officials what is in effect a monopoly in the function of cost control, actually interferes with true competition. My objective in this paper is therefore to illustrate what competition means or ought to mean, to argue that it can work effectively in medical markets, and to show which of the arrangements labeled "competition" are most like the real thing.

HOW TO ANALYZE MARKETS

There are two important points to keep in mind when analyzing any market. One is the definition of objectives, and the other is the practical choice among strategies.

Efficiency and equity are two standards against which market outcomes can be measured. As we will see, efficiency can be impeded if some transactions are restricted, or if markets in beneficial activities fail to exist. On the question of equity, economists have less to say but we can be sure that not all efficient markets are necessarily equitable.

In choosing among alternative strategies for achieving these objectives, it is most important to be realistic. This counsel is so obvious that one may wonder why it is mentioned. Yet arguments are frequently made—both by advocates of competition and advocates of regulation—that compare the actual imperfect practice of the alternative they oppose to an idealized version of the scheme they favor. For example, it is commonplace to observe that medical markets are not now, and probably cannot be, exactly like the economist's ideal of perfect competition. Since any deviation from perfect competition implies inefficiency, it is often argued that regulation is needed. Of course, the regulation being described is always good regulation, not the regulation by imperfect men in an imperfect world that we so often find in practice; health care regulation, it is said, will be different. And, of course, ideal regulation beats imperfect competition every time.

The non sequitur here is obvious: Regulation is an alternative to an imperfect market only if perfect regulation is really feasible—and we have no evidence that it is. The relevant comparison is between imperfect markets and imperfect regulation. But then armchair theorizing cannot settle the matter; the policy choice cannot be made so cheaply, but requires that one actually try to observe and compare feasible real-world markets with real-world regulation and regulators.

It will nevertheless be useful to list the possible market failures in the medical market, since such failure is necessary (if not sufficient) for regulation to be superior to the market.

Moral Hazard and Flat-of-the-Curve Medicine. The failure of the medical care sector to convey value for money is commonly blamed on the incentives inherent in conventional forms of health insurance coverage. The primary problem with such coverage is that, compared to a no-coverage situation, it greatly attenuates the incentives to patient and provider to weigh the costs of additional care against its benefits. Conventional health insurance warps the price system. This problem is called *moral hazard* in the insurance literature. It arises because the linking of benefit payments to the use of medical care makes it appear that this care is free, or of zero cost, at the point of use, with consequent incentives to use care of low marginal benefit.

One way to think about the effect of moral hazard is to imagine a curve plotting the relationship between the quantity of medical care used and the level of health achieved. The first units of medical care a person consumes will produce large improvements in health, so the curve will rise steeply. Compared to no medical care, the opportunity to see a physician can make the difference between life and death. The first diagnostic tests can yield a great deal of information. At some point, however, the curve flattens out: Additional doctor visits yield only a little bit of benefit (in the form of reassurance), and an additional lab test rarely detects anything new. The point is that, because of the effect of moral hazard, people may well be on this flat part of the curve. From the perspective of a patient with a generous insurance policy, it may make sense to agree to that last lab test or to come in for that "reassurance" visit, because the care is virtually free.

Of course, medical care is not free, and additional use must eventually show up as higher insurance premiums. But to the individual consumer, whose premium is independent of his use, care does appear to be free. The result of this set of incentives is that consumers will desire, and be willing to pay for, care on the flat of the curve. From the viewpoint of the physician as well, the welfare of an individual patient is improved by recommending care of low but positive additional benefit; he may feel that he would be failing his responsibility to his patients if he failed to recommend such care or to approve its use.

As a result of this set of incentives, people will use care in volumes that are too high in the sense that the benefit, although positive, is below the real cost. At the limit, where insurance covers all of the cost, the additional benefit may become infinitesimally small. Just as insurance encourages the extra hospital day or the extra doctor visit, it also induces patient and provider to consume additional costly services per day and per visit, thus adding a qualitative dimension to the quantitative one. But greater intensity of service requires higher unit price. The consequence is a double-barreled incentive to push up expenditures, one that works on both price and quantity.

This failure of the market to choose the appropriate level of quantity and quality of care is a fundamental problem. Many of the arguments for regulation are, in effect, attempts to mitigate the problem of moral hazard in health insurance.

Undersupply of Cost-Containment Devices.   There do exist possible features of insurance policies that are known to be, or thought to be, effective in controlling medical care costs. Until recently, however, insurers were reluctant to include these features in their policies, and when they were included, consumers showed little interest in them. Whatever the cause, it was the case that attempting to bargain for lower prices, utilization review, mandatory second surgical opinions, preadmission screening, and a host of other such devices were not common in private insurance policies. Although there has recently been a boom in the introduction of such devices, they are still far from universal.

Certainly in the past, and perhaps continuing up to the present, the insurance market supplied little in the way of direct cost containment. There was a failure of the market to provide these devices even when, on balance, they were beneficial. One of the justifications for regulation then was (and to some extent still is) the failure of the market to furnish such devices.

Consumer Information Imperfections.   Consumers have a difficult time judging the quality of medical care. Moreover, they are often ignorant about the quantity of medical care needed to cure or palliate a particular health problem. Indeed, a person often seeks medical care simply to buy information about what to do next. Because he is poorly informed, the consumer turns over some of the decision-making power to physicians and other professionals, that is, he hires an agent. However, it may not be possible to guarantee that the agent will always

act in the consumer's best interest, particularly if the agent who provides information on the need for services is the same as the one who
will eventually sell those services.

There are two potential market defects traceable to imperfect consumer information. If the consumer cannot judge price and quality
differences among sellers, sellers can profitably raise their prices above
the competitive level (for a given level of quality), or choose a lower
and less costly (but more profitable) level of quality at a given price.
In addition, imperfect information may make it possible for the provider in the dual role of seller of information and services to "induce"
the demand for excessive levels of services—not just services of zero
additional benefit, but even those with some chance of harming the
patient. In short, there can be unnecessary use of medical services.

Regulation is often offered as a cure for the adverse effects of consumer information imperfections. Regulation of either price or quality
might be justified on this basis.

Another aspect of consumer (and producer) ignorance has arisen in
connection with the recent upsurge in private cost-control devices,
such as managed care and utilization review. In the ideal state, the
consumer should receive medical care up to the point where marginal
cost just equals marginal benefit. This equation should be observed
for both quantity and quality. Under conventional insurance, there is
a financial incentive to go beyond this point, and the new interest of
conventional, health maintenance organization (HMO), and preferred
provider organization (PPO) insurers in cost containment is serving
to limit quantity and quality. But if good things are to be limited, at
what point should the limit be set? If one begins from the excessive
cost level of conventional insurance, one can probably cut cost for a
while just by eliminating activities of minimal marginal benefit—true
waste. But at some point it may be difficult to excise only the fat.
How are consumers to judge whether a PPO or a preadmission screening program has chosen the right point on the steep part of the curve,
the right point over the range of cost/quality trade-offs? Indeed, given
current knowledge, how are providers and insurance plans to judge?
Can regulation be of use in markets for products distinguished primarily by price and quality of a total benefits package?

Redistribution of Income from the Sick to the Well.   Illness obviously
increases the demand (and the "need," if only one knew what the

term meant) for medical care. In and of itself, the uneven incidence of illness causes no particular problem for the functioning of markets if insurance is available to cover the cost of unexpectedly high expenses and if the market for insurance is not itself distorted. By means of insurance, the irregular pattern of illness can be converted into a regular pattern of uniform insurance premiums. I will consider the market for insurance itself below, but a different (though related) problem arises when the pattern of illness is not entirely unexpected. For example, one can forecast with considerable confidence that someone with diabetes, or someone with a previous heart attack, or even someone with a family history of cancer, will have above-average medical expenses. Indeed, insurers do sometimes make these kinds of forecasts (though less frequently than one might expect), and such persons are then charged higher-than-average premiums. In extreme cases like Alzheimer's disease or already diagnosed cancer, the premium can be very high indeed.

To some people, this form of market functioning represents an unacceptable redistribution of income from the ill to the well. Of course, whether it represents *re*distribution depends on what one regards as a neutral distribution, but it certainly represents a different distribution from the one that would occur if all people paid the same insurance premiums. Oftentimes regulation is used to try to bring about a situation of identical premiums for identical coverage—so-called community rating—even among people who differ greatly in expected losses. For example, community rating was required as a condition for receiving federal qualification under the HMO Act.

It also sometimes happens that insurers cannot (or will not) distinguish among people at different levels of risk, even though the people themselves know their risk level. But this still does not mean that all will end up paying the same premiums. If insurers offer policies with several different levels of coverage, the high-coverage policies will tend to be more attractive to people with higher expected expense, while the low-coverage policies will be more attractive to people who expect to spend less. In some cases the situation can arise in which different risk groups are separated by the types of policies they buy, with high risks paying high premiums for the high-coverage policies they choose, premiums that are much higher than would have been charged if people at all risk levels had bought that kind of policy and their losses had been averaged. This kind of adverse selection is also sometimes felt to be a problem with market functioning.

Excess Capacity, Excess Cost, and the Technological Imperative. Hospital beds stand empty with increasing frequency. Open heart surgery units are used at only a small fraction of their capacity, even while many hospitals have such units. Hospitals provide ambulatory care in their outpatient departments at twice the per-visit price of a physician's office. To many people these phenomena are obvious examples of inefficiency calling for regulation as a solution. Indeed, we do have regulation of capital expenditures, designed to reduce the proliferation of underused facilities, and some states (Michigan and Maryland, for example) have begun programs to cut down on excess hospital beds.

Such obvious examples of waste are, for many people (including coalitions of employers and others concerned about hospital costs), prima facie evidence of market failure. And they are the plain-as-the-nose-on-your-face reason for the introduction of regulation of hospital capital expenditures—via the Certificate of Need (CON) program nationwide—and for the regulation of hospital costs and charges in an increasing number of states.

One of the hallmarks of modern medicine has been the widespread introduction of beneficial, complex, but costly procedures usually associated with the purchase of new types of capital equipment. Although it is important not to overemphasize the importance of complex technology in raising costs—costs also rose rapidly at smaller hospitals that did not buy fancy machines—it is nevertheless probably true that the introduction and diffusion of new technology have contributed to hospital cost. In itself, this statement is something of a paradox; in other industries we usually credit modern technology with offering us better products at lower prices. But in the medical care sector, technological change has been cost-increasing rather than cost-saving over time. Quality, in the sense of being able to perform new diagnostic and therapeutic procedures, has also surely increased, but the question is whether the benefits have been worth the cost and whether beneficial new technology has been introduced where it is (to use an undefinable word) needed.

In other industries, not every quality-improving invention reaches the marketing stage. Both firms and market processes themselves perform a kind of comparison of the benefits and costs of all potential innovations; the successful ones are those that cut costs without compromising quality, or that provide quality whose value exceeds its cost. In the medical care industry, it has been suggested that this kind of comparison of costs and benefits does not happen; instead, in striving for prestige and better patient care, hospitals and physicians feel they must have the latest in technology—must offer their patients the most up-to-date equipment in the most modern facilities. There is, it is alleged, an almost inexorable pressure on hospital administrators (especially, but not only, from their medical staffs) to have the best of the new. This phenomenon has been labeled the *technological imperative*.

The view that the market fails to lead to proper choices about new technology in medicine has led to a number of regulatory interventions. The CON laws are intended to slow down the growth of new technology. Some states are proposing to decide whether or not hospitals can provide organ transplants. And the federal government funds programs intended to "assess" new technology and to determine (somehow) whether it is worth it.

Squeezing the Poor.   Under ideal competition, the price for any good or service will come to reflect its marginal cost under the most efficient production technology available. In the absence of competition, price can exceed marginal cost. Ordinarily this excess monopoly rent is raked off by for-profit firms as profit, but that need not be the only use. For one thing, a regulator may in effect order a regulated for-profit firm to make profits on one service or on one set of customers and then use such expected profits to make it feasible for other services to be priced below cost. Cross-subsidization in a competitive for-profit industry would usually require regulation, since it is not consistent with profit maximization per se. (Of course, if the monopolist can price-discriminate, it may well maximize profits by choosing different margins above marginal cost, but that is not the same as cross-subsidization, though it may be hard to distinguish in practice. The monopolist may also choose to cross-subsidize complementary goods purchased by the same person, as, for example, in the case of loss leaders.)

With the health care industry dominated by not-for-profit firms, however, there may be a kind of cross-subsidization even in the absence of regulatory intervention. Firms may choose to reduce the price for certain services (or to certain customers) below cost in pursuit of their objectives, but still break even by setting other prices above cost. It is as if they turned the monopoly profits they could have earned in some submarkets into a subsidy for the prices in other submarkets.

While the empirical evidence is, as we shall see, not entirely con-clusive on the matter, not-for-profit health care firms, especially hos-pitals, are generally thought to cross-subsidize when they have the (market) power to do so. Some of the subsidy goes to research or teaching, some to higher-prestige types of care, but some of it almost surely goes to cover the cost of care rendered to those who do not pay the full price. It is undeniably the case that a higher proportion of low-income people not eligible for Medicaid receive this uncom-pensated care, although it is also the case that many of those receiving such care are above the poverty line.

Competition makes continued practice of this cross-subsidization more difficult for not-for-profit hospitals because it puts pressure on monopoly rents. The possibility that competition will then mean some reduction in the well-being of the poor is thought to be a major defect (at this writing, probably *the* major defect) of competition. It is the possibility of injury to the poor and the sick that now furnishes much of the case for retaining regulation or introducing further controls on hospital behavior.

THE MEANING OF COMPETITION IN THE MEDICAL CARE SECTOR

Since this chapter discusses the ways in which competition or regu-lation will deal with the problems just discussed, it is important to define or describe what I mean by *competition* in this context. *Com-petition* is a word that, at least in the United States, has a favorable connotation. After all, no one is in favor of monopoly, and compe-tition (unless preceded by the adjective *cutthroat*) generally describes a situation that results in low prices, adaptability to changing con-sumer demands, and the absence of government bureaucracy—all American virtues.

However, while people tend to favor competition in the abstract, in concrete contexts (and depending on their own interests), they tend to describe it in a variety of ways. The definition I will use in this paper is one based on economics, as opposed to one based, for ex-ample, on marketing or public relations. What I will mean by *com-petition* is generally captured by the notion of free entry and potential entrants willing to offer goods and services to consumers, with no one firm large enough to have an important influence on levels of price or quality.

Competition in this sense does not enshrine any particular way of organizing, producing, or financing medical care as superior in principle; superiority depends on the ability to please consumers (with regard to both price and quality). The implicit test of that superiority is the ability to survive in a competitive market in which consumers know what they are buying and where there is no subsidy or favor for one firm over another.

For the medical care industry, there are two important aspects of this discussion. First, currently existing arrangements that offer particular avantages to particular types of firms would not be present in a fully competitive situation. Licensing restrictions on entry, favorable tax treatment of Blue Cross/Blue Shield insurance plans, and limits on the expansion of for-profit firms, whatever other rationales they may have, all serve to insulate their beneficiaries from the full force of competition.

Second, competition in an economic sense does not prejudge the superiority of one form of organizing medical care over another. In particular, the presence of large numbers of HMOs is neither necessary nor sufficient for competition. To be sure, it is likely that HMOs will appeal to some consumers, and they should surely not be restricted from entry by regulation or collusion of fee-for-service providers (and there is some sad history of both practices). But an economic notion of competition would not favor HMO-type coverage, under the rubric of fair competition, to the detriment of conventional insurance plans with other types of cost-containment features (such as high co-payment), or even to the detriment of first-dollar coverage, if that is what consumers choose to buy.

MORAL HAZARD AND FLAT-OF-THE-CURVE MEDICINE

Conventional forms of health insurance provide the patient with a user price that is below the market price (and presumably the true cost) of medical care. Why is this so? (Does it have to be so?) Are there regulatory alternatives to the problems caused by this form of insurance? Is this kind of moral hazard necessarily an inefficiency that must be corrected? How might markets deal with moral hazard? Are there currently impediments to their doing so in the most efficient fashion?

Moral hazard arises as the unintended side effect of a good thing—insurance coverage against risky events. It comes about, as noted earlier, because conventional forms of health insurance lower the apparent price the insured has to pay when he uses an additional medical service or opts for a more expensive service. Of course, all insureds eventually have to pay higher prices in the form of higher insurance premiums, but the critical point is that, from the viewpoint of any individual, his use of an additional unit of medical care or his choice of a higher quality or more expensive provider does not in itself raise his premium by a perceptible amount; the additional cost is spread over the premiums of all others who purchase insurance from the same insurer. The fundamental problem with health insurance is that it induces people to use medical care that is worth less to them than its cost.

Why does this problem arise in health insurance when it does not seem to be a problem (at least to the same degree) in other types of insurance? The reason ultimately goes back to the difficulty of defining in an insurance policy the event that determines whether benefits should be paid, and in what amounts. The clearest case is life insurance; the event there is the death of the insured, which is usually easily observable, and the amount is determined by the size of the policy. Other "loss coverage" types of insurance policies also define the event independently (for example, the occurrence of an auto accident) and base the benefits on an estimate of the damages. The insured is then free to spend those benefits however he likes.

In contrast, health insurance defines the event that triggers benefit payments as the incurring of a health care bill, and makes the level of payments depend, not on some independent estimate of damage, but on the size of the bills incurred. It is as if one purchased automobile collision insurance that would pay whatever body repair bills one chose to incur, as long as the owner of the car and the body shop repairman agreed that they were needed. Excessive price and "overrepair" of bumps and dents would be a predictable outcome. Health insurance policies have presumably taken this form because of the difficulty in (1) defining an independent event on the basis of which payment would be made, (2) assessing the cost of repairing damage before receipt of care, and (3) limiting the amount of payment that would be made. Presumably the risk of losing benefits altogether from a real and painful illness that is not apparent to an insurance benefits estimator and the difficulty of seeking estimates in advance make health insurance coverage rational nevertheless.

Some checks on use and cost are still needed, however. Of course, some restriction is implied by the fact that medical care takes time and may be uncomfortable, even if it is free. Further restriction is most frequently provided by policies that leave some part of the total expense uncovered via deductibles and copayments. The price of containing cost in this fashion is exposure to a larger amount of risk.

So moral hazard in itself is undesirable. But does that provide a case for regulatory intervention? The answer is, only if regulation makes it possible to control the use of care with value below cost in ways that are not available to the market. If such advantages are not possible, then moral hazard becomes a regrettable fact of life, like original sin and mosquitoes, which one must deal with the best one can. In particular, those who buy greater insurance coverage presumably face a trade-off between more protection from risk and more distorted incentives to overuse. Unless there are some other distortions (resulting, for example, from a tax loophole or some other type of market imperfection), consumers will presumably make that choice as well as it can be made, taking into account their attitudes toward risk and the benefits from medical care. They would presumably choose the optimal amount of moral hazard.

The strongest case for regulation is therefore based on the hope that it can somehow attenuate moral hazard, somehow cope with the incentives to overuse care. This overuse can take several forms. The most obvious is quantitative overuse of care—too many office visits, too many hernia repairs, too many urinalyses and chest films. By controlling the supply of inputs used to produce output, primarily through CON laws, it may be possible to bring use down, and closer to the point at which care is worth what it really costs. Overuse can also take a qualitative form—using an expensive specialist, an expensive teaching hospital, or an expensive new machine when a less costly form would be much cheaper and not too much lower in terms of both clinical quality and patient amenity. By controlling hospital costs via hospital rate (price) regulation, there may again be a supply-side constraint that mitigates some of the effects of moral hazard.

This discussion only explores the realm of the possible; to make the case for real-world regulation, however, one needs to be able to show that (1) actual regulation does indeed control the consequences of moral hazard in an appropriate way, and (2) it does so in a way not available to the private market. Since there is relatively more evidence available on the first topic, I will deal with it at length; I will then turn to speculation about the second topic in the next section.

Of the two major kinds of regulation, the capital investment controls embodied in CON programs have a longer history. They also present less evidence of doing any good. Early work on CON programs, which compared states that had already enacted the laws with those that did not, failed to find any effect on total capital investment. The surveys did find evidence that the form of investment was altered, away from beds toward other facilities, and that the consequence of restricted supply was higher unit price.[1] There is also considerable evidence to suggest that CON programs tended to be "captured," or dominated by the hospitals they were intended to regulate, and that those hospitals used regulation to keep out competition. There is some evidence that mature programs, which have been in place for a number of years, can depress capital investment. But there is still little evidence that they reduce total health care spending.

Rate regulation, on the other hand, does seem to be able to slow the growth of spending, at least in some states with mature programs.[2] More recent evidence suggests that the impact is not uniform—it ranges from minimal in New York to strong in Massachusetts and Minnesota.[3] Indeed, it would be surprising if explicit regulation of hospital charges did not eventually reduce hospital revenues. But this is not the same as saying that the effects have been beneficial on balance, or that they have been more beneficial than other alternatives that might have been tried.

In particular, as a result of their requirement that all consumers be treated the same, state regulatory programs fail to recognize potential differences among consumers in the extent to which they would like costs cut. If what is ultimately sought is some restriction on consumer choice at the point of service (in return for lower health insurance premiums), it is not at all obvious why this control needs to be imposed uniformly, and on all consumers. The function of controlling

---

1. David Salkever and Thomas W. Bice, *Hospital Certificate of Need Controls: Impact on Investment, Costs, and Use* (Washington, D.C.: American Enterprise Institute, 1979).

2. Paul L. Joskow, *Controlling Hospital Costs* (Cambridge, Mass.: MIT Press, 1981).

3. David Dranove and Kenneth Cone, "Do State Rate Setting Regulations Really Lower Hospital Expenses?" *Journal of Health Economics* 4, no. 2 (June 1985): 159–66.

or limiting consumer choice is a service, and it would seem that there should be a market in and for such services.

UNDERSUPPLY OF COST-CONTAINMENT DEVICES

In fact, there is plenty of evidence to suggest that the market is currently able and willing to sell cost and use controls to those who desire them. The HMO, for example, achieves most of its savings by limiting quantitative use, particularly of expensive hospital admissions and procedures. It is illuminating to view the HMO as an integrated package of full-coverage insurance and cost control. Of course, non-price rationing cannot cater perfectly to individual consumer tastes, but by choosing among HMOs (as well as non-HMO alternatives), consumers can in effect buy the kind of cost control they want; they can hire the regulator or the set of regulatory rules and procedures they most prefer. Similar comments apply to the newly emerging PPOs, which often provide utilization review as well as lower unit prices.

The interest of the private sector in cost containment is relatively recent. Indeed, most of the regulatory structures currently in place date from an era in which there was virtually no such movement in the private sector. Until about 1980, employers, who nominally pay for 80 percent of all private insurance, were very reluctant to tamper with fringe benefit health insurance. To some extent this reluctance was a reaction to the hostile reception given by providers—especially physicians—to past attempts to control prices and costs. The best-known example of such hostility was the long-standing opposition of organized medicine to prepaid group practice (now HMO) firms. Another instructive example was the formation of Blue Shield plans as a way of eliminating competition from the "hospital plans" on the West Coast, which tried to deny benefits for services deemed excessive.[4]

Even after the courts prevented the harassment of HMOs, however, there was a long period in which there was still little movement toward private-sector cost control. Then, beginning about 1980, everything changed. HMOs, PPOs, and benefit limitations spread, to such an extent that some employers are now mandating HMO or PPO membership.

4. Lawrence G. Goldberg and Warren Greenberg, "The Effect of Physician-Controlled Health Insurance: *United States vs. Oregon Medical Society," Journal of Health Politics, Policy, and Law* 2, no. 1 (Spring 1977): 48–78.

Why the change? Surely employer reaction to an automatically increasing part of their labor cost was part of the reason, even though these increases had been occurring for the past twenty years, during which time little had been done. The softening of the labor market in the early 1980s probably also contributed, as did the surge in the number of new physicians, which made all doctors more willing to consider working in organizational structures that had previously been labeled unethical. It was probably also true that the ten-year romance with national health insurance inhibited the private sector from taking steps on its own.

Whatever the reason, the fact is that cost containment is now a high priority—often the highest—in the private sector. The form of cost containment in vogue changes from time to time—now HMOs, now utilization review, now copayments, and now PPOs—but what is left behind is a wide variety of devices from which insurance purchasers can choose.

What advantage does government regulation have over these private-sector alternatives in dealing with moral hazard? If providers resist attempts to limit the use they prescribe, it is possible that political muscle may be needed. This may have been a legitimate argument at certain times. The American Medical Association and the local county associations resisted HMO development for many years, until they lost an antitrust suit. And insurers may at some point have been squeamish about questioning physician decisions. But the rise of surgical second-opinion programs, not to mention utilization review and preadmission screening, suggests that this type of reticence is no longer a problem.

In short, it no longer appears that there is failure in the market for moral hazard control devices. With less market failure, there is less case for regulation. But, one may object, don't many people (even if a shrinking fraction) still buy the old type of health insurance, and thus need someone, even the government, to control moral hazard? Such an argument may have been valid in the past, but in today's market it must surely be the case that, in many areas, those who buy insurance with greater moral hazard do so because they think such insurance yields them larger benefits in some other way. They could have had restriction, but chose not to do so. It does not seem sensible, then, for government regulation to force on them what they had specifically considered and rejected although there would be a governmental role in providing information to assist in their choice. People who do not shop intelligently for health insurance may still make mistakes, but their number is probably small, since employers "pre-screen" most options.

What are the market solutions to the problem of moral hazard, and are there any impediments to their spread? As I noted above, moral hazard arises because the event of illness cannot be defined precisely, making it necessary for insurance benefits to be linked to the amount of expenditure rather than to the amount of loss. There may be some circumstances, however, in which the event can be defined, or at least defined well enough. The classic device for providing full coverage of risk without moral hazard is the indemnity insurance contract, which pays a fixed dollar amount regardless of the level of expenditure, and which depends only on the occurrence of the loss-producing event. While such perfect indemnities are not feasible in health insurance, approximations are possible.

Probably the best-known recent approximation is the diagnosis-related group (DRG) method of paying hospitals. Initially developed for the public Medicare program, it has also been adopted by a number of Blue Cross plans (for example, in Kansas and Pennsylvania). In essence, the DRG mechanism pays a fixed dollar benefit conditional only on the occurrence of a hospital admission with a particular diagnosis. The variability of severity, and therefore cost, with a given diagnosis is handled by having the hospital pool the risk across all patients covered by the insurer, so that the not-so-sick balance off the extra sick. While a full discussion of the DRG method is not appropriate here, and while it is subject to certain limitations (for example, the hospital must have a total volume large enough to permit pooling), the important point to be noted is that it does limit the moral hazard associated with the additional use of services by a hospitalized patient. It does not offer incentives to keep down hospitalizations, but it does constrain cost per hospital visit.

Another emerging marketing device that can usefully be viewed as a form of indemnity is the PPO. Until the mid-sixties, a conventional form of health insurance benefit was the per-unit indemnity, a contract that paid a fixed number of dollars per hospital day, per normal delivery, and so forth. Such a contract does control the moral hazard associated with using a high-cost provider, since the insured with full coverage would still have to pay out of pocket for a provider who charged more than the indemnity level. Then hospitalization insurance, even that provided by commercial insurers, moved toward cost-based, first-dollar coverage. One can view the PPO as nothing more than a return to a set of indemnity benefits linked to the prices of a particular set of providers. A PPO that provides full benefits if preferred hospital X is used, but that requires the insured to pay if he uses a more expensive hospital, is like an indemnity plan whose benefits are equal to hospital X's price levels and that provides the information that hospital X has agreed to accept the indemnity benefit as payment in full.

Of course, the parallel between PPOs and indemnity benefits is not perfect; under an indemnity plan, the patient paid just one dollar out of pocket if he used a provider who was one dollar more expensive than the indemnity benefit, while under a PPO plan the use of a more expensive, nonpreferred provider will often cause a reduction in the dollar value of benefits, so that it costs more than a dollar to buy from someone who is a dollar more expensive. The point, however, is that PPOs (and indemnities of the conventional type, which are also experiencing something of a resurgence in the form of prudent purchaser plans) control the "more expensive provider" type of moral hazard.

Finally, even the HMO can be viewed as a device to control moral hazard by limiting the consumer's benefits. In this case, the implicit indemnity payment if illness occurs is defined by the HMO's standard care protocols. Adding to the level of care the HMO is willing to pay for is usually possible, although doing so sometimes requires the patient to forgo any insurance benefits. Nevertheless, here again we have a kind of per-illness payment device that can control moral hazard.

The array of other cost-control devices—utilization review, surgical second-opinion programs, preadmission screening, special requirements to use ambulatory surgery for some procedures, and all the other emerging rules—can also be viewed as market substitutes for universal regulation; that is, as a kind of voluntarily chosen set of regulatory controls. The virtue of a market in which people choose before the fact how much they will be constrained after the fact is that it permits diversity, while at the same time permitting people to make whatever trade-offs they prefer between freedom of choice after the fact and the cost induced by the moral hazard associated with free choice and full coverage.

One final point about market responses to moral hazard: In order for the insurance purchaser to choose the optimal level of cost control—whether via copayment or limitation of choice—he must face effective prices for insurance that really do reflect its cost. That is, in choosing whether or not to buy insurance coverage associated with another dollar of expected loss, the purchaser should face a price of an extra dollar of insurance premiums (plus administrative costs). There is one important area in which this condition is not met, in which the price is distorted. In the case of employer-provided group health insurance, there is a tax subsidy that makes the price of insurance excessively low. When additional insurance is bought by the employer on behalf of the employees, cash wages must be reduced if the employer's labor cost is to stay the same. But since the reduction in cash wages reduces employees' tax liability, the net cost of a dollar's worth of insurance coverage is less than a dollar. By moving health care costs from out-of-pocket payments to employer-provided health insurance, net costs can be lower because the insurance premiums are shielded from taxation.

The predictable consequences of subsidizing insurance premiums are excessive insurance coverage, excessive moral hazard, and excessive health care costs. Even a choice that includes devices such as HMOs and PPOs is probably distorted, because the employee pays tax on any premium savings he recovers as cash wages but has to pay the "inconvenience costs" without a subsidy.

In short, while there is substantial evidence that the market can and will supply devices to control moral hazard—devices that are often superior to those regulation can provide—there are still some distortions in the market for private insurance that probably lead to undersupply of cost control. The remedy is obviously to remove the distortion, since it is caused by government, rather than to call for yet more regulation to clean up the mess.

CONSUMER INFORMATION IMPERFECTIONS AND DEMAND CREATION

There is no doubt that consumers lack perfect information about medical services. Indeed, the reason for purchasing such services is often uncertainty about the nature of an illness one might have or the appropriate course of treatment. Because illnesses are so variable and so infrequent, it is difficult for consumers to judge the quality of different providers, and therefore difficult to evaluate price differences, even when those prices can be known beforehand. In essence, the medical care market is in large part a market for information itself, or a market for a combination of services and information.

It is here that the point about government imperfection comes to the fore. There is no use arguing that all medical markets are, or could be, consistent with the full competitive ideal of perfectly informed consumers choosing among many alternatives. There can often be many alternatives, but consumers will never be perfectly informed about everything—if they were, they would have much less need for medical care. What we can discuss, however, is whether there are information deficiencies that government regulation—feasible government regulation—can correct.

Since government is imperfect, it would seem reasonable to suppose that medical markets in which conditions do come within hailing distance of those required for consumers to be reasonably well informed might be left unregulated. Frequent purchase, ability to observe whether the outcome the seller asserts does in fact occur, and frequent exchange of information among family and friends would characterize such markets. Primary care physicians' services, especially pediatric care, routine dental care, and care for normal obstetrical cases, might all be said to have these characteristics, and such services account for about a fifth to a quarter of all medical expenses. If care in nursing homes and for chronic illnesses, which are by definition repetitive, are added, the fraction rises to about a third.

It is the nonroutine types of care that pose the greatest information difficulty to consumers. These are primarily in-hospital services; many of them involve care of acute and serious illnesses such as trauma and heart attacks, although others, especially the common, nonemergency surgical treatments such as hysterectomies, gall bladder surgery, and the like, do not require hurried decisions. There is little doubt that consumers currently find it difficult to obtain the information they want about such services; in true emergencies, they could probably not use the information effectively even if they had it.

Thus a *potential* problem does currently exist, one that regulation might help. But will it help, or are there other ways in which the market may cope? There are some possible answers to this question, although they are at the moment rather speculative. The problem with much of medical care is that good advice and good outcomes are hard to detect. An appendectomy patient will feel the same after surgery—whether his appendix was diseased or something else caused the original problem. What is needed is some way of accumulating a larger stock of information than one person can obtain on the relationship between advice or procedures and results—in jargon, large sample data is needed, since mistakes are hard to detect except by looking at the totals.

To some extent, people try to accumulate such a data base privately, by asking their friends and family about experience with a particular doctor or hospital. Work by sociologists does indeed show that this is the conventional way to shop for medical care. It is also easy to see that reputations do develop as consumers exchange information among themselves, and the possibility of damage to his reputation may deter an overeager surgeon even if his patient has already said, "You're the doctor." There has been some fairly advanced work in economic theory on this subject that suggests what common sense may have already hinted—that such a mechanism can support the quality of physician or dentist advice, but that it will not necessarily work perfectly. People forget; the number of friends is limited; and the probability of error can be very important even if it is low and therefore hard to detect.

There have recently appeared on the scene a number of devices that may supplement the social network in developing information about particular doctors and hospitals. As part of its new method for paying hospitals, the government has created peer review organizations (PROs) across the country. One of the jobs a PRO performs is to collect the data on Medicare patients that would allow one to compare hospitals on length of stay, excessive admissions, mortality and readmission rates, and other similar proxy measures for quality. To be sure, these data (like all data) do not speak for themselves, but it is hard to argue that they would be worthless to a consumer trying to pick a hospital. Since the PROs will now make public the information they collect, that information can supplement the other buyers' guides to hospitals and doctors that help consumers make better choices.

The development of these new types of cost-control measures does raise different kinds of information problems, both for consumers and producers. The problem for producers is that of determining what level of quality of intensity of service to provide. Surely there are some examples of utterly unnecessary care—costly care that in no sense improves consumer well-being. But it is just as surely a mistake to conclude that such examples are widespread, or that providers will agree that they are providing unnecessary care. The "unnecessary" hospital day is likely to be one that benefits a family not too eager to provide convalescent care, and the "unnecessary" hospital admission may be a substitute for a long and uncomfortable period of out-of-hospital treatment. The common cases and the more difficult cases are ones in which there is some benefit—at least in terms of comfort or peace of mind—from additional costly care. The challenge to providers, then, is to choose how much quality of this type they wish to provide, and at what cost. The challenge to purchasers is to find a way to pay providers to get them to supply the quality the buyers want.

The knowledge base for meeting that challenge is currently not very good. Even for some of the most common medical procedures— routine surgeries like hysterectomies or cholecystectomies, or admissions for pneumonia—there is little definitive medical evidence on the relationship between care and the expected level and distribution of health outcomes. Even less is known about how consumers of different types may value an outcome that usually involves a blend of risk, discomfort, and average level of health achieved. And finally, how much all of this is worth in terms of dollars—for benefits must be converted to dollars if they are to be compared with costs—is the greatest mystery of all.

One should not be overly pessimistic here. The school of hard knocks we call competition will eventually give surviving providers some intuitive knowledge of what consumers seem to want. Nevertheless, it would seem that more information about health outcomes, values, and costs would be highly useful.

Moreover, one should be realistic about the benefit such information will provide, and how it can be used. The controversy surrounding the question of whether elderly people are being discharged "quicker and sicker" after the introduction of the Medicare prospective payment mechanism provides a good example of an unrealistic approach. That controversy seemed to be directed at finding out whether hospitals were discharging some patients earlier than before, with adverse effects on patient well-being, and then fiscally punishing the culprits. The unrealistic expectation was the hope that Medicare could control costs with its new payment mechanism without reducing quality. That is, politicians and lobbyists for beneficiaries argued that largely not-for-profit hospitals could be paid less and still be forced to deliver the same quality of care. This could occur only if one assumed that there was a substantial amount of pure waste in hospital production and that it was possible to compel hospitals to cut only the waste. This assumption is surely unproven and probably implausible, despite the recent increase in the "profits" of nonprofit hospitals. Hospitals were induced to cut costs under the new system, but such lower costs certainly involved at least some reduction in quality. The relevant question is not how to ensure that quality will not change, but rather how to ensure that buyers will get the quality they want and are willing to pay for.

If there is a problem on the provider end in setting protocols for HMOs, PPOs, and cost-control devices in conventional insurance, there is also a problem consumers face. To be sure, the choice of which HMO to join or which PPO insurance to buy can usually be made in a calmer atmosphere than that which surrounds an on-the-spot decision about fee-for-service care. It is easier to think clearly when you are well than when you are sick. One should not, however, overemphasize this difference, because the great bulk of fee-for-service care is rendered in nonemergency situations. But in another sense, choosing among such plans is much more difficult than a typical choice in the fee-for-service system. In picking an HMO or PPO, one is really choosing the style of care one will receive in virtually all medical circumstances. The HMO, for example, agrees to render all needed care, but uses its protocols and rules of thumb to say how much is needed. The consumer must not only learn what these protocols are, but must imagine what he would choose in all the possible adverse health events that might happen to him. In contrast, fee for service allows choice to be postponed unless and until illness strikes, and then requires choice only concerning that particular illness.

The point is that the choice among plans is extraordinarily complex, and there would seem to be some public role in making available the information that might assist in that choice. Exposés of plans denying "needed" care are not of much help because of the ambiguity of the notion of need and because efficiency requires that beneficial care sometimes be withheld. What would be useful would be some more direct information, perhaps in terms of a set of scenarios about how a consumer would expect to be treated in a number of illness situations. The generosity, aggressiveness, and cost of those treatments could then be compared.

While direct provision of consumer information can be a solution to some of the problems of information imperfection, that imperfection potentially makes it possible for providers of medical care to affect the demand for their services. And the possibility of demand creation does call into question the efficiency of the unregulated market. The regulatory remedies for demand creation, if the latter does occur, tend to take two forms. The direct remedy is to try to limit the quantity of care to that which is thought to be necessary. This limitation can take the form of either specifying protocols for treatment, much as we have discussed earlier, or monitoring and punishing overtreatment. The indirect remedy is to identify the cause of demand creation and try to deal with *it*. The most frequently discussed cause is the stock of inputs to produce care—physicians and hospital beds—but other remedies could include altering the level of fees or substituting salary or capitation for fee for service.

The most persuasive evidence that there is a problem with demand manipulation is the well-documented finding that rates of use of medical procedures, such as surgical treatments or hospital admissions, vary across populations that appear to be fairly similar in terms of age and other proxies for health status. Some rates vary more than others—rates for hip replacement surgery vary less than those for tonsillectomy, for instance—but it is by no means true that the variation occurs only for elective or discretionary surgery. Appendectomy rates, for instance, also display fairly wide variation.

One frequently suggested cause for this variation in rates of use is the variation in physician and hospital-bed stock across areas. Recent empirical evidence is not, however, very supportive of this idea. For ambulatory physician services—office visits and the like—the impact of physician stock on use (when other determinants of demand, such as insurance coverage and health status, are held constant) is almost surely very small, and may well be zero. Wilensky and Rossiter find, for instance, that an increase of 10 percent in the number of physicians will increase the volume of physician-initiated office visits by only 1 percent.[5] For surgical inpatient episodes, there is again some

---

5. Gail Wilensky and Louis Rossiter, "The Relative Importance of Physician-Induced Demand in the Demand for Medical Care," in *Milbank Memorial Fund Quarterly* 61 (Spring 1983): 252–77.

evidence for no availability effect when health status is held constant. Even when health status is not held constant, the effect appears to be modest. A typical study would find, for example, that increasing the number of surgical specialists in a town (population held constant) by 10 percent would lead to only a 2 to 3 percent increase in surgery rates. Since many conditions can be treated about equally well with or without surgery, this variation seems within the margin of opinion in physician judgment about the course of therapy. The presence of conventional insurance does make expensive surgery and cheap medical treatment equally cheap from the patient's perspective, but it is hardly the fault or the obligation of patient or physician to be custodian of insurance company finances.

Hospital beds seem to have a somewhat more consistent, though again not especially strong, impact on use. Here the story is fairly straightforward. Hospitals, even ones with low average occupancy rates, do fill up on occasion, and then the best strategy may be to use an outpatient method of treatment, especially for borderline cases. Here again the patient is about equally well off, but the insurer sometimes gains if ambulatory care is used. And a situation in which people are continually turned away from crowded hospitals can hardly be an equilibrium.

One potentially important consequence of increased numbers of producers of a service is the possibility that more sellers make it difficult for the consumer to shop. However, one solution here—as in the case of some of the demand-creation phenomena—would be to provide information to consumers rather than to regulate suppliers. In any case, limiting supply may well do as much harm as good, given that the problem of demand creation and price inflation is fairly mild to begin with.

But if the availability of physicians and hospital beds accounts, at best, for only a small fraction of the observed variation in procedure rates, what accounts for the rest? John Wennberg, who has studied this question for the longest time, offers "physician practice style" as a proximate cause, and the inherent uncertainty, even among the best-trained physicians, about the most effective therapy as the ultimate cause.[6] When medical opinion differs on the desirability of a surgical

6. John E. Wennberg, "Dealing with Medical Practice Variations: A Proposal for Action," *Health Affairs* 3, no. 2 (Summer 1984): 6–32.

procedure, it should not be surprising that practicing physicians will look to their local colleagues for guidance; different practice styles may thus develop in different areas.

The practice-style theory explains the nonrandom variation, but as a positive theory it is little more than a label for our ignorance about why different physicians treat the same medical problem differently. As a normative theory it is useless, because it does not tell us which practice style is best—certainly the cheapest is not necessarily the best. Here again an alternative to regulation is information—we should do the studies required to determine clinical indications for various forms of therapy. But rather than use this information to set a uniform standard, it would be better to communicate it to patients and physicians, since patients may well place different values on various outcomes.

In summary, regulation is often an inferior solution to problems of consumer information. Market functioning would be improved if consumers were given the information to help them judge the quality of care.

REDISTRIBUTION OF INCOME FROM THE SICK TO THE WELL

The incidence of illness is uncertain. If the market for medical care is approximately competitive, risk-averse individuals will demand insurance, and competitive insurance markets will supply it. The purpose of insurance against the cost of medical care is to convert risky large expenses into smaller but certain payments. Since the main (but not the only) reason for incurring large medical expenses is illness, the effect of insurance purchase is to reduce the money one has available to spend on other things in times when illness does not occur, and to increase the money available when serious illness strikes. In effect, wealth is redistributed to those who unexpectedly become ill from those who stay well, and all parties to the transaction are made better off in the bargain.

All of this is belaboring the obvious (and complicating the simple), so why then do some critics think that competitive markets in insurance can be defective—so defective that regulation is needed? There are really two distinct reasons.

When competitive markets for insurance work as they should, the premium that will be charged to any buyer of insurance will vary with the probability and average size of the loss he faces. If I have a less fire-resistant frame house, or if my house is worth more, then my fire insurance premiums will be higher. In the case of medical insurance, this means that people who have higher expected expenses will be charged higher premiums, whether those higher expenses come from living in a market where medical care costs are high, from seeking coverage against the cost of higher amenity but more expensive care, or from having a current level of health associated with a greater chance of higher expenses in the period of coverage.

This type of risk rating will mean that those who are expected to be ill will pay higher insurance premiums than those who are expected to be well. If we were discussing fire insurance—and the financial impact of a fire is surely many times larger than that of illness, even a serious illness—no one would object to the person with the higher expected loss paying the higher premium. But in health insurance, it may not seem fair that the diabetic should pay more than the non-diabetic and that the person with a stroke should pay the most. Does the market thus fail?

At one level, the objection seems to arise from a misconception about the function of insurance. The purpose of insurance is to pool risky events so that each person can pay a certain premium, *equal to the expected loss he faces*, rather than face the probability distribution with the same expected or average value but much larger variability. If people are risk averse, they will gain by choosing the certain loss over the risky loss. They will always be able to afford the insurance as opposed to bearing the loss. Among a set of people with the same expected loss at the beginning of a time period, insurance redistributes wealth away from those who are lucky enough to stay well to those unlucky enough to get sick. But it does not, and should not be expected to, redistribute from those known to be well at the beginning of the period to those known to be sick at the beginning of the period.

Not only is it not the function of insurance to engage in such a redistribution, using regulation of insurance premiums to do so will lead to inefficiency. Suppose one mandates insurance premiums that are community rated—the same premiums are charged to all. One of two things will then happen. Perhaps insurers will refuse to (or at least avoid) selling coverage to high risks—which clearly makes high risks worse off than when they were charged more but allowed to buy. Or perhaps insurers will be compelled to accept all applicants (assuming this could be enforced); high risks will then buy too much coverage and—even worse—low risks will buy too little, perhaps choosing to go without coverage altogether because the price they must pay is too high relative to their potential losses.

Many would probably agree, however, that on equity grounds one would not want the insult of exorbitant insurance premiums added to the injury of serious illness. Even in this case one may question whether it is desirable to subsidize the wealthy ill at the expense of the healthy poor, but some transfer could surely be justified. The main point is that regulation of insurance premiums is an inferior way to accomplish such a transfer. The better method is an explicit subsidy financed by explicit and nondistortive taxes.

Moreover, there are devices available to insure against the adverse event of high insurance premiums. Both guaranteed renewability and the purchase of convertible insurance in an employment group in effect provide this type of coverage. To be sure, there is probably some role for a public catastrophic backup, but here again explicit subsidies, explicit tax finance, and explicit criteria for eligibility would all seem to be desirable.

The most serious problem for the working of a competitive market occurs when expected losses differ but insurers *cannot distinguish among risk levels*. What they can do, and would be expected to do where there is free entry into insurance markets, is try to get the high- and low-risk individuals—who are assumed to know their own levels of risk—to identify themselves. Obviously, no high-risk person would identify himself directly. But such persons can be induced into doing so indirectly by an insurer who takes advantage of the fact that, at a premium that is an average of the group's loss levels, high-risk people will try to buy more insurance coverage than will low-risk people. If an insurer can observe the total amount of insurance a person buys (something that sometimes, but not always, occurs in health insurance), then it will be possible to "pick off" the low risks by offering a low-coverage policy at a premium closer to the loss experience of the low risks under that policy. The low risks will find a policy with low coverage and a low premium attractive, while the high risks will want to stay with the old, more extensive policy at a premium based on the average.

Of course, once the low risks are picked off, then the old policy can no longer be sold profitably at the "average" premium. Economic models of this situation now become even more complicated, because two outcomes are possible. It may be that, even when the premium of the old, full-coverage policy is raised to cover the losses experienced by the high risks, they will still prefer that policy to the low-premium-but-low-coverage policy the low risks are buying. However, it may also happen that, as the premium of the high-coverage policy rises, the high risks flood in to join the low risks in the low-coverage policy, and the break-even premium again comes to reflect the average loss experience. When that happens, then both types of risks would prefer a more extensive policy—the high risks because they want more coverage anyway, and the low risks because the low premium, which was the main advantage of the low-coverage policy, has now disappeared. But then the cycle starts all over again. The surprising thing is that in this kind of market there is no equilibrium at all—things just keep churning.

All of this has been discussed extensively by economic theorists, who have tried to think of something that would—conceptually at least—stop the cycle. The most common trick is to assume that insurers anticipate; that is, that they refrain from the "pick off" strategy because they know that the separate policies cannot last. Another, more recent explanation is to assume that people display persistence—that they do not switch the moment a more attractive policy is put on the market. The third type of explanation supposes that the same insurer must offer both types of policies, but is only concerned with overall profits. Since the "pick off" strategy would create profits on the low-coverage policies only at the expense of losses on the high-coverage policies, the strategy may not be followed.

What does all this theorizing about adverse selection—for that is the name of the phenomenon we are discussing—have to do with real health insurance markets? All insurers worry about adverse selection, and there are some experiences in health insurance that suggest it has occurred. For instance, federal employees who can choose among a wide variety of insurance plans have in recent years been deserting the conventional high-option, first-dollar Blue Cross plan, with the result that premiums for that plan have leaped. Only older workers and those with large families continue to purchase it. Of course, the experience of federal employees does not really prove that adverse selection has to be a problem; it arises because Blue Cross is not allowed to vary its premium sufficiently with age and family size, and might well disappear in an unconstrained competitive market. Moreover, when (and if) all the high risks switch to the low-option and HMO plans, it may well be possible to reintroduce the high option at premiums that many find attractive. So we really do not know whether adverse selection has to be a problem in this market.

Why would adverse selection be a problem in any case, and how is regulation a solution? One nonreason is similar to that discussed earlier as risk rating. If the good risks get picked off, then the bad risks pay more than if no such strategy were available. But this kind of distributional effect is not necessarily bad, since such a premium is closer to the bad risks' expected losses, and would in any case be cured more appropriately by direct subsidies. The real problem with adverse selection is not what it does to the high risks; they are treated fairly. Rather, it is what it does to the low risks, for it causes them to purchase excessively small policies in order to keep the package unattractive enough to dissuade the high risks from flooding in.

There is some circumstantial evidence (although it is far from conclusive) to suggest that this may be a real problem in health insurance. About 30 million Americans have no health insurance. But these uninsured are not predominantly bad risks. Instead, they tend to be healthy (at least relative to the under-65 population as a whole), largely because they are young (under 25). They tend to rate their health lower than others of the same age, but have fewer days on which they cannot perform their usual functions. They also tend to have low incomes, and are more likely than average to be nonwhite. Why don't these people buy the individual insurance coverage that Blue Cross and the commercial insurers would be willing to sell them? One answer is the rather high administrative cost built into the premiums for individual insurance. But another answer is surely that such insurance is a bad deal. Since a 20-year-old is quite unlikely to use the hospital, insurance will correctly seem to him to be a waste of money at the price he has to pay, even if he knows that there is some chance that he will need to be hospitalized. The fact that any private insurance must be used before public subsidies can be used also helps to discourage purchase.

What solutions are there to the problem of adverse selection? It is surely *possible* that a regulated solution would be superior to the market outcome, although the information problem the government would need to solve in order to pick out a superior solution is quite formidable. And, as noted above, it is by no means obvious that there really is a serious problem to begin with. Moreover, the market has developed tools to use on adverse selection. The most obvious one is the linkage of insurance purchase to employment by means of group insurance. Approximately 80 percent of private insurance is provided in this way, and the number of choices employees have is typically limited, if there is any choice at all. By tying the amount of insurance to employment, adverse selection is reduced (though probably not eliminated). A second aspect of employment-related insurance is that the employer, or the union, or even the insurer, usually wants to avoid the consequences of adverse selection. One way to do that is to offer a somewhat more extensive low coverage policy to low risks, but then subsidize the premium for the high-coverage option enough to keep the high risks from flooding into the lower-coverage option. In fact, it has been shown that such a subsidy can still be consistent with break-even on the set of policies offered to a group, and that the final outcome is optimal.[7]

The safest statement on this complex subject is that the specter of adverse selection alone does not furnish an a priori case for regulation. To be sure, when adverse selection occurs, the competitive market is imperfect, but the ability of governments to improve on matters is just as surely open to question. Moreover, given the existence of group insurance as a way of dealing with adverse selection, and given the absence of any good evidence that adverse selection is a serious problem, it seems unlikely that actual governments can improve on the situation.

EXCESS CAPACITY, EXCESS COST, AND THE TECHNOLOGICAL IMPERATIVE

In this section we will analyze the two arguments for Certificate of Need regulation. One argument is based on the view that, in the absence of control of bed supply or other hospital capital investment, such investment will occur and then remain unused. The other argument is that new technology, even very expensive technology, will

---

7. Jonathan Cave, "Subsidy Equilibrium and Multiple-Option Insurance Markets," in Richard Scheffler and Louis Rossiter, eds., *Advances in Health Economics and Health,* vol. 6 (Greenwich, Conn.: JAI Press, 1986), pp. 27–35.

be adopted and used even if it is not worth the cost, unless the adoption process is controlled by regulation.

Evaluation of capital investment regulation is in a state of flux, largely because of changes in the form of insurance reimbursement. Under cost-based reimbursement, it was surely possible that hospitals would invest in rarely used capital facilities or in expensive technology simply because insurance would pay for it. Empirical studies suggest that regulation was ineffective in controlling such investment even in that period, at least in terms of its money total, although regulation may have affected the form of investment. As discussed above, when CON concentrated on the number of beds, investment per bed surged. When it concentrated on large projects, hospitals assembled a large number of small investments. And in a development that still seems to be occurring, when it concentrated on hospitals, investment moved to nonhospital substitutes like million-dollar diagnostic equipment on trailers as a way of avoiding regulatory controls.

The problem with using regulation of capital input to control cost was, of course, that as long as revenues could be generated by incurring costs, holding down one part of cost—that associated with capital—just made costs balloon out elsewhere. But now there are increasingly severe constraints on the revenues hospitals can collect, either because of Medicare's prospective payment system or because of increased competitive pressures on private insurance. Capital is about to be included in the DRG system. With revenues limited in this way, hospitals have a strong incentive to limit costs as well. In such an environment, CON is at best excess baggage, and can even be an impediment to efficiency. As a result of increased competition in the final product market, input regulation has changed from a theoretically plausible idea that could not be carried out in practice to an influence that is very likely to be pernicious.

A number of states have now ended or are planning to end their CON programs as controls on total capital investment. Nevertheless, considerable interest remains in using such rules to restrict the introduction of modern technology that is judged to be unnecessarily expensive or of uncertain effectiveness. Here again regulation seems to be an inferior alternative to the use of the market.

To begin with, it is important to note that cost containment in and of itself is not an appropriate objective for any medical care financing system. Rather, the overall objective of maximizing consumer welfare really breaks down into two parts: (1) ensuring value for money; i.e., that whatever services are obtained are produced at the least cost, and (2) choosing the mix and scope of service that consumers view as worth the cost.

Obviously, then, a capital investment that reduces costs without reducing quality will always be desirable. But what about a new technology that adds both to cost and quality? The answer is that someone must make the trade-off. The market permits individuals to make their own trade-offs, which will reflect the diversity of preferences people unquestionably have for how they want to spend their money. One person may prefer an expensive and risky operation rather than suffer some disability; another may prefer to avoid risk and conserve cash, even at the cost of some sacrifice in ability to perform physical activities. The genius of the market is that, at least in principle, it allows both of these preferences to be satisfied simultaneously: the defect of regulation is that it will inevitably frustrate one of the two types of people.

Similar comments apply to state hospital revenue regulation, also discussed above. Such regulation undoubtedly can contain cost, although it is instructive that states with such regulation tended to start out with a higher-than-average cost level. Given the effects of moral hazard, it is likely that even a blunt instrument can be effective for a while. But the problem arises when the easy-to-dispose-of fat has been eliminated. Then political regulation will, by its very nature, leave some consumers unnecessarily frustrated.

There is another reason, discussed in the next section, that is now being advanced for the retention of CON laws. Some argue that they should be used to compel hospitals to provide free or reduced-price care to the poor; the reward to the hospital administrator for agreeing to keep his expensive and money-losing ambulatory care clinic in operation would be his certificate of need for his most recent technological wish.

It is easy to see that using capital controls is an inferior way to provide subsidized care for the poor. This carrot will be meaningful only to those hospitals that want to invest; there is no stick to prod hospitals to do more. In addition, the hospital may not be the best site for rendering charity care. The answers sometimes given to these serious objections is that the political process will not approve direct and efficient subsidies to the poor; hence the use of the CON backdoor method is a means justified by its ends. But such an answer implies that policies rejected by the voters' representatives when they are presented directly still ought to be enacted. This topic too will be discussed in the next section.

SQUEEZING THE POOR

The most frequently cited objection to competitive arrangements for hospital care is their potential impact on low-income individuals. The conceptual argument here is straightforward and surely valid. Competition tends to force price down to equal cost for each person who buys a good or service. Hospitals have typically provided care to some individuals at prices below cost, often making care free of charge altogether. Sometimes (though by no means always) the recipient of this uncompensated care has been a low-income person whom the hospital chose as a recipient of charity. When competition was weak, not-for-profit hospitals could in principle use some of the resources that might in other circumstances have represented profits, or have been used to indulge in perquisites, to cover the cost of such care. With the advent of for-profit firms whose owners did not choose to exercise their charity in this way, and with the strengthening of competitive pressures on not-for-profit firms, this kind of cross-subsidy becomes more difficult.

All of this is impeccable economic logic, as far as it goes. It describes a potential impact of competition. But to turn this theory into recommendations for public policy, two important questions need to be answered: (1) Does competition in fact limit the amount of care consumed by low-income individuals, and (2) if it does, is that limitation appropriate or inappropriate?

Let us begin by considering the second question. Presumably medical care for the poor is a social concern because of the impact that care can have on health. Although the desired health level for low-income people is a matter of political choice, deprivation of care affecting that level appreciably would be a cause for concern. Indeed, both one's evaluation of the current performance of the market and one's choice of remedies for any flaws would seem to require evidence that the poor are being deprived of care that is beneficial. Since not all inpatient care is beneficial—this is the main message of HMO performance—one must be careful to distinguish.

There is little evidence that competition causes hospitals to ration care with increasing stringency and that the care thus cut is care the poor really need in the sense that the marginal value of the care exceeds the marginal cost. (This is not, I hasten to add, the same thing as saying that we know that the health of the poor has not been or would not be harmed; we just don't know.) Since the need for hospital care is usually fairly manifest, it would seem to be difficult to deny care on a priori grounds, although news stories reporting ambulances being turned away from some hospitals show that it is not impossible. Moreover, even the patient turned away once may eventually find care.

What evidence we do have suggests that insurance coverage has some impact on use by the poor; moral hazard does exist. In comparisons of unadjusted population means, the uninsured use substantially less care than do the insured. The differences are about the same whether one compares all uninsured with the insured, or just the uninsured poor. Physician visits and the chances of having several physician visits during a year's time are about 30 to 40 percent lower for the uninsured, and their hospital admission rates are only about half that for the insured. These differentials continue to hold when self-reported health status is held constant. The most recent study by Blendon et al. compared use rates between poor people in states with generous Medicaid programs and those in states with less generous programs or no programs, and found that higher use matched with higher coverage.[8] All of this only shows that with less coverage, use is less; it does not permit an estimate of the impact on health of increased use caused by greater financial capacity.

There is evidence that some hospitals (like some physicians) require evidence of financial capacity before admitting a patient for elective surgery. Indeed, this practice has occurred for years, antedating competition by decades. However, that some hospitals in a market area choose not to provide charity care is not the same thing as saying that no such care is available. It may be available at other hospitals in the area—those that have a stronger taste for such services, that receive larger philanthropic donations, or that can turn to taxpayer support.

8. Robert Blendon, et al., "Uncompensated Care by Hospitals or Public Insurance for the Poor: Does It Make a Difference?" *New England Journal of Medicine* 314 (May 1, 1986): 1160–63.

No conclusive evidence is available as yet on the extent to which such competition-induced rationing affects the health levels finally achieved. This is in large part because there is also little evidence on the first question—whether competition has caused an actual reduction in the consumption of any care (whether needed or not). The evidence cited in this discussion is either highly circumstantial or strongly anecdotal.

There is, for example, fairly convincing evidence that the share of the population with third-party coverage declined in the early 1980s. The evidence is not conclusive, but there were probably two (and possibly three) reasons for this change. One was an increase in the unemployment rate, which caused the loss of private coverage; the other was a tightening by states of eligibility for their Medicaid programs. The third possible reason is that high costs for medical care resulted in a loss of private coverage. (More about this below.) But translating shallower coverage into deprivation of care requires a few more steps. And even if those steps can be made, it is still not possible to blame competition per se; the cause is rather government policy, either through sins of commission—deciding to cut Medicaid—or sins of omission—mismanaging the macroeconomy and throwing people out of work.

The logical link between less coverage and less use is furnished by moral hazard. With less coverage there should be some reduction in use, although hospital care is unlikely to feel the brunt of this kind of impact. Especially for low-income people, however, there is another important possibility that mitigates the sting of moral hazard. Hospital care is usually rendered before it is paid for. There are several reasons for this, but one important one is that people who eventually will pay do not like having to pay up front; it is not good marketing strategy to require cash on the barrelhead. But then bad debts become possible; in fact, eliminating bad debts is probably impossible. People with less insurance coverage are more likely to incur bad debts, and the chance of doing so presumably varies inversely with a person's assets (or income to attach). Hence, even the absence of insurance coverage need not be an insurmountable impediment to care.

The most frequently cited piece of evidence on health effects of recent deprivation of care for the poor is based on trends in infant mortality rates. For both whites and nonwhites, infant mortality rates have been declining for the past twenty years, though they are still higher in the United States than in some other countries. However, in recent years the rates have not fallen as rapidly for nonwhites as for whites, despite the fact that it should be easier to produce a given percentage reduction in the higher rate. At the same time, there has been a cut in the fraction of people below the poverty line on Medicaid, an event that should have a disproportionately greater effect on nonwhites because of their lower incomes.

Of course, there could be other reasons for the differential fall in rates, reasons having nothing to do with access to medical care. There has, for example, been an increase in the number of black babies born into female-headed households, where the rate tends to be greater. But even if one grants that there is a relationship between lower access and infant mortality, the relevance of this health indicator to the questions of uncompensated care and competition is unclear. For one thing, prenatal care, which many believe influences infant mortality, is not a hospital-based activity. Hospitals do save babies' lives with neonatal care—and much of the decline in the infant mortality rate has occurred because of lower birthweight-specific mortality rates, not because of higher-birthweight babies that are supposedly the result of better prenatal care. There has been no evidence of denial of access to neonatal care. Moreover, while there probably has been some effect, it is virtually certain that the effect has been caused by the cutback in Medicaid—an action of government—rather than by competition per se.

Finally, and most important: Is the slowdown in the rate of decline in the infant mortality rate appropriate or inappropriate? Political rhetoric aside, it is obvious that in some sense the taxpayers *chose* to put less than they could (though more than they had been spending) into Medicaid in a period when the number of officially poor was growing. Does this represent an informed expression of their political choice, a desire not to spend more even though it might do some good (with both *might* and *some* worthy of emphasis)? Put somewhat differently, Are we observing nothing more than the politician's ploy of spending less on public services and then blaming the private sector for not supplying more? Or is there some more subtle defect in the political process? I will discuss these issues further below.

What is obvious is that the relationship of competition to this problem has not been established. It is not known, for example, whether the level of consumption of hospital care by low-income people is lower in areas characterized by stronger competition. Nor is it known, other than by anecdote, that stronger competition is related to less uncompensated care. It *is* known that the absolute amount of uncompensated care furnished by hospitals, far from having fallen, has in fact increased over the period of increasing competition. But what happened was that, when the number of people below the poverty line increased, the hospital sector did not increase the amount of uncompensated care proportionately. Private not-for-profit hospitals maintained about the same level of such care, while public hospitals increased their levels—but not by enough to lead to an increase proportionate to the increase in numbers of people without insurance or below the poverty line.

In short, recent years have been marked not by reductions in the level of assistance hospitals give to the poor, but rather by cutbacks in publicly funded support (at the federal and state levels) that hospitals were unable or unwilling to offset. To be sure, hospitals have earned high profits in the post-DRG era, and they apparently are using those profits to hedge against a cut in revenues (from both Medicare and private sources), which many hospitals believe to be inevitable. Hospitals have not done all that would be financially feasible in the short run, but more fundamentally the real cause of the problem is the failure of the public sector—of taxpayers or their representatives—to increase the level of public support when the number of people who might benefit from that support rose.

So the actual contribution of competition to the problem is unknown; it is not even known with any precision whether there is a problem of underconsumption of hospital care by low-income people. (Some evidence exists that there are types of health-improving care that low-income people do not obtain. Pregnancy care and care for hypertension are two major examples; these types of care, however, as well as most other effective therapies that are underconsumed, are not provided by hospitals. They are provided by physicians in the ambulatory care sector, where complaints of competitive pressure on willingness to provide care for the indigent have not been heard.)

The fact of ignorance has not, however, deterred either arguments or policies. Indeed, some states have instituted new programs to tax hospital care for the nonpoor to finance hospital-provided care for the poor, while other states have used the needs of the poor as a justification for the continuation of regulation. The problem with such stopgap measures is, of course, that they are likely to be inefficient and inequitable ways of solving the problem if it does exist. How, then, might one design an ideal policy, and what are the problems with the commonly advocated solutions?

To begin to answer this question, we need to return to the major unknowns. Without knowing which types of beneficial care poor people lack, and without knowing how the greater availability of funds to hospitals will induce hospitals to behave, it is hard to know what to recommend. The absence of information on what health care the poor need most—and the sneaking suspicion that hospitals are singularly inappropriate to provide it—makes it hard to favor direct transfers to hospitals. One can, of course, make transfers to hospitals with strings attached that are intended to induce them to do what may be more efficient, such as provide the ambulatory care the poor really need. But in addition to being hard to push with, such strings seem to be tied in the wrong place, since hospitals are quite inefficient sources of ambulatory care.

To be blunt, hospitals, especially private not-for-profit hospitals, seem to be poor instruments to fund if one wants to improve the health of the poor. Attempts to do so in the past—for example, the attempt to require hospitals to render charity care in return for Hill-Burton capital subsidies—have floundered. Private teaching hospitals especially are likely to divert such funds to projects—teaching and research—rather than to efficiently supplying the care the poor really need. Some benefit may spill over to the poor, but surely much less than could have been provided by the same resources had they been used in a more explicit and better-targeted way.

The best way to target subsidies to effective care for those in need is to do so directly. Medicaid, especially if freed from federal minimum benefit rules, is one method of doing so. Using private organizations that bid for Medicaid contracts, as has been done in Arizona and California, is one way of accomplishing this targeting, although one must always remember that the outcome cannot exceed what is feasible with the funds allotted to the program, and that even that maximum requires constant vigilance to make sure that the contractors do not skimp. Furnishing a small amount of resources and then looking the other way is a recipe for a dangerous rip-off.

A second way to target subsidies is to use public-sector production, by means of public clinics and public hospitals where inpatient care is appropriate. Here again the quality of the outcome will depend largely on the resources provided and the level of supervision.

Even with the best possible Medicaid or public hospital program, targeting will be imperfect. Not all, not even a majority of persons who lack insurance are below the poverty line. Most of the uninsured, and probably most of the recipients of uncompensated care, have incomes above the poverty line. They often have good reasons for low coverage or failure to pay, but those reasons do not always justify direct tax support. The problem, in short, is not really uncompensated care; it is underconsumption by low-income people. Much of uncompensated care is simply a natural consequence of doing business on a credit basis. Once subsidies for the poor are set at socially appropriate levels, any remaining problem of uncompensated care would not really be a problem of public policy; it would be a problem of the private business of hospitals. To the extent that competition exacerbates this problem, hospitals would be expected to respond by increasing collection efforts and seeking ways to avoid rendering care to people who are not poor but who are unwilling to pay. Refusal to render care is one method, and it may sometimes be the only way. In a perfect world, such action would not be necessary, but the actual world is imperfect.

What is needed is some way to make sure that such revenue collection techniques do not reduce social welfare. First, one needs to be sure that persons being denied care are not the poor who need help. Second, since nonpoor bad debts are not distributed uniformly across hospitals, one needs to make sure that adaptation to the situation is as efficient as possible.

Neither task is easy. An income-conditioned subsidy program can deal with the poor, but what is one to do about the improvident, self-employed middle-income individual who seeks care for a genuine illness, who will undoubtedly be worse off without care, but who is unlikely to pay the bill? Possibly there can be some public assistance in attaching assets or income; after this, it would seem that holding individuals to the consequences of their acts is the only sensible policy.

The second problem is no simpler. An efficiently run hospital can experience financial difficulty, even bankruptcy, if its nonpoor clientele have a high bad-debt ratio. Raising charges to those who do pay may help in some (probably many) situations, but it can in principle be self-defeating. There seems to be no solution to this problem once the hospital has exhausted all avenues for collecting revenue. Having an above-average percentage of customers who do not pay their bills is one of a number of adverse events that can befall an efficiently run business; the business needs to reexamine its policies to avoid these events. Sometimes the exit of the hospital, and redistribution of its bad debts among other firms, may be the only solution.

Financing Uncompensated Care.   Let us return to the case in which uncompensated care is rendered to the poor. We have argued that the best solution is one that targets subsidy funds toward the poor rather than toward hospitals, and toward the care that is needed. One other characteristic of a best solution is that the taxes used to raise this subsidy should be efficient and equitable. While no tax is perfect on both scores, it is likely that broad-based revenue measures, such as income or sales taxes, will work best.

What of the schemes that raise money through taxes on health insurance or on hospital care? Both such tax instruments have some serious problems.

The practical problems with insurance taxation (or its analogue, a pool for the uninsured financed by assessments) are easy to see. Such a tax induces people to take steps to avoid it, and those steps will be distortive. To the extent that some succeed in avoiding the tax, equity is also reduced. The most obvious way to avoid an insurance tax and still spread risk is for an employee group to self-insure. Even if some stop-loss insurance is purchased (and taxed), a sizable chunk of the tax base can be eroded in this way. Not only is it unfair that groups that find self-insurance feasible can avoid paying their fair share of a social responsibility, the tax would also lead to an inefficiently excessive use of self-insurance. Moreover, high-income people can self-insure even without a group, and thus avoid taxation. Finally, taxing insurance will reduce the demand for insurance—another distortion.

It is true that at present some insurance—that paid for by employers—is currently subject to a tax subsidy. Removing the subsidy and using the proceeds to pay for uncompensated care to low-income persons could be efficiency improving. However, an ad valorem excise tax on insurance (or on hospital care) does not match the income tax–based subsidy to employer-provided coverage. Some people buy insurance without employer assistance; there is no tax subsidy for them, and an excise tax would be pure distortion. Indeed, the tax could induce some people at the margin to become uninsured as a way of avoiding the tax, thus further aggravating the problem it is intended to cure.

The alternative strategy is to tax hospital care. Such a tax is more difficult to avoid than a tax on insurance. However, the tax will have distortive effects, causing people to use less hospital care and to use ambulatory care in order to avoid the tax. At least some of this shift will be inefficient. Moreover, the tax will be highly inequitable, at least when judged by the usual standards of equity. Hospital expenditures do rise with income, but not very strongly. Hence, a tax on hospital expenditures will be highly regressive, something many people would find objectionable. One might argue that this public tax really just replaces the private tax inherent in cross-subsidies, so that there really is no redistribution. One problem with this argument is that cross-subsidization is not the only way hospitals cover the cost of uncompensated care. Historically, philanthropy has been a vehicle, and some hospitals have simply eaten into the endowment furnished by the donations of the past. A second problem is that one could equally well argue that since it was Medicaid cutbacks that caused the problem, the tax not collected is the broad-based Medicaid tax. Indeed, as noted above, there has as yet been no hospital reduction in the level of uncompensated care. It is not that some group has stopped paying; it is that no group has stepped forward to deal with the new poor. In any case, raising funds from a hospital tax just to replace hospital-provided uncompensated care might help some hospitals (while hurting others), but the poor will only be helped if total resources devoted to their care are increased. By definition, there is no group that used to pay for this care.

Political Choice and Support for the Poor.   The discussion of what taxes might be used raises what is in some sense the most troublesome question about uncompensated care. Most people who support programs to tax hospital care, or other equally bizarre indirect methods of finance, do not do so because they would prefer those methods to an explicit and targeted subsidy financed by broad-based taxes. An improved Medicaid program would probably be at the top of almost everyone's list of preferred policies. The reason for the excursion into the fiscally baroque is that, as Gail Wilensky has put it, direct methods are not politically feasible.

This approach to developing policy is troublesome in the extreme.

There would be no problem if the optimal level of support for the poor had already been determined and the only issue was how to entice a reluctant political system into supporting it. In that case one would, based on Machiavelli's advice, advise the prince to find what works. The problem is that in a democracy we rely on the political system to fix the appropriate level of support as well as making that support possible. This necessary reliance on public choice is even more essential to this problem than to others, since there are few objective technical facts that can determine how much care is appropriate or who is sufficiently poor to be a deserving recipient.

The problem, then, can be stated as follows: If only a relatively low level of support is politically feasible when the support program is presented explicitly and when appropriate taxes are used, on what basis do we judge that a higher level of support is desirable and therefore *ought* to be made politically feasible? If a program can only be enacted with subterfuge and deceit, how can one judge that program to be appropriate? I personally would prefer a much higher level of support for the poor than is currently provided in my state, but if I cannot persuade my fellow citizens to support my preferences, it would not seem that my preferences then have any special legitimacy. Certainly I would not be justified (as an analyst) in suggesting that appropriate public policy is one that seeks ways to make my preferred outcomes politically feasible. Those who oppose expansion of Medicaid when the proposal is made explicit would probably be worse off if taxation of hospital care or insurance, either directly or by regulatory fiat, were substituted.

On the other hand, one strong conclusion from economic theory is that conventional methods of political choice, whether direct referendum with majority rule or representative government, do not necessarily pick the best outcomes. The crucial question to be answered in the case of medical care for the poor is *why* the indirect methods are thought to be politically feasible when the explicit decision is not. If the reason is that voters and legislators tend to overlook decisions made by regulators, or to view those decisions incorrectly as matters of technical fact rather than political choice, then the indirect methods would not seem to be appropriate. If, as James Buchanan has argued, taxes that are much more difficult for a voter/taxpayer to detect lead to inappropriate voter choices because they disguise the trade-off between public goods and the price paid for them—and a tax on hospital care, which is only rarely used and which, when translated back into group insurance premiums, is thought to be paid by the employer (or perhaps by the hospital) is certainly one of these—then again the appeal to political feasibility would be inappropriate.[9] If, however, the use of taxes on hospitals or health insurance allows some citizens with high demands for the public good to pay a large share, so that those with weaker demands can be induced by lower taxes to support a program from which all benefit, then the move would be desirable.

Judgments in this case are hardly rock-solid; indeed, the judgment that explicit expansion of Medicaid is infeasible while indirect strategies will work ultimately rests on some amateur assessments of the political game. Nevertheless, I believe that the improved feasibility under the indirect methods is based on political flim-flam—hiding the costs off budget, disguising taxation as regulation, and insulating the choice by moving the locus of choice from the legislature to the bureaucracy. Facts would help here: Do voters with typical preferences but good information really favor expanding programs to cover hospital costs for the poor? Do they favor the regressive tax structure embodied in hospital services taxation? If the answer is negative, as I believe it would be, it would appear that the movement toward indirect methods of support pushes the medical economy toward an imperfect system financed in an inefficient way.

If the solution does not lie in taxing hospital care to support hospitals, what is the answer? Slowing down competition is not an answer, since that imposes an even higher tax on the nonpoor in return for a more elusive benefit for the poor. One possible solution is to reexamine the explicit solution. Has a program of selective expansion of public subsidy financed by general taxes really been proposed and found wanting, or has it never really been proposed? To be sure, federal support for Medicaid is likely to prove difficult to expand, but there is much that states could do with their own finances, particularly since doing so might permit them to target benefits to population groups and types of care more selectively. The result might not be a bail-out of hospitals—which helps to explain why hospitals are easy to convince that this strategy is not politically feasible—but it might be salable to the voters if the case can be made strongly enough.

9. James Buchanan, *Public Finance in Democratic Process* (Chapel Hill, N.C.: University of North Carolina Press, 1968).

The case also requires more than just anecdotes about turning ambulances away or hailing a taxi for someone hooked to intravenous tubes; it requires showing what additional care would be made available with the subsidy, to whom, and what the effect would be on levels of health achieved. My earlier discussion was not meant to convey the impression that we know the poor get all the care they need or that they are not deprived of care that would produce large improvements; it was meant to indicate that, even after a review of the research literature, one does not know whether more care would do much good. Here is where the issue of documenting the health impacts of uncompensated care, or any additional care for the poor, is important. If one adopts the view that desirable social policy seeks an appropriate level of care for the poor—rather than the level at which additional care will provide no more benefit—it is critical to determine what the marginal benefits are, and to convince politicians and taxpayers of their importance. People who work in the health field assume all too often that they only need to show that someone is sometimes being deprived of care of some benefit to convince voters/taxpayers that there is a problem. But politicians and voters know that they have objectives in addition to health, that trade-offs will have to be made. Debate (and assistance for the poor) is not advanced by assuming that need is self-evident based on some fragmentary statistics or journalistic anecdotes. People who are concerned about the use of health care by low-income people need to find better ways and better information to convince others of the desirability of increased support. They need to find the kind of information that will be persuasive to voters and taxpayers.

An ideal solution would probably imply insurance coverage of a catastrophic form, as Danzon has suggested, rather than first-dollar coverage, especially if lower-middle-income persons are to be included.[10] That solution is not without problems of its own. Probably the most serious is that of targeting the subsidy. As noted above, most of the uninsured and the recipients of uncompensated care are not poor, and most low- and middle-income families already have insurance and therefore do not receive uncompensated care. Danzon has

10. Patricia Danzon and C. Conover, *Health Care for the Uninsured Poor of North Carolina* (Durham, N.C.: Duke University Center for Health Policy Research and Education, August 1985).

stated the dilemma well. If low income is made the criterion for eligibility, many of the public dollars will simply replace funds that individuals or their employers would have spent in the private sector. If eligibility is based on inadequate insurance coverage, many of the tax dollars would flow to people who are not poor. In either case, incentives would be distorted—either there would be incentives to have a low income/wealth level, or to drop insurance coverage in order to qualify for the subsidy. My own view (and hope), however, is that politicians and voters would be willing to override these difficulties and provide care where it is needed. One consolation is that the replacement of private contributions by the poor who do pay would at least improve equity among the poor.

While such a solution would deal with the fundmental issue—the health and dignity of low-income people—it would not wholly cure the hospital's problem of uncompensated care. The volume of such care would be reduced, but since there are still nonpoor people who do not pay their bills, the problem of bad debts remains. In market terms, these shortfalls between billed and paid charges are part of doing business and will need to be built into the nominal price structure. Doing so will be a problem for hospitals, a serious one for some, but there does not seem to be any remaining case for public intervention. Hospitals will at least have incentives to do the best they can. In my view, they will be successful.

PART II

THE HOSPITAL INDUSTRY

2

AN ECONOMIC HISTORY OF AMERICAN HOSPITALS

Peter Temin

The modern hospital is less than a century old. It was born in conditions far different from those that exist today, and it has passed through several transitions in its brief history. Yet it has acquired a place of such centrality in modern medical care that it is impossible for many people to conceive of medical care without the current dominance of the hospital. This chapter attempts to place the current role of hospitals in historical perspective to suggest both how the existing institutions were created and how they might be modified by future conditions.

While hospitals will be the focus of this inquiry, it is clear that they cannot be studied in isolation. Changes in the roles of hospitals were connected, on the one hand, to alterations in the practice of medicine, and on the other to events in society at large, including, most notably but not exclusively, the development of government programs for health and welfare. One of the tasks of this chapter will be the assessment of the relative influence of these two disparate factors.

OVERVIEW

Table 2–1 shows the number of hospital beds per 1,000 population during the twentieth century. General hospitals were the analogue of short-term hospitals, although the earlier category was a bit more in-

Table 2–1.   Hospital Beds, 1909–1980 (Per 1,000 Population).

	Total	General	Short Term
1909	4.7		
1920	7.7	2.9	
1930	7.8	3.0	
1940	9.3	3.5	
1950	9.6	3.9	3.3
1960	9.3		3.6
1970	8.0		4.2
1980	6.0		4.6

SOURCES: U.S. Bureau of the Census, *Historical Statistics of the United States* (Washington, D.C.: Government Printing Office, 1975), p. 78; American Hospital Association, *Hospital Statistics* (Chicago: AHA, 1981), pp. 14–15; *Economic Report of the President, 1983* (Washington, D.C.: Government Printing Office, 1983), p. 195.

clusive (as the overlapping data for 1950 reveal). Other hospitals cared for long-term patients, whether the mentally ill, the incurably ill, or (earlier) the tubercular or indigent. The total number of hospital beds rose faster than the population up to mid-century and has risen more slowly since. The number of short-term beds, by contrast, has continued to rise slowly throughout the whole period. The current decline in per capita hospital beds is entirely due to the fall in long-term beds; there is no hint of a decline in the growth of short-term beds. After growing at more or less the same rate as the population until about 1960, the number of long-term hospital beds began a precipitous decline. This fall is in large part the result of our current policy to deinstitutionalize mental patients.

National health expenditures are broken down into a few categories in Table 2–2. The share of hospital expenditures has more than doubled since 1929, reaching 40 percent of the total in 1980. The share of nursing home care has also risen, showing one reason for the decline in long-term hospital beds: Many aged people who formerly would be in hospitals are now in nursing homes. As we will see, the boundary between hospital and other care has shifted greatly over time.

The share of the gross national product (GNP) expended on medical care has also grown during these years. It was 3.5 percent in 1929 and 9.4 percent in 1980. The share of the GNP spent on hospital care (calculated as the product of the share of health expenditures in GNP and the share of hospital care in health expenditures) has risen

Table 2–2. Percentage Shares of National Health Expenditures, 1929–1980.

	1929	1940	1950	1960	1970	1980
Hospital care	18	25	30	34	37	40
Physicians' services	28	24	22	21	19	19
Drugs and medical sundries	17	16	14	14	11	8
Nursing home care	—	1	2	2	6	8
Dentists' services	13	11	8	7	6	6
Other	24	23	24	22	21	19

SOURCES: Robert Gibson, "National Health Expenditures, 1979," *Health Care Financing Review* 2, no. 1 (1980): 1–36; "National Health Expenditures," *Health Care Financing Trends* 2, no. 5 (1982): 1–9.

from about 0.5 percent in 1929 to almost 4 percent in 1980. A second task of this chapter is to explain why hospital expenditures have risen much faster than GNP while the number of hospital beds has risen only as fast as the population.

Hospital expenditures are not the same as direct patient payments, and most of the cost of hospital care currently is not paid by the patient at the time of his or her hospital stay. Table 2–3 shows the share of personal health expenditures and two of its components that are paid for directly by patients at the time of service. The share of direct payments has been falling continuously and dramatically since the Depression. While almost all personal health expenditures were paid for directly in 1929, less than one third are paid that way now. And the share of hospital expenditures paid for directly has been smaller in each year for which there are data than the share of personal health

Table 2–3. Direct Payments as a Percentage of Total Hospital Costs, 1929–1980.

	1929	1940	1950	1960	1970	1980
Personal health expenditures	88	81	66	60	40	32
Hospital care			30	20	10	9
Physicians' services			83	65	44	37

SOURCES: Robert Gibson, "National Health Expenditures, 1979," *Health Care Financing Review* 2, no. 1 (1980): 1–36; Robert Gibson and Daniel Waldo, "National Health Expenditures, 1980," *Health Care Financing Review* 3, no. 1 (1981): 1–54.

expenditures as a whole. It has fallen rapidly in the past few decades to only 9 percent in 1980 as public programs like Medicare and Medicaid have supplemented private hospital insurance.

The distribution of short-term hospital beds among hospitals of different sizes and ownership is shown in Table 2–4. While two-thirds of short-term hospital beds are in nongovernment, nonprofit hospitals, these are not the only type of hospital. In particular, the share of for-profit hospitals is rising, although it remains small. It can be seen from Table 2–4 that the for-profit hospitals are smaller than the nonprofit ones, so that they account for a smaller share of hospital beds than of hospitals. Almost all large short-term hospitals—and therefore almost all teaching hospitals—are nonprofit. The final task of this chapter is to explain how this came about and whether the growth of for-profit hospitals will affect it.

The following sections of this chapter will approach these tasks from a historical perspective. The first section will describe the origins of the modern hospital before the Depression. The next section will describe the effect of the Depression and the growth of government health policies on the growth of hospitals. The following section will analyze the growing costs about the rate of increase in hospital costs, and the final section will discuss recent changes in the regulation and growth of hospitals.

ORIGINS OF THE MODERN HOSPITAL

Hospitals were primarily nonmedical institutions throughout most of the nineteenth century. They existed for the care of marginal members

Table 2–4.   Hospital Beds, 1980 (In Thousands).

Hospital Size in No. of Beds	Nongov't. Nonprofit	For Profit	State & Local Gov't.	Total
6–24	2	1	3	5
25–49	14	5	19	38
50–99	46	14	38	98
100–199	114	32	38	183
200–299	121	22	25	168
300–399	113	8	17	138
400–499	93	4	20	117
500+	170	1	42	213
Total	673	87	200	960

SOURCE: American Hospital Association, *Hospital Statistics* (Chicago: AHA, 1981), p. 14.

of society, whether old, poor, or medically or psychologically deviant. Medicine was practiced outside the hospital, and the medical staffs of hospitals were small. Hospitals were charitable institutions, and they looked for moral rather than physical improvement in their patients.

The nineteenth-century role of hospitals conformed to the theory of disease current at the time.[1] The theory was based on a view that saw healthy people in equilibrium with their environment. There were no specific diseases, but rather disequilibrium, either within individuals or between people and their environments. It followed that the purpose of medical treatment was to alter the relationship between these components in an attempt to restore the healthy equilibrium. In particular, drugs were used to change the balance between internal and external forces, and drugs were evaluated by their effects on the intake and outflow of the various nutrients and excretions of the body. Drugs were sought whose effects could be seen, since the visible alteration of the patient was an index of the efficacy of the treatment. Mercury was a popular drug because of its dramatic physiological effects, although it surely did far more harm than good to the hapless patients.

Medicine was typically practiced at people's homes. Drugs could be administered as easily at home as in the hospital, and the balance of internal and external forces could be maintained and monitored better in a familiar environment. Doctors, who were not then the practitioners of an exalted science, traveled to patients' homes. The time had not yet come when people journeyed to see the doctor. Hospital patients were those who lacked homes in which to be treated, or who lacked the resources to pay a doctor to come in their homes and treat them. Hospital patients were the poor and the homeless.[2]

The holistic view of medicine carried with it the conviction that the moral and the physical lives of patients were also interconnected. And while hospitals lacked the means to act directly on most parts of the body, they could attempt to alter the moral character of the sick and the poor. Regimentation, paternalism, order, and Christian atti-

---

1. Charles E. Rosenberg, "The Therapeutic Revolution: Medicine, Meaning, and Social Change in Nineteenth-Century America," in Morris J. Vogel and Charles E. Rosenberg, eds., *The Therapeutic Revolution: Essays in the Social History of American Medicine* (Philadelphia: University of Pennsylvania Press, 1979).

2. Charles E. Rosenberg, "And Heal the Sick: The Hospital and Patient in 19th Century America," *Journal of Social History* 10 (1977): 483–97.

tudes were enlisted to this end. Charity on both the financial and the conceptual planes was the controlling ethic.

In short, the nineteenth-century hospital was closer to an almshouse than to a modern hospital. Many municipal hospitals, like Philadelphia General Hospital, were explicitly almshouses, while others, like Boston City Hospital, were less explicitly tied to this model. The Baltimore City Hospital was named the Baltimore Almshouse until 1912, when it became an asylum, acquiring the appellation of hospital only in 1924.[3]

The funds for all these hospitals came from public contributions. Municipal hospitals like the two just named were supported largely by tax revenues. Other hospitals were public in the sense of being for the public as opposed to having a fixed claim on the public purse. They were supported primarily by private charities, often closely related to church organizations.

This old style of hospital was replaced by the modern type in the years following 1880. The changes were produced by three separate, albeit not entirely independent, forces: the development of the germ theory of disease, new hospital technologies, and increased urbanization. These in turn produced radical changes in the organization and financing of both medicine in general and hospitals in particular.

The germ theory of disease was articulated by Louis Pasteur in 1870 and began to be adopted among medical practitioners a decade later. Pasteur isolated the cause of disease as a specific identifiable organism separate from the ailing individual. The separation of the disease from the sick person was a radical change in the fundamental conception of illness and the beginning of the path to the dehumanized medical care of today. Instead of seeing people as unitary, this approach saw them as a collection of distinct activities. Instead of seeing them in equilibrium with their environment, it saw them as hosts to specific parasites. And instead of seeing health as a reflection of moral character, it saw health as part of the neutral evolutionary environment. Medicine was changing from synthetic to analytic, from holistic to reductionistic.

Diphtheria antitoxin, which became available in the mid-1890s, was a dramatic demonstration of the power of the germ theory. The in-

3. Toba Schwaber Kerson, "Almshouse to Municipal Hospital: The Baltimore Experience," *Bulletin of the History of Medicine* 55 (1981): 203–20.

cidence of diphtheria in Boston fell from 30 per 10,000 in the years before 1895 to 5 per 10,000 in 1899. Citywide mortality from this disease fell from 18 per 10,000 population in 1894 to 5 per 10,000 in 1899. And the diphtheria mortality rate at Boston City Hospital fell from almost 46 percent in the two decades before 1894 to 10 percent in 1899.[4] The antitoxin enhanced the prestige both of medicine and of the new view of medicine.

It also gave rise to a demand for regulation. Unlike previous drugs, the antitoxin had no immediate physiological effects. Its purpose was not to change the overall interaction between the patient and his environment, but to offset the effects of specific toxic agents. It therefore could not be evaluated by the consumer on the basis of its initial impact. It was one of the first modern medicines, and the demand for its regulation anticipated the modern regulation of drugs.

But while the benefits were not apparent to the layman and did not arrive immediately, dangerous aspects of drugs—harmful side effects—soon became obvious. Actual regulation, in the form of the Biologics Control Act of 1902, arose in response to contaminated diphtheria antitoxin that fatally infected thirteen children with tetanus.[5] The legislative response to a medical tragedy also foreshadowed the path of drug regulation to come. The political forces generated by health disasters continued to be stronger than the less tangible and more theoretical benefits of drugs.

The spread of the germ theory led to the rise of clinical laboratories and their integration with hospitals. Doctors who had practiced happily without laboratory tests began to find them necessary to their diagnoses. Medical care had been separated from hospitals in the nineteenth century, but the need for centralized diagnostic facilities was a factor in bringing them together at the end of the century. The identification of medicine with science was beginning.

Surgical technology was also being improved by a series of innovations in the late nineteenth century. Ether was introduced in 1846, allowing operations to be conducted under anesthesia. But while this

4. Morris J. Vogel, *The Invention of the Modern Hospital: Boston, 1870–1930* (Chicago: University of Chicago Press, 1980), pp. 62–63.

5. Ramunas A. Kondratas, "The Biologics Control Act of 1902," in *The Early Years of Federal Food and Drug Control* (Madison, Wis.: American Institute of the History of Pharmacy, 1982).

discovery was a great boon to patients undergoing surgery, it did not affect the appallingly high mortality resulting from infection. One such infection, gangrene, was a frequent consequence of an operation, and even when amputation was performed, death was a frequent outcome. Lister's carbolic acid introduced antisepsis to hospitals in 1867, but its spread was slow. Antisepsis involved an attitude in addition to the spray, an attitude that developed slowly and only in conjunction with the germ theory of disease.

Antisepsis was also an intellectually hybrid measure, and the change in attitude—when it came—produced the adoption of asepsis rather than antisepsis. Given the germ theory of disease, it was better to avoid the infection altogether than to attempt to combat it after it had begun. It was also much easier on the patient. Aseptic procedures— which we often refer to today as antiseptic ones—vastly reduced the mortality rate inside hospitals. They also made the hospital a far more pleasant place to be, free of the dirt and smells that were offensive as well as harmful.

The introduction of X-rays around the turn of the century improved the ability of doctors to diagnose injury without surgery. X-rays made surgery more effective, both by targeting it more precisely and by eliminating some exploratory operations. Like clinical laboratories, X-rays also increased the scope of the centralized facilities of hospitals, making the support of the hospital itself an important adjunct to medical care. As medical care and centralized medical facilities became more central to hospital activities, the need to support these facilities was added to the previously existing need to feed and house patients.

The University of Virginia Hospital was opened in 1901 and enlarged to 100 beds by 1907. It was a modern hospital of its day. Typical of the new-style hospitals, it was primarily a place to perform surgery. In 1907–1911 it served 70 percent of its patients in the surgical ward and only 20 percent in the medical ward, compared to 42 percent and 35 percent respectively in 1973–74.[6]

The third factor that was transforming hospitals was only tangentially medical. Increasing urbanization led many working people to

6. George Moore and Wilhelm Moll, "Changing Practices and Disease Patterns at the University of Virginia Hospital since 1907," *Bulletin of the History of Medicine* 52 (1978): 571–78.

live apart from their families. Poorer and younger people took lodgings, or rooms without board. They ate at cafeterias and restaurants, which sprang up to serve them, and took their laundry to separate establishments. More affluent people came to live in apartments, the product of both rising urban land values and the invention of the elevator. The division of labor and monetization of services typical of urban life expanded greatly around the turn of the century. People increasingly lived apart both from their family of origin and from the houses in which they were raised.

It follows that when these people took ill, they could not be treated at home. Often no one was there to look after them. Just as eating and doing laundry had become separated from the home, so too had medical care. These middle-class people needed a place to be sick or to recover, even though they—unlike the previous hospital patients—were neither homeless nor socially marginal. Hospital patients were changing from the objects of charity to a cross section of the population. The new middle-class patients came to the hospital both because of the new hospital technology and because of their need for a specialized place in which to be sick or convalescent.[7] And the same improvements in urban transportation that enabled cities to expand at the turn of the century also increased access to hospitals located in those cities.

The growth of the middle-class hospital was part of a process that had been going on since the eighteenth century. The family had been a multipurpose institution in the colonial period, providing a framework for virtually all activities of life except worship. In the late eighteenth and nineteenth centuries, household functions were increasingly split off from the family by free-standing operations. It proved cheaper and easier to buy clothing, do business, and finally care for the sick in specialized institutions than in the family.

The change in the demographic composition of the hospital population created a crisis in hospital finance. As long as hospitals treated only dependent members of society, philanthropy could be counted on to provide the physical resources, while physicians donated their services to the care of the poor and the helpless. But when hospitals came to be used by ordinary members of the community, the appeal

7. Vogel, *The Invention of the Modern Hospital*, pp. 97–119.

for philanthropy was harder to hear. In addition, physicians not affiliated with hospitals accused their hospital-based colleagues of stealing their paying patients by offering free care in the hospital.

Private hospitals, which were small and associated with individual doctors, grew to serve the middle-class trade. But the public hospitals did not wish to see the middle-class cases go, and the resident physicians did not want to have these patients cut off from their practice. So the public hospitals opened special facilities for paying patients to segregate them administratively and physically from the charity cases. Massachusetts General Hospital opened Phillips House in 1917, replete with all the comforts of home. Going to Phillips House carried no taint of accepting charity or even of mingling with those who did. New York hospitals advertised for paying patients, stressing the identification of hospitals with hotels.[8]

At the same time, workmen's compensation, introduced in Massachusetts in 1911, began to change the financial arrangements for the workingman. According to this law, hospital care for injured workmen was paid by the state. The care was no longer a matter of charity; it had become a public obligation implemented through formal assessments. Workmen's compensation paid the hospital for the patient's accommodations, but it did not pay the attending physician. Medical care in the hospital continued to be free, although physicians became increasingly unhappy about their exemption from the public funds. An initial compromise allowed the attending physician to be paid for his "aftercare," the follow-up after the patient left the hospital. But this indirect payment was soon superseded by a more direct one.

Workmen's compensation also provides the first example of insurance causing a rise in hospital rates. The growth of demand from middle-class patients had led to the creation of paying patients; their rate at Boston City Hospital was initially a dollar a day. When the advent of workmen's compensation introduced a new class of patients to the hospital, the hospital's trustees set a rate of three dollars a day for them. The Industrial Accident Board, which administered workmen's compensation, protested that no more should be charged for an injured man employed by an insured firm than for a similarly injured man not employed by an insured firm. The hospital and the

8. David Rosner, *A Once Charitable Enterprise: Hospitals and Medical Care in Brooklyn and New York, 1885–1915* (New York: Cambridge University Press, 1982), pp. 77–80.

board negotiated a rate of $10 a week for insured workmen, but the board remained unhappy. Under renewed pressure to equalize the two rates, the hospital trustees raised the rate for paying patients to the rate for workmen's compensation cases. Massachusetts General Hospital did not try to protect its ward patients; it took the opportunity presented by the introduction of insurance to raise its general ward rate to $15 a week for insured and uninsured patients alike.[9]

As increasing numbers of patients fell into the paying or insured classes, hospitals began paying their operating expenses out of fees rather than contributions. The hospitals' need for philanthropic contributions consequently changed from covering operating expenses to the financing of capital expansion and research. As the hospital began to shift from a caring to a curing place, its fund-raising shifted from financing care to supporting the facilities and the acquisition of knowledge needed to cure increasing numbers of patients.

In 1903, nonprofit and ecclesiastical hospitals derived their income from three sources in roughly equal parts: government support, philanthropy and endowment income, and patient fees. The contribution of the first two categories fell to two-fifths of the total by the mid-1930s, leaving patient fees to cover the remainder.[10] Paying beds grew from 12 percent of total beds in Brooklyn Hospital in 1892 to 58 percent in 1917.[11] From no contribution at all in the days of charitable support, patient fees had grown to constitute one-third of hospital income by the turn of the century and well over half by the onset of the Depression.

The change in financing led to a change in the hospitals' internal balance of power as well. When the primary source of income was philanthropy, the trustees who generated and managed those funds were the locus of control. But as patient fees grew ever larger in hospital budgets, the doctors who attracted the patients assumed more authority. They had become the key to a hospital's success, and they consequently acquired control over its direction.[12]

One index of the changing role of doctors was the integration of hospitals and medical education. Just as hospitals had been largely

9. Vogel, *The Invention of the Modern Hospital*, p. 122.

10. Rosemary Stevens, "'A Poor Sort of Memory': Voluntary Hospitals and Government before the Depression," *Milbank Memorial Fund Quarterly* 60 (1982): 551–84.

11. Rosner, *A Once Charitable Enterprise*, p. 85.

12. Paul Starr, *The Social Transformation of American Medicine*, vol. 1 (New York: Basic Books, 1982), pp. 161–62; Rosner, *A Once Charitable Enterprise*, pp. 103–8.

innocent of medicine in the nineteenth century, so medical education had been quite independent of hospital care. Hospitals, in fact, actively excluded medical students as disruptive, making them pay fees to attend ward walks with doctors or to obtain patients for courses. Johns Hopkins built its own hospital for teaching purposes, foreshadowing the future of medical education and providing the exception that proves the general nineteenth-century rule.

The Flexner Report of 1910 stimulated a general reform of medical education in which science held a prominent place. Increased clinical education was also desired, although it came more slowly. The growth of interest in laboratory results and active medical intervention in both hospitals and medical schools helped bring science and clinical education together. Medical schools found it possible to renegotiate agreements with their affiliated hospitals to provide student access to them. The decade following the Flexner Report saw the introduction of the modern teaching hospital and the spread of "clerkships," the forerunner of modern internships.[13]

THE DEPRESSION AND HOSPITAL INSURANCE

The modern hospital that emerged in the early years of the twentieth century was not a static institution. It continued to change in response to economic events and public policies as the century developed. The onset of the Depression produced a crisis in hospital financing, which led to the creation of effective hospital insurance. After World War II, the government became progressively more involved in the operations of hospitals, under a variety of different programs. And because some of the largest government programs were administered through the existing providers of hospital insurance, the two developments were closely interrelated.

Hospitals had come to rely on patient payments as an important source of income by the end of the 1920s. The onset of the Depression therefore had an immediate effect on hospital revenues. Average hospital receipts per patient fell from $236 to $59 between 1929 and 1930; occupancy fell from 71 percent to 64 percent; and average deficits rose from 15 percent to 20 percent of disbursements.[14] Private

13. Kenneth M. Ludmerer, "Reform at Harvard Medical School, 1869–1909," *Bulletin of the History of Medicine* 55 (1980): 343–70.
14. Sylvia A. Law, *Blue Cross: What Went Wrong?* 2d ed. (New Haven: Yale University Press, 1976), p. 6.

expenditures for hospital construction fell from $96 million in 1927 to just $6 million in 1932.[15] That same year the president of the American Hospital Association warned of "the possible breakdown of the voluntary hospital system in America."[16] Having made the transition from charitable institutions dealing with the societally marginal to providers of services to the population as a whole, hospitals faced the task of maintaining the demand for their services in the face of economic disaster. They worked both to increase their attractiveness to potential patients and to ease the financial burden of hospital stays.

The internal changes in the hospital can be seen through the changing role of nurses. Trained nurses were not used in hospitals before the Depression. Nursing was done by either student nurses or unskilled help. When they graduated from nursing school, nurses went out into the community to practice, setting themselves up in competition with hospitals. Nursing education, it might be noted, was not yet in its modern mode. A 1928 reform in nursing education played the same role that Flexner's famous report of 1910 played in the education of doctors, except that nursing schools were already located near hospitals where the students could get training and assist the hospital at the same time. Prior to 1928, in other words, hospitals were training their competitors, not their staff.

The Depression markedly reduced the demand for nursing care outside hospitals at the same time that it reduced hospital patients' ability to pay. Hospitals were faced with the dual task of convincing patients who could pay that they should use hospitals and convincing those who could not that the hospital was no longer the almshouse of the nineteenth century. They sought to accomplish both of these objectives in several ways, one of which was to employ graduate nurses. They were helped in this campaign by the economic problems of nurses, which encouraged nurses to become complements rather than competitors to hospital medical care. But they were hampered by the poor working conditions in hospitals and the nurses' memories of the paternalism and discipline of their student years. The upshot was a slow transition of nursing to a hospital-based activity in which working conditions remained bad during the excess supply of nurses during

15. Arthur C. Bachmeyer and Gerhard Hartman, eds., *The Hospital in Modern Society* (New York: Commonwealth Fund, 1943), p. 62.
16. Michael M. Davis and C. Rufus Rorem, *The Crisis in Hospital Finance* (Chicago: University of Chicago Press, 1932), p. 3.

the Depression, improving only when nurses became scarce during World War II and the years following.[17]

Hospitals did not stop with internal reform. They also took an active part in increasing patients' ability to pay their bills. The model was taken from a plan instituted at Baylor University in Dallas, Texas, in 1929. There it was noted that the university medical facilities had many unpaid bills from schoolteachers. In order to alleviate this problem, the university enrolled more than a thousand teachers in a plan whereby they paid fifty cents a month for twenty-one days of semiprivate hospitalization at Baylor University Hospital.[18]

Other hospitals adopted this idea when the economic downturn put many patients in the same position as the Dallas schoolteachers. And in the early 1930s several plans were organized that allowed free choice among the hospitals in a given city. The American Hospital Association (AHA) drafted enabling legislation for these plans in 1933. The legislation proposed separate, nonprofit hospital service corporations that would be exempt from the normal insurance and antitrust laws. The argument was that these corporations would be offering public services, not competing with commercial insurers. They would pay hospitals directly, as opposed to reimbursing subscribers for their expenditures. In retrospect this appears to be a distinction without a difference, but it was sufficient to allow the plans to achieve their favored status.

The AHA coined the name Blue Cross for its hospital plans and vigorously promoted their expansion. It coordinated the organizations in separate states until 1960, when a separate Blue Cross Association was formed. But the continuing close coordination of the two associations is illustrated by the fact that the AHA owned the Blue Cross name and insignia for more than a decade after the creation of the Blue Cross Association.

Blue Cross plans enjoyed a virtual monopoly of hospital insurance in the 1930s. All but 0.1 million of the 1.5 million people who had hospital insurance in 1938 belonged to Blue Cross plans.[19] These plans charged the same rate for all people, irrespective of current status or

17. Susan Reverby, "The Search for the Hospital Yardstick: Nursing and the Rationalization of Hospital Work," in Susan Reverby and David Rosner, eds., *Health Care in America: Essays in Social History* (Philadelphia: Temple University Press, 1979).

18. Law, *Blue Cross*, p. 7.

19. Ibid., p. 11.

previous history. This was called *community rating* and corresponded to the public service component of Blue Cross. Payment for insurance was not yet effected by means of payroll deductions; that came only after Social Security taxes and union dues had become integral parts of paychecks. Hospital insurance quickly became a matter for collective bargaining, and unions too supported the growth of Blue Cross.

Competition in hospital insurance arose only during the war. Blue Cross accounted for only two-thirds of hospital insurance by the war's close, and it had less than half the market in the 1950s and 1960s. Community rating was a casualty of competition. Merit rating, in which different rates were established for different groups, spread among Blue Cross plans in the 1950s, foreshadowing even greater differentiation among groups in the 1980s.

Blue Cross was highly successful in tiding hospitals over during the Depression, and it set the pattern for hospital insurance after the war. As hospital creations, Blue Cross plans were designed to provide funds for hospitals, not to monitor hospital functions or expenses. Increases in costs were passed on to subscribers. At the same time, the proportion of costs paid by patients at the time of their hospitalization decreased. (See Table 2–3.)

The Hill-Burton Act of 1946 actively involved the federal government in the provision of hospital care, echoing the earlier involvement of local government in nineteenth-century hospitals. Funds were provided to replace and expand the aging hospital facilities resulting from the virtual absence of hospital construction during the Depression and the war. In order to qualify for federal grants, states had to create a unit that would inventory and plan hospital facilities in the state. The program emphasized rural construction and introduced standards for hospital construction for the first time. By 1971 Hill-Burton expenditures exceeded $12 billion, slightly more than one-quarter of which was federal money. This amounted to about 30 percent of all hospital construction from 1946 to 1971.[20] The program's emphasis on statewide plans foreshadowed current efforts to limit hospital construction through state planning.

Regression analysis of the change in hospital beds per 1,000 pop-

20. Judith R. Lave and Lester B. Lave, *The Hospital Construction Act: An Evaluation of the Hill-Burton Program, 1948–1973* (Washington, D.C.: American Enterprise Institute, 1974), p. 13.

ulation suggests that the Hill-Burton program increased the number of beds per capita. For an average state, the best available estimate is that the subsidy increased the rise in total hospital beds by almost 30 percent, and the rise in short-term beds by 6 percent, between 1947 and 1970.[21] These numbers are hard to interpret, since the total number of hospital beds per capita peaked before 1970, as shown in Table 2–1, but the figures are probably accurate in indicating that the increase in short-term beds was largely independent of the Hill-Burton program.

The program also initiated a limited program of hospital licensing. Doctors have been licensed in all states since the late nineteenth century, before the introduction of the modern hospital. Hospital accreditation by medical societies has its roots in the early twentieth century, when the American College of Surgeons set requirements for Fellows that involved surveying records of 100 patients on whom the prospective Fellow had operated. The college quickly discovered that the requirements were unrealistic because hospitals rarely kept records, and in 1918 it formulated a set of minimum standards for hospitals. Included were requirements that the hospital have clinical laboratories and X-ray facilities for diagnostic purposes, and that it have an organized medical staff and periodic staff conference to review clinical work. The standards also mandated complete medical record-keeping—the initial motivation for the standards—and the elimination of fee-splitting. Only 13 percent of the hospitals surveyed in 1918 were approved while 94 percent of those surveyed were approved in 1945.[22] The Hill-Burton Act required states to institute state licensing of hospitals in order to receive federal funds. The AHA, which began to share support of the College of Surgeon's accreditation program in 1952, supplied a model licensing law that was widely adopted. And when the Medicare program began to certify institutions for receipt of its funds in 1966, it too followed the lines of the surgeons' accreditation.

The Medicare and Medicaid laws were passed with the support of Blue Cross and the AHA. The AHA broke ranks with the American Medical Association (AMA) at the beginning of 1962 and supported

21. Lave and Lave, *The Hospital Construction Act,* pp. 29–38.
22. Anne R. Somers, *Hospital Regulation: The Dilemma of Public Policy* (Princeton, N.J.: Industrial Relations Section, Princeton University, 1969), p. 105.

a national health program on the condition that it be administered by Blue Cross. The administration had tailored its bill to get the support of these organizations, providing for a "fiscal intermediary" chosen by the receiving hospitals to administer Medicare. This provision prevented a clash between the government and the hospitals, and even a possible boycott of the program, at the cost of giving control of the program to the hospitals and their agents. Since the fiscal intermediary controlled the flow of information from the hospitals to the government, there was no possibility of independent action by the government.

The AHA nominated the Blue Cross Association, from which it had only recently been separated, as fiscal intermediary for Medicare. Almost 7,000 of the 8,000 hospitals participating in Medicare did likewise. Formally, the federal government contracts with the Blue Cross Association, which subcontracts the actual administration of Medicare to its member Blue Cross plans. The resulting many-layered structure makes communication between hospitals and the government extremely tenuous; it also gives control of the individual plans to the Blue Cross Association rather than the government.[23]

There was no provision for fiscal intermediaries in Medicaid. Instead, states were to designate a single agency to administer the program in the state. Many Blue Cross plans requested participation in the administration of Medicaid, and they were involved in roughly half the states. The Federal Employee Benefit Program, established in 1959 with the support of Blue Cross, also provided for Blue Cross participation through specifications that were met only by Blue Cross. As a result of all these programs, Blue Cross offset its loss of private subscribers with massive involvement in public programs, thereby regaining its dominant position in the financing of hospital expenditures.

As the hospitals' advocate, Blue Cross has succeeded in having these various government programs adopt an expansive definition of costs. Depreciation is an allowable cost, despite the absence of a requirement that a fund be established for this purpose. Hospitals therefore have used the depreciation reimbursement for operating expenses and have raised money independently—frequently through Hill-Burton—for capital projects. A "plus factor" of 2 percent was originally added to allowable costs for interest on equity capital and other un-

23. Law, *Blue Cross*, pp. 41–44.

specified costs. After continual controversy, it was replaced in 1969 by a nursing cost differential that provides for extra payments scaled on the use of nursing services. Administrative costs also were eligible for reimbursement, with few restrictions. Hospitals and Blue Cross could get repayment, for example, for advertising and other attempts to sway public opinion.

The implementation of these definitions has also favored hospitals. Charges for different services were set by hospitals on terms that they chose. There were no standardized cost data or other guidelines to constrain them. Charges for Medicare patients were the same as for all patients, even though older patients often have longer hospital stays and therefore incur fewer costs during the later stages of their stays. Hospitals were also given the choice of two accounting methods, so that they could use whichever yielded higher payments to them.

According to one prominent observer: "The picture that emerges is one of total unaccountability. Hospitals are paid in advance for whatever they claim."[24]

THE RISE OF HOSPITAL RATES

The preceding section has shown how the existing structure of hospital payments under public programs has led to hospital charges that may easily be higher than they would be under alternative methods of hospital support. But it does not explain why hospital charges should have been rising over time, although it could explain a jump in or around 1966 at the start of Medicare or Medicaid. Martin Feldstein, formerly chairman of the President's Council of Economic Advisers, has constructed an argument to explain the high rate of inflation in hospital charges. His discussion of the issue is the most sophisticated to date and deserves careful scrutiny.[25]

The argument starts with the data in Tables 2–2 and 2–3. Both the cost of hospital care (Table 2–2) and the share of that care covered by insurance (Table 2–3) have risen dramatically since World War II. Relying on more detailed calculations, Feldstein cites the increases

24. Ibid., p. 96.
25. Martin S. Feldstein, *The Rising Cost of Hospital Care* (Washington, D.C.: Information Resources Press, 1971); idem., *Hospital Costs and Health Insurance* (Cambridge: Harvard University Press, 1981).

between 1950 and 1975 to illustrate his point. In 1950 the average hospital cost per patient-day was $16. Public and private insurance paid about half that amount according to his estimate, making the net cost to the consumer $8. By 1975, average daily costs had jumped to $152, and the share paid by insurance had risen to 88 percent. This means that the net cost to patients had only risen from $8 to $18. Since the price level rose by slightly more than double during that period, the net cost to patients did not rise at all in real terms.[26]

The rise in hospital costs and the rise in hospital insurance are clearly related. A rise in costs gives rise to an increased demand for insurance to cover the higher costs. And a rise in insurance induces a rise in costs by hiding the price that people pay; that is, by lowering the effective or net cost. Feldstein argues that the influence of insurance on costs is much stronger than the influence of costs on insurance. His argument is not about the numbers—over which there can be little dispute—but rather about the direction of causation. Is hospital insurance the savior of individual solvency, or the villain of high medical costs?

Feldstein's theory rests on three functional relationships. The first is the demand curve for hospital care. An important assumption in the analysis is that the demand for hospital care, like the demand for most goods, is negatively related to its price. This assumption appears innocuous to an economist, but it is critical to the argument. There are reasons to at least suspect that the price sensitivity of the demand for hospital care might be very low, as much of hospital care is not elective in nature; it is in response to a health emergency. Accidents, heart attacks, and cancers give rise to hospitalization under conditions in which price is not likely to be an important consideration. And to the extent to which doctors make the decision about hospital care for the patient, the response to price may be small. The assumption of price sensitivity can be raised as a matter of theory, but it must be settled empirically.

The second functional relationship is between hospital costs and hospital quality. Feldstein is no more successful than others in defining hospital quality, falling back on perceptions by administrators or patients. But even without a precise definition, it is clear that hospital care today is different from what it was a generation ago. And the

---

26. Feldstein, *Hospital Costs*, p. 2.

increase in costs has had to be channeled somewhere. It is too large to have gone into profits, and most hospitals are nonprofit in any case. It is also too large to be explained by massive decreases in efficiency in hospital operations. The increase in costs has been at least in part an increase in care, which we can refer to as an increase in quality.

Caution must be exercised in the use of this rather amorphous concept of hospital quality. We normally define the quality of a service in terms of its results. The relevant results of hospital care would be health status or life expectancy. But even though life expectancy and some other indexes of health status have improved over time, they have neither changed with changes in hospital costs nor been the result of hospital expansion alone. Hospital quality is consequently measured by the inputs to medical care rather than by the outputs. Those people who see quality improvements equate the increase in care with an increase in health by some definition. Those who fail to see as much increase in quality question whether all the increases in costs—all the tests, all the operations—have a beneficial effect on health. It is worth noting that this issue cannot be settled with data on hospital operations.

Taking the two relationships together—the demand for hospital care and the cost of hospital quality—Feldstein derives a trade-off between the quantity of hospital care, measured by the number of beds, and its quality, measured by the cost. The location of the trade-off is determined by the demand curve, which shows the willingness of people to pay for hospital care. But the existence of a trade-off is not sufficient to determine how society will choose, given the mix of quality and quantity; only to reveal that a choice must be made. The third functional relationship describes hospitals' preferences, and locates them at a point along the trade-off between quality and quantity.

These three functional relationships provide a model of how hospitals decide how many beds to have and how much care to include with them. They can be used to show the effect of hospital insurance on this decision. An increase in insurance raises the demand curve. At a given price charged by the hospital, more insurance lowers the price paid by consumers and therefore increases the quantity of care demanded. Raising the demand curve also raises the trade-off between hospital quality and quantity, resulting—if preferences for hospital care are like preferences for other goods and services—in an increase in both. Increasing hospital insurance is the exogenous force that increases both the number of hospital beds and their cost.[27]

The importance of the price elasticity of demand can now be seen. If the demand for hospital care is not responsive to price, then the presumed shift of the demand curve owing to increasing insurance could not have taken place. Insurance is supposed to have increased the quantity of hospitalization demanded by lowering its net price. If lowering the price has no effect, then increasing insurance has none as well.

Insurance has its presumed effect because of the relationship between an individual's hospitalization and the cost of his or her hospital insurance. Insurance rates rise when the cost of hospitalization rises. But the fate of any single individual does not have a significant impact on the rate of hospitalization of the population as a whole. The actions of people have little impact on the cost of insurance; people are consequently guided by the net cost of hospitalization, not the total cost.

Only one of the three fundamental relationships can be estimated. Without an independent measure of quality, the relationship between cost and quality is largely definitional; the preferences of individuals are simply assumed to exist. The demand for hospital care, however, can be estimated empirically. Feldstein found that the price elasticity of demand for hospitalization is less than one-half but clearly greater than zero. He also found that the number of hospital beds in a state increased the demand for hospitalization; that is, supply created its own demand. Approximately half of any increase in the number of beds was used up by the induced demand, reducing any effect of bed availability on price by half.[28]

The existence of a downward-sloping demand curve supports the contention that the growth of insurance has shifted the demand curve and increased the cost of hospital care. It also has unhappy implications, however, for the relationship between cost and quality. For if the increase in cost comes about because people do not have to pay for it, then there is reason to doubt that the increased cost provides an equivalent increase in quality. Phrased differently, we would expect hospitals to incur costs with decreasing benefits as consumers

27. Ibid., p. 187.
28. Ibid., pp. 118–30.

paid a decreasing share of the costs. As the share that consumers pay goes to zero, the ratio of marginal benefits to marginal costs of a hospital expenditure should go to zero also.[29] Feldstein's argument about the cost of hospital care thus needs amendment: The implication is that not all of the increased cost is equally beneficial to consumers.

Insurance therefore stands as a double villain in Feldstein's story. It increases the cost of hospital care, and it decreases the ratio of benefits to costs in that care. But it is hard to cast insurance in this role by itself, since people appear to want hospital insurance very much. Feldstein therefore carries the argument a step further, insisting that people want insurance largely because of its preferred tax status. Medical insurance is excluded from taxable income when it is supplied by employers or when income tax deductions are itemized. It is therefore cheaper than it would be in the absence of the tax break. More insurance is demanded as a result.

This part of the argument is reminiscent of that used to explain the growth of Blue Cross during World War II, namely, that health insurance increased because it was outside the limits of the wage control board. It is also parallel to the first part of Feldstein's argument in its insistence on the importance of a factor that cheapens the net cost of an activity to the consumer. And like the first part of the argument, it depends on an estimated demand curve: the demand for insurance itself.

But here the story hits a snag. Feldstein's demand curve for insurance fails to show a significant effect of price on demand.[30] Moreover, interviews with corporate officers have shown that large corporations are not interested in reducing the costs of health insurance granted to workers as part of collective-bargaining agreements, suggesting limited price sensitivity in the demand for health insurance.[31]

A recent estimate of the demand for health insurance, however, might save the day. A health insurance experiment run by the Rand Corporation generated new data on the consumption of medical care. Placing families in groups with different forms of health insurance and observing their consumption of medical services, the Rand in-

29. Louise B. Russell, *Technology in Hospitals* (Washington, D.C.: Brookings Institution, 1979).

30. Feldstein, *Hospital Costs,* p. 184.

31. Harvey M. Sapolsky et al., "Corporate Attitudes toward Health Care Costs," *Milbank Memorial Fund Quarterly* 59 (1981): 561–85.

vestigators found a significant price effect on the use of medical resources. The difference, however, was primarily in the subjects' use of ambulatory care. Individuals whose medical expenses were fully covered had more hospital admissions than did the others, but the number of hospital admissions was not affected by the extent of insurance coverage once the subject had to pay any part of the cost. And the cost of hospital stays was totally unrelated to the subjects' cost.[32] The jury is still out on the question of whether the demand for hospital care—not the demand for total medical care—is responsive to price and the extent of insurance coverage.

An alternative way to stop the rising cost of hospitalization, in Feldstein's scheme, is to mandate a different kind of insurance. Feldstein has taken this step, advocating health insurance that pays for major medical expenses but does not offer first-dollar coverage.[33] It would be like automobile or house insurance with a deductible. Presumably, some way would have to be found of keeping first-dollar insurance from creeping back into the market if it turned out that people wanted it on top of disaster insurance. Like the use of the tax structure to reduce the demand for health insurance, this proposal too uses a price incentive to discourage the demand for health care. It can be effective only if the demand for hospital care is responsive to the nature of insurance coverage.

Feldstein's analysis, persuasive though many parts of it are, has not yet found much of an audience among policy-makers. Its reliance on the deterrent effect of price has not been seen as desirable in the medical area. Although it may yet come to be implemented, so far attempts to contain the growth of hospital costs have been aimed at hospital rather than consumer behavior.

RECENT CHANGES IN HISTORICAL PERSPECTIVE

Comprehensive hospital planning began with the Hill-Burton program's requirement that states institute a licensing and planning process. The Comprehensive Health Planning Act of 1966 institutionalized this process by creating state health-planning agencies. This

---

32. Joseph P. Newhouse, Willard Manning et al., "Some Interim Results from a Controlled Trial of Cost Sharing in Health Insurance," *New England Journal of Medicine* 305 (1981): 1501–7.

33. Feldstein, *Hospital Costs*, pp. 252–56.

act, with its mix of state and federal funding and its insistence on consumer representation, added complexity to the health care sector without much effect. Its purposes were never articulated, and the planning agencies functioned as lobbyists for federal funds for their state as much as anything else.

The National Health Planning and Resource Development Act of 1974 replaced these planning agencies with a national network of Health System Agencies that were concerned for the first time with cost containment. States were required to institute Certificate of Need (CON) programs, in which hospital capital expenditures required approval by a state agency before they could be undertaken. The CON was to be the mechanism by which planning agencies initially designed to encourage the growth of hospitals were to be transformed into agencies for the control of hospital costs.

One of the chief goals of the CON requirement was to avoid duplication of hospital facilities. One efficient unit was to replace two small, inefficient, and possibly underutilized units. Despite the attractiveness of the goal, the gains from avoiding or removing this duplication of facilities are small.[34] It is unlikely that much of the hospital cost inflation of the past few decades can be accounted for by the costs of duplication. Certificates of Need are required only for certain kinds of hospital expenditures—capital expenditures over a specified minimum—and therefore may miss other costs or even create perverse incentives for hospitals to expand other costs, such as operating costs, in place of seeking capital expansion. And the CON process itself is very costly. It requires a lot of information for each decision and a complex bureaucracy to process this information. The net gain from the program is only the hospital cost savings minus the cost of administering the program.

Certificates of Need might be used for more ambitious goals as well. They could try to counter the rise in demand for hospital care that comes from the prevalence of insurance by restricting the supply, in the style of the British National Health System. But without some directives and some political backing to counter the strong forces on the demand side, it is highly unlikely that programs originated to ex-

---

34. William B. Schwartz and Paul L. Joskow, "Duplicated Hospital Facilities—How Much Can We Save by Consolidating Them?" *New England Journal of Medicine* 303 (1980): 1449–57.

pand hospital facilities can be transformed into effective constraints on the growth of the hospital system as a whole.

Approximately half the states had CON regulations before the federal requirement was introduced in 1974, and the remainder were required to institute them by the end of 1980, although the law has since been changed to permit discontinuation. A variety of investigators have tried to discover what effect these programs have had. Regression analyses from the first half of the 1970s generally indicated that states with CON regulations had smaller increases in the number of hospital beds than other states, but not smaller increases in hospital expenditures.[35] They therefore suggest that Certificates of Need have altered hospital incentives without affecting the growth of the system, although they are based on only the first few years of the CON requirement.

More recent analysis has had to take account of hospital reimbursement regulation, which also developed gradually in the 1970s. With this approach, states express their concern with rising hospital costs by regulating these costs directly. Hospital rate regulation has the attraction of drawing on the states' long experience of public utility rate regulation. But this apparent bonus shows its weakness, for hospitals are not public utilities in the traditional sense. Public utilities tended to be natural monopolies, and the concern of regulators was to prevent them from charging monopoly prices. The problem with hospital costs is not one of excess profits deriving from market power. Even if extra hospital revenues generated higher costs—the analogue of higher profits in a nonprofit corporation—utility regulation is not indicated since it bases rates on costs.

Utility regulators also typically dealt with small numbers of utilities, since the economies of scale that gave the utilities their market power restricted their number. Hospital regulators, by contrast, have to deal with myriad, often diverse hospitals. In addition to having a less clear mandate than traditional utility regulators, hospital rate regulators also have much more serious informational needs. Their effectiveness may consequently be limited.[36]

35. For example, D. C. Salkever and T. W. Bice, "The Impact of Certificate-of-Need Controls on Hospital Investment," *Milbank Memorial Fund Quarterly* 54 (1976): 185–214.

36. Paul L. Joskow, *Controlling Hospital Costs: The Role of Government Regulation* (Cambridge: MIT Press, 1981), pp. 100–4.

A comparison between the eight states with mandatory rate regulation in 1980 and other states shows that the former have had a slower rate of growth of hospital expenditures and unit costs than have the other states. The comparison also shows, however, that the states that instituted this regulation had the highest hospital costs and the most sophisticated hospital equipment before the regulation was imposed. Consequently it is not clear whether rate regulation decreased the growth of hospital costs in these states or whether these states were initially outliers whose costs have now been brought back into line with other states by natural processes, such as the other states catching up. When both rate regulation and CON regulation are used in regressions explaining the growth rate of hospital expenditures by state, only the rate regulation has a statistically significant effect. And this effect is small and subject to the difficulty of interpretation just mentioned. Only in New York does rate regulation seem to have been stringent enough to have had a major impact on hospital expenditures.[37]

The federal government took a new approach in 1982. Congress directed the Department of Health and Human Services to develop a prospective payment system for government-financed hospital care. The plan was adopted in 1983 as part of the Social Security amendments of that year. It was based on the concept of diagnosis related groups, or DRGs, which had been in experimental use in New Jersey for about two years.[38]

Under such a system, all patients are classified into one of 467 DRGs. Reimbursement is calculated on the basis of a hospital's DRG mix, not on the basis of the actual care given to patients. After an initial phase-in period, Congress envisioned a single national standard for reimbursement, distinguishing only between urban and rural hospitals. The aim of the program is to change the incentives facing hospital administrators. Instead of being reimbursed for whatever costs they incur, hospitals will be reimbursed in the future according to the problems presented to them. They will not be able to recover "excess" expenditures, and they will be able to keep at least part of any reductions in costs they achieve.

37. Joskow, *Controlling Hospital Costs*, pp. 142–62.
38. John K. Iglehart, "New Jersey's Experiment with DRG-Based Hospital Reimbursement," *New England Journal of Medicine* 307 (1982): 1655–60; idem., "Medicare Begins Prospective Payment of Hospitals," *New England Journal of Medicine* 308 (1983): 1428–32.

Setting reimbursement rates on the basis of medical problems rather than on the basis of incurred costs is an attractive idea. There are, however, some reasons to doubt that it will be the cure-all that its supporters hope. The experience in New Jersey was too short to give any reading on whether the DRG system reduced costs. In fact, it increased costs in the short run, a phenomenon that was explained by the need to get hospital acquiescence in the plan. The DRGs, while quite detailed, clearly cannot describe the diversity of patient problems. If the patient mix within a DRG was the same in different hospitals, this would not be a cause of concern. But there is some suspicion that large teaching hospitals may get more difficult—and hence more costly—cases than other hospitals. And the single national standard has problems as well. Hospital rates vary regionally for reasons that do not seem the same as the variation within a single geographic area. In addition to shifting revenue within local areas to the less costly hospitals, the national DRG system will shift revenues interregionally in ways that are unrelated to efficient hospital management.

Only time will tell if the DRG prospective reimbursement system will be implemented nationally and, if it is, what its effect will be. The short history of government attempts to limit the magnitude of hospital cost inflation by regulating hospitals suggests that some skepticism about the ability of this plan to reduce the inflation rate is appropriate.

The DRG-based reimbursement system may affect aspects of hospital operation that are less in the public eye but no less important than the rate of cost inflation on the conduct of hospital affairs. The incentives to cut costs created by the DRG system may well increase the power of hospital administrators relative to medical staff. The need for complex equipment and centralized control of many hospital functions has allowed administrators to gain back some of the power they lost to doctors early in the century, but they have remained the lesser partner till now.[39] The need for cost control, however, may make administrators the senior partners, just as the ability to attract paying patients made doctors the senior partners in the Edwardian era.

Some evidence is emerging that suggests that proprietary hospitals

---

39. Jeffrey E. Harris, "The Internal Organization of Hospitals: Some Economic Implications," *Bell Journal of Economics* 8 (1977): 467–82.

make their profits by being more efficient at using the reimbursement system than by increased efficiency in the delivery of medical care. Despite equal or greater operating costs, proprietary hospitals seem to earn greater "profit" from their services than do nonprofit institutions. In particular, they have higher rates for ancillary services and higher utilization rates for profitable ancillary services than do nonprofit and public hospitals. This effect is most noticeable for proprietary hospitals in multi-institutional systems, the number of which has been increasing rapidly (they now account for more than half of all proprietary hospitals in the United States).[40]

If effective use of the reimbursement system is the source of profit and therefore the stimulus to the growth of proprietary hospital chains, then it is appropriate to ask whether the change to a DRG-based reimbursement system will arrest the growth of these chains. The question is really whether these hospitals have arisen because of opportunities presented by the current method of reimbursement or whether they have grown due to their superior skill at exploiting reimbursement schemes in general. In other words, can they change as the incentives change? As the editor of the *New England Journal of Medicine* said, "It will be interesting to see what happens."[41]

The only sure prediction is that the role of hospitals in American health care will continue to evolve. In the space of a century, hospitals have gone from being peripheral to being central to medical care. With this change has come a shift in the locus of power within the hospital and an enormous increase in the price of hospital services. The latter phenomenon is providing the current impetus for change. The problem is to end a price inflation most probably caused by the increase in hospital insurance without decreasing the insurance. Recent efforts have had little effect. The current analysis suggests that effects will come only when they are coupled with changes in the organization and administration of the hospital itself.

40. Robert V. Pattison and Hallie M. Katz, "Investor-Owned and Not-For-Profit Hospitals: A Comparison Based on California Data," *New England Journal of Medicine* 309 (1983): 347–53.

41. Arnold S. Relman, "Investor-Owned Hospitals and Health-Care Costs," *New England Journal of Medicine* 309 (1983): 370–72.

3

PROPERTY RIGHTS
IN THE HOSPITAL INDUSTRY

Frank A. Sloan

INTRODUCTION

The hospital industry provides a useful setting for comparing the behavior of organizations having different ownership forms. In 1982,
only 13 percent of nonfederal, short-stay hospitals (hereafter termed
"community hospitals") were organized on a for-profit basis.[1] By
contrast, 57 percent of such hospitals were private, not-for-profit (or
"voluntary") hospitals, and the remaining 30 percent were operated
by state and local governments. The share of the hospital market held
by the voluntaries understates the importance of this ownership form,
since voluntary hospitals tend to be larger than for-profit and public
community hospitals. The percentage distribution of hospitals by
ownership type has remained remarkably constant during the past two
decades.

There are major differences in the percentage distribution of
community hospitals by ownership type. For-profit hospitals have
substantial market shares in a few states, such as California, Texas,
Tennessee, and Florida. Yet, as of late 1982, there was not even one
in most of the New England states, Delaware, Iowa, or Wisconsin.

---

1. American Hospital Association, *Hospital Statistics, 1983* (Chicago: AHA, 1983).

103

In some states—Alabama, Arkansas, Georgia, Idaho, Iowa, Louisiana, Mississippi, Oklahoma, Texas, and Wyoming—public hospitals had the largest share of the three ownership forms.[2]

Some dramatic organizational changes, however, have occurred. For one, the industry, which is still largely composed of independent hospitals, is rapidly consolidating into multihospital systems.[3] Although the growth of for-profit hospital chains has received the most publicity,[4] voluntary hospital chains have been increasing at a rapid pace as well. Between 1978 and 1982, the number of for-profit chain hospitals grew by 5.3 percent per year, compared to an annual growth of 11.4 percent for voluntary chain hospitals.[5] Many free-standing hospitals are being acquired by chains of the same ownership form. The stability of hospital distribution by ownership type obscures an important change occurring in hospital control.

The growth of for-profit chains in particular has elicited substantial concern among many persons in the health field that horizontal integration of this type under the aegis of powerful corporations will mean higher-priced (and lower-quality) care that is generally inaccessible to the poor and the severely ill. This view stands in sharp contrast to the majority position among economists and much of the public—that profit-seeking organizations typically are more efficient, albeit perhaps less responsive to society's distributional preferences than are their counterparts organized as private not-for-profit or public enterprises. Some economists would not agree that not-for-profit organizations are better in redistributing services to the poor and needy, but rather have hypothesized that profits are directed in ways that benefit highly paid administrators and others (such as doctors in the community).[6]

2. Ibid.

3. Dan Ermann and Jon Gabel, "Multihospital Systems: Issues and Empirical Findings," *Health Affairs* 3, no. 1 (Spring 1984):50–64.

4. See, for example, Arnold S. Relman, "The New Medical-Industrial Complex," *New England Journal of Medicine* 303, no. 17 (October 23, 1980):963–70; and Paul Starr, *The Social Transformation of American Medicine* (New York: Basic Books, 1982).

5. Ermann and Gabel, "Multihospital Systems."

6. See, for example, Maw Lin Lee, "A Conspicuous Production Theory of Hospital Behavior," *Southern Economic Journal* 38, no. 1 (July 1971):48–58; and Joseph P. Newhouse, "Toward a Theory of Nonprofit Institutions: An Economic Model of a Hospital," *American Economic Review* 60, no. 1 (March 1970):64–74.

A number of important public policy issues are emerging from this debate. First, given that the rise in real expenditures for hospital care during the past two decades has been substantial by any standard,[7] will the increased market share of the multi-unit hospital corporation contribute to hospital cost containment, or instead contribute to still higher rates of increase in real expenditures for hospital care? Second, do hospitals under the control of these companies provide higher- or lower-quality hospital care? Third, are the patient acceptance practices of the for-profits markedly different from those of the others? If so, what are the implications for financing the care of the indigent and persons with catastrophic illnesses? Fourth, to the extent that such hospitals do not engage in teaching and research yet compete with hospitals that cross-subsidize these activities, will competition from profit-seeking hospitals lead to a deterioration of medical education and research in the United States? Some observers, not affiliated with the medical education–research establishment, place such a high value on making current subsidies explicit that they seem willing to allow the medical education–research system to deteriorate if taxpayers are not willing to appropriate explicit subsidies to maintain the status quo. The insiders argue, however, that these taxpayers may be sorry when they see the results, and it would take years to rebuild the system.

The second section discusses the rationale for not-for-profit organizations in the hospital sector, both private and public. The third section describes alternative models of organizational behavior pertinent to analysis of hospital behavior. The fourth section reviews studies that have compared the efficiency of hospitals under various ownership forms. Nursing home care is also provided by for-profit, public, and private not-for-profit firms. Especially because the empirical evidence on efficiency in that industry points in a different direction than that in hospital care, research results from nursing home studies are also reviewed in this section. The fifth section evaluates findings on other dimensions of hospital performance—product mix, types of patients treated, and quality. The sixth section provides further discussion of results and develops public policy implications based on the literature on property rights in the hospital industry.

7. Robert M. Gibson, Daniel R. Waldo, and Katharine R. Levit, "National Health Expenditures," 1982, *Health Care Financing Review* 5, no. 1 (Fall 1983):1–31.

RATIONALE FOR NOT-FOR-PROFIT HOSPITALS

Several reasons have been advanced for the dominance of the not-for-profit form of organization in the hospital sector. There is no consensus about which are the more important ones.

Legal Distinctions

The principal distinction between for-profit and private not-for-profit organizations is in the distribution of accounting profit. The latter organizations do not distribute such profit to individual equity owners. Ideally, the sponsoring group and/or its designees receive a dividend in the form of some public good. In principle, the community, however defined, is the equity holder of the private not-for-profit organization. In practice, there are no rules requiring such organizations to define their "community," although many choose to do so. Also, there are no requirements specifying the form the community dividend should take, or, for that matter, that a community dividend should be paid. Incorporation laws do not prevent such organizations from paying economic rents to employees or persons who exercise control over them, unless perhaps such rents are blatantly large. There are no statutory limitations on the profit a private not-for-profit organization can make. Some states allow such organizations to engage in any noncriminal activity. Others require that such institutions limit themselves to a specific set of activities.[8]

Private not-for-profits enjoy some specific state-conferred advantages, such as exemption from corporate income and property taxes, better access to tax-exempt debt-financing, favored treatment under antitrust laws, and eligibility for private and public donations. However, the Economic Recovery Tax Act of 1981 appears to have reduced substantially the competitive advantage stemming from the corporate income tax exemption. For-profit firms can obtain debt capital through the sale of industrial revenue bonds, which are tax exempt, and some for-profit hospital chains have obtained appreciable amounts of debt capital from this source.[9] Although ability to receive

8. Henry B. Hansmann, "The Role of Nonprofit Enterprise," *The Yale Law Journal* 89, no. 5 (April 1980):835–901, especially p. 839.

9. See, for example, Hospital Corporation of America, *Form 10-K for Fiscal Year Ended December 31, 1983* (Nashville, Tenn.: Hospital Corporation of America, April 27, 1984).

donations gives them one type of advantage in equity markets, private not-for-profit organizations also face an important disadvantage—namely their inability to raise equity capital through the sale of stock.

Potential sources of revenue differ markedly between for-profit and not-for-profit enterprises. Whereas the former receive revenue exclusively from sales of goods and services, the latter have the following potential revenue sources in addition to such sales. They may derive revenue in monetary form from private donations, government grants, and fees imposed on members. In-kind subsidies may come from private donations in the form of services given at below-market (often zero) prices, or from the government in the form of tax breaks or free or subsidized services.[10] Not-for-profit institutions vary in their dependence on these sources.[11]

Another important legal distinction concerns the election of boards of directors. Since private not-for-profits do not have shareholders, there must be an alternative mechanism for selecting the board. The boards of such organizations are sometimes selected by the organization's membership. Alternatively, the board may be self-perpetuating. Until recently, many Blue Cross and Blue Shield plans (private not-for-profit health insurers) allowed hospital and physician organizations to select members of their boards.[12] Whether or not boards truly influence what organizations do is an important behavioral rather than a legal issue.

In many respects, public enterprises resemble private not-for-profits. In the case of public enterprise, the equity owner is clearly the sponsoring government. Dividends are paid to the community through this government, which is often a net subsidizer of the enterprise. Government bureaucracy monitors output and appoints the directors of the enterprise.

The public enterprise has many of the competitive advantages accorded private not-for-profits, with one important exception. Al-

10. Burton A. Weisbrod and Stephen H. Long, "The Size of the Voluntary Nonprofit Sector: Concepts and Measures," in Burton A. Weisbrod, *The Voluntary Nonprofit Sector: an Economic Analysis* (Lexington, Mass: Heath-Lexington Books, 1977), pp. 11–40, especially p. 14.

11. Hansmann, "The Role of Nonprofit Enterprise."

12. Federal Trade Commission, Bureau of Competition, *Medical Participation in Control of Blue Shield and Certain Other Open-Panel Medical Prepayment Plans,* Staff Report to the Federal Trade Commission and Proposed Trade Regulation Rule (Washington, D.C.: FTC, April 1979).

though it has the advantage of better access to public subsidies, the public enterprise often has less autonomy. This is often the case in personnel matters, such as compensation and employment practices, but often external groups may seek to monitor output as well. In the hospital field, for example, an outside authority is far more likely to monitor the record of a public than a private not-for-profit hospital in accepting indigent patients for treatment.

Reasons for Dominance of the Not-for-Profit Form

In the vast majority of U.S. industries, including some in health care, profit-seeking firms dominate. Several experts have provided ex post facto justifications for the minority position of for-profit hospitals.

Fiduciary Relationship between Patients and Physicians.   Some assert that medical care is nearly unique in that patients are unable to judge the quality and appropriateness of the services they receive or ought to receive. As a consequence, patients expect physicians to give priority to their health needs without regard to pecuniary gain. Providers are well positioned to dupe consumers, and health businesses can make considerable profits by doing so.[13] Patients would therefore rather deal with hospitals that do not have profit-making as an objective.[14]

A recent article by David Easley and Maureen O'Hara extended this notion, arguing that the not-for-profit may be superior to the for-profit organizational form in cases where output cannot be closely observed.[15] They drew the motivation for their formal analysis from Henry Hansmann, who used the following as an example of what would lead to "contract failure" if output were exclusively supplied by for-profits: When one buys food for one's own consumption, output is obviously easy to observe. But suppose one wishes to feed the hungry in Ethiopia. Travel to that country is costly, at least for North Americans. For that reason, a profit-maximizing firm might sell the food rather than give it to the hungry. Because of its nondistribution

13. Relman, "The New Medical-Industrial Complex."

14. Kenneth J. Arrow, "Uncertainty and the Welfare Economics of Medical Care," *American Economic Review* 53, no. 5 (December 1963):941–73

15. David Easley and Maureen O'Hara, "The Economic Role of the Nonprofit Firm," *Bell Journal of Economics* 14, no. 2 (Autumn 1983):531–38.

constraint, managers of a not-for-profit organization would not be similarly tempted.[16]

Unfortunately, it is possible to stand this argument on its head. If the managers of a not-for-profit have no stake in the organization's profits, might they not make money by selling output to black marketeers at some location distant from the donors? Are such activities unknown in countries where the means of production are in the hands of the state?

The asymmetric information argument has at least two fatal flaws as applied to hospitals. First, if one accepts consumer ignorance as a rationale for the existence of not-for-profit hospitals, then how does one explain the fact that most physicians, dentists, optometrists, and pharmacists work for proprietary firms, that many nursing homes are for-profit, or that drugs and medical devices are manufactured by such firms? Would it not make more sense to organize physicians' practices on a not-for-profit basis so that these physician agents might protect the public against exploitation by for-profit hospitals? Doctors appear to prefer not-for-profit hospitals to not-for-profit physician practices for reasons that are not too difficult to comprehend. Second, if the not-for-profit hospital is an institution designed to cope with supplier-induced demand in the face of asymmetric information, why is the fee-for-service payment system, which generously rewards the physician for admitting more patients to hospitals, dominant? Physicians earn far more per hour when they work in hospitals than when they work in their offices.[17]

Implicit Subsidies. A profit-seeking organization accomplishes its objective by setting output so as to equate marginal revenue with marginal cost for each output type. Strict application of profit-maximizing criteria allegedly leads to the wrong constellation of outputs. A profit-seeking hospital surely would not engage in much unsponsored biomedical research or in medical education, since marginal cost exceeds marginal revenue at any output level. Such activities would be undertaken only for their advertising or prestige value. A for-profit hospital would undersupply public health measures such as inocula-

---

16. Hansmann, "The Role of Nonprofit Enterprise."

17. Ira L. Burney et al., "Medicare and Medicaid Physician Payment Incentives," *Health Care Financing Review* 1, no. 1 (Summer 1979):62–78.

tions against contagious disease, since private demand curves do not reflect the external effects of being inoculated. Furthermore, such a hospital would not treat patients who are unlikely to pay their bills (or have their bills paid by a third party). Since all of the above activities are desired by society, it is preferable to have hospitals that desire to perform these good acts.

This set of justifications is also not without weaknesses. First, there is some question whether implicit cross-subsidies are the most efficient and equitable way to achieve socially desirable objectives. There is some question whether decision-makers of voluntary hospitals are particularly astute in reading society's preferences, other than those that are manifest through the normal workings of the market. Implicit subsidies generally do not rank well in terms of either horizontal or vertical equity. Taxing paying patients at an inner-city hospital to cover the cost of uncompensated care while allowing patients at a suburban hospital to escape the tax because few no-pay patients go there is one major type of inequity. However, there may be a case for such subsidies in the hospital field on second-best grounds.[18]

Second, as a practical matter, no state to date has linked not-for-profit tax status (501-C3) to the constellation of outputs provided. The vast majority of hospitals, irrespective of ownership type, do not engage in research or teaching, and although public and teaching hospitals provide considerable amounts of uncompensated care (defined as the sum of charity care plus bad debts), ratios of such care to charges are almost identical for nonteaching voluntary and for-profit hospitals.[19] This justification has much greater relevance for public and major teaching hospitals, which are a distinct minority. Most voluntary hospitals are not known for their efforts in the public health field. At least until recently, few promoted immunizations, screening programs, or programs to encourage healthy lifestyles. The presence of important externalities in public health is beyond dispute, but it seems unlikely that most voluntary hospitals do or would engage in such activities without an explicit payment.

18. Jeffrey E. Harris, "Pricing Rules for Hospitals," *Bell Journal of Economics* 10, no. 1 (Spring 1979):224–43.

19. Frank A. Sloan, Joseph Valvona, and Ross Mullner, "Identifying the Issues: A Statistical Profile," in Frank A. Sloan, James F. Blumstein, and James M. Perrin, eds., *Uncompensated Hospital Care: Rights and Responsibilities* (Baltimore, Md.: Johns Hopkins Press, 1986), pp. 16–53.

Explicit Subsidies.   There is a market for private and public donations.[20] Suppliers of gifts would not want to give funds to profit-seeking firms because the donors desire to increase certain outputs beyond their profit-maximizing levels, not to maximize the wealth of the recipient firm's owners.[21] This argument once had merit, more than it does at present. Since the enactment of Medicare and Medicaid, the major public subsidy for hospital care takes the form of payment per unit of patient service; for-profit hospitals, like the other ownership types, receive such subsidies. There has been a secular decline in private giving to hospitals; as of 1981, only about one-tenth of funds for hospital construction came from private charity.[22] This estimate excludes for-profit hospitals that are not eligible to receive gifts for which a donor can claim a tax deduction. Unfortunately, there are no data on the value of private donations used to cover operating expenses. Judging from data on "other hospital revenue," an item that includes revenue from gift shops, parking lots, and other sources in addition to charity, charitable giving could amount to no more than 2 percent of operating revenue of voluntary hospitals, if this much.

Cartel Theory.   Mark Pauly and Michael Redisch and Sol Shalit have argued that hospitals are operated in the interest of a physician cartel.[23] This notion has considerable intuitive appeal and is consistent with some commonplace institutional arrangements. The combination of closed medical staffing and barriers to hospital entry that Certificate of Need (CON) programs establish may serve the interest of physicians already located in an area. Hospital care is an input in the production of the health care service that consumers demand. Even if patients are able to make informed judgments about attributes of the product they purchase, they are likely to be pleased if their doctors select the appropriate input mix.

20. Henry Hansman, "Nonprofit Enterprise in the Peforming Arts," *Bell Journal of Economics* 12, no. 2 (Autumn 1981):341–61.
21. H. E. Frech III, "The Property Rights Theory of the Firm: Empirical Results from a Natural Experiment," *Journal of Political Economy,* 84, no. 1 (February 1976):143–52.
22. Ross Mullner et al., "Funding Aspects of Construction in U.S. Hospitals (1973–1979)," *Hospital Financial Management* 35, no. 11 (1981):30–34.
23. Mark V. Pauly and Michael Redisch, "The Not-for-Profit Hospital as a Physicians' Cooperative," *American Economic Review* 63, no. 1 (March 1973):87–99; Sol S. Shalit, "A Doctor-Hospital Cartel Theory," *Journal of Business* 50, no. 1 (January 1977):1–20.

To link cartelization with the predominance of the private not-for-profit hospital, one must explain why doctors choose to organize most often at voluntary rather than at for-profit hospitals. The argument that physicians prefer slack seems implausible. Why would doctors want to squander their income on "perks" for managers or pay hospital employees more than the minimum pay level required to hire them, as Martin Feldstein has claimed is the case (his "philanthropic wage hypothesis"[24])? If doctors want to give to charity, why would they not collect the maximum amount possible from their practices and then be free to give to the charities of their choice? The tax laws allow both types of charity to be deducted from taxable income.

Robert Clark has suggested several reasons why doctors may prefer to deal with voluntary hospitals.[25] First, physicians may find it easier to divide the profits of a nonprofit than a for-profit corporation. In for-profits, doctors have to share profits with equity holders, whereas they would prefer to split the profit in proportion to the amount of business brought in, much as in a profit-seeking partnership. They may see a nonprofit hospital as a substitute for such a partnership. As Clark himself noted, this is not a particularly strong argument. For one, why is such a substitute needed? Also, in the long run, refusing to compensate equity holders would put the doctors at a competitive disadvantage. Of course, doctors may have been fooled up to now by the notion that they do not "need" externally supplied equity other than from philanthropy, and the growth of the hospital chains is a market response that is proving them wrong.

Second, physicians may avoid the for-profit form to exploit the tax advantages of nonprofit hospitals. Why should one share one's profit with the government when a good nontaxpaying organizational substitute is available?

Third, the not-for-profit form may facilitate physican control over membership in the hospital medical staff. Local physicians might have much more difficulty exercising such control if the hospital were owned and operated by a publicly held for-profit corporation. There is unquestionably something to be said for this argument. Potential loss of

24. Martin S. Feldstein, *The Rising Cost of Hospital Care* (Washington, D.C.: Information Resources Press, 1971).

25. Robert Clark, "Does the Nonprofit Form Fit the Hospital Industry?" *Harvard Law Review* 93, no. 7 (May 1980):1416–89.

local physician autonomy provides a rationale for physician anxiety about, and opposition to, the growth of investor-owned hospital chains. To date, in order to attract physician referrals and reduce local opposition, these companies have taken several important actions to preserve local physician autonomy, such as appointing several local doctors to the boards of their hospitals.[26] However, with increased physician supply, such policies may change—to the disadvantage of local physicians.

Fourth, Clark reasons that physicians may prefer voluntary to for-profit hospitals because patients believe a profit-seeking hospital will exploit them. As emphasized above, the trust argument has important weaknesses. On balance, Clark's second and third reasons for the predominance of the not-for-profit form in this industry are more persuasive.

All voluntary hospitals do not fit perfectly into the cartel mold. For example, the fit is not at all good for hospitals with a close university affiliation. Such hospitals are not controlled by community doctors; in fact, "town" and "gown" doctors are increasingly competing for patients. Nevertheless, the notion that many hospitals are run in the financial interests of local doctors has intuitive appeal and is consistent with several institutional arrangements common to the industry. To the extent that this is the case, the voluntary hospital is only a profit-seeking hospital in disguise, and there is no reason to expect it to behave much differently.

ALTERNATIVE MODELS OF ORGANIZATIONAL BEHAVIOR

Two alternative models, property rights and public choice, predict that for-profit organizations will be more efficient. However, they arrive at this common conclusion in different ways.

The Property Rights Approach

The owner of a profit-seeking firm will seek to maximize utility by selecting the levels of money and nonpecuniary benefits (pleasant work environment, prestige, etc.) necessary to achieve such maximization,

---

26. Frank A. Sloan, "The Internal Organization of Hospitals: A Descriptive Study," *Health Services Research* 15, no. 3 (Fall 1980):203–30.

recognizing that nonpecuniary benefits must be "paid" in the form of lost money income. Under conditions that attenuate property rights, the price of nonpecuniary benefits is reduced, leading the decision-maker to purchase more of such benefits. Since less effort in supervision of personnel and in purchasing both labor and nonlabor inputs, and more perquisites for management—such as nice offices—tend to be important among the nonpecuniary items purchased, property rights theory predicts that for-profit firms will be more efficient than firms under other types of sponsorship.

Organizations of all types face the problem of monitoring the performance of managers. The owners may solve the problem in part by instituting various rules and regulations by which appointed managers must abide. However, when performance is difficult to monitor by outsiders, owners of a profit-seeking firm may assign some of the residual claim to managers, the amount being contingent on the profitability of the firm.

Furthermore, managers face competition from potential replacements. Trustees of nonproprietary organizations may want to monitor their managers, but they face two important constraints. First, it is more difficult to set up a profit-sharing compensation scheme as a "carrot" to management, since the trustees themselves are not residual claimants. This leaves them with only "sticks." But the managers may have tenure or political constituencies of their own, especially in the public sector, and as a consequence the sticks may not work very well, either.[27] Thus, even if nonproprietary organizations do not want to purchase a mix oriented to nonpecuniary benefits, they may end up doing so for lack of alternative inducements.

Although the matter is rarely discussed in the property rights literature, one may suppose that nonpecuniary benefits include charitable acts, teaching, and research, especially when the top decision-makers are likely to receive credit for engaging in such activities. This suggests a two-way empirical test of property rights theory. Not only should profit-seeking firms be more efficient, but they should be less likely to sell nonremunerative outputs.

If profit-seeking firms are superior in terms of technical and allocative efficiency—both input and output—why do other types of firms

27. Kenneth W. Clarkson, "Some Implications of Property Rights in Hospital Management," *Journal of Law and Economics* 15, no. 2 (October 1972):363–84.

continue to exist? The answer by proponents of property rights theory is that nonproprietary firms enjoy important competitive advantages. Presumably, if these advantages were removed, they would soon convert to proprietary firms—or eventually disappear.

An extensive body of empirical evidence has accumulated from a variety of industries and countries in support of property rights theory.[28] Comparisons between profit-seeking and private not-for-profit enterprises and between profit-seeking and public enterprises have spanned such diverse sectors as air and rail transport, electric and water utilities, banking, hospitals, fire protection, and refuse collection.

Reasons have been given for the few results inconsistent with standard property rights theory—either special characteristics of the market or poor methodology. Important among the special characteristics is intense competition among firms with different ownership forms and competition between these firms and firms in other industries selling a product that is a close substitute. Such a seeming contradiction may be more apparent than real. Even the most fervent advocate of property rights theory would admit that if the private not-for-profit or public enterprise has no competitive advantage, it had better act like its profit-seeking competitor—actual or potential—or fold. One case in which competition has existed is between the Canadian National (CN), a public railroad, and the Canadian Pacific, a for-profit railroad. Richard Caves and Laurits Christensen found the two firms to be about equally efficient.[29] Because the Canadian government has limited the subsidy to CN, the authors concluded that it has had to behave like a profit-seeking firm.

Public Choice Approach

The public choice approach reaches some of the same types of conclusions as the property rights approach, but it focuses more directly on bureaucratic behavior as well as interactions among various public actors—the bureaucracy (including employee unions), the legislature,

28. Th. E. Borcherding, W. W. Pommerehne, and F. Schneider, "Comparing the Efficiency of Private and Public Production: The Evidence from Five Countries," *Zeitschrift für Nationalökonomie/Journal of Economics: Public Production,* Supplement 2 (1982):127–56.

29. Douglas W. Caves and Laurits R. Christensen, "The Relative Efficiency of Public and Private Firms in a Competitive Environment: The Case of Canadian Railroads," *Journal of Political Economy* 88, no. 5 (October 1980):958–76.

and special interest groups.[30] This view also predicts that public enterprise will tend to be less efficient than private enterprise, but adds that, as bureaucrats and their allies act in their self-interest, publicly supplied outputs may exceed socially optimal levels, and wage rates of public employees may be pushed well above competitive rates.

The difference between the property rights and the public choice approaches is more a matter of style than substance. Some studies, such as the one by Martin Feldstein that maintained that hospitals are wage philanthropists (that is, they pay their employees more than competitive wages), do not specifically claim allegiance to either school.[31] Actually, however, they belong to both.

The "Bottom Line"

Although both views have some intuitive appeal, and certainly considerable empirical backing, some aspects of the two approaches are unsettling. First, as Borcherding and coauthors emphasized, these studies put economists—who use the idea that waste will be minimized as the cornerstone of their thinking—in a rather awkward position.[32] If society wants to minimize waste, defined as both technical and allocative inefficiency, why does it continue to tolerate institutional arrangements that perpetuate its existence? Borcherding and coauthors answered this question by raising the possibility that transactions cost, and ultimately total cost, would be still higher if regulated for-profit firms were asked to produce the outputs produced by firms under other ownership forms. Another possibility is that allowing the other ownership forms to persist represents a mechanism for effecting an in-kind transfer. Let us suppose, for example, that society believes every person between the ages of 18 and 65 ought to have a job; public enterprise may then be the cost-minimizing way of achieving this objective. Finally, the view that waste will be minimized need not hold at every point in time, but rather economists may only be expressing their optimism that, in the long run, the more efficient arrangements will prevail.

30. Borcherding, Pommerehne, and Schneider, "Comparing the Efficiency of Private and Public Production."

31. Feldstein, "Rising Cost of Hospital Care."

32. Borcherding, Pommerehne, and Schneider, "Comparing the Efficiency of Private and Public Production."

There are a number of specific reasons to question the applicability of standard property rights theory to the U.S. hospital industry. In the main, these are criticisms of the application of the theory to this industry rather than criticisms of the theory itself.

First, if one believes that the cartel theory has some applicability, the private not-for-profit hospital is really a for-profit hospital in disguise. Any competitive advantage such hospitals enjoy by reason of their legal status is ultimately appropriated by doctors. Many small rural hospitals, though legally "public," are in reality operated like private not-for-profit hospitals. In particular, they deliver very little charity care.[33] Such hospitals too may possibly be described by the cartel theory.

Second, inefficient hospitals are prime candidates for acquisition by for-profit hospital chains. Hospitals are much more likely to be subject to acquisition than are public libraries, fire stations, and nationalized airlines. This mechanism for weeding out inefficient producers has become especially important in recent years. The management contract whereby a hospital chain manages a free-standing hospital is another such mechanism.

Third, up to now, competition on the basis of price has not been a dominant force in the hospital industry. Even so, cross-price elasticities among neighboring hospitals are not zero, which places some limit on inefficiency. Very recently, price competition among hospitals has become fierce in some locations, but this development is too recent to be reflected in the data used in past studies.

COMPARATIVE EFFICIENCY OF DIFFERENT OWNERSHIP FORMS

A number of empirical studies have appeared in recent years, both descriptive and multivariate, that have sought to compare the relative efficiency of alternative organizational forms of hospitals. Many of these have been descriptive. A few have employed regression analysis. Although they attempt to hold factors other than ownership constant by means of a "matched pairs" methodology or by regression analysis, even the more careful studies have one major Achilles' heel: their failure to control adequately for variations among hospitals in

---

33. Sloan, Valvona, and Mullner, "Identifying the Issues."

quality and amenities. Especially because potential quality-amenity differences are always lurking in the background, it is advisable not to make too much of small differences in the variables used to compare efficiency. Comparisons of the management process by ownership type do not suffer from this deficiency.

As will be seen below, efficiency has been measured in several ways. Some studies have compared the management process of hospitals under different ownership forms. Some have compared levels of input use and wage rates. Others have focused on cost per unit of output. In some, a cost function was estimated to permit comparisons of efficiency among hospital types. In these, input prices were considered to be exogenous. In several cases, the study's primary objective was not to compare hospitals of various ownership types. But since binary variables for ownership were included as explanatory variables in these studies, this review takes advantage of their data. Because very little pertinent empirical analysis on the subject appeared before the early 1970s, this review is limited to studies written from 1972 to the present.

Descriptive Studies

Clarkson (1972).   Kenneth Clarkson made two types of comparisons. First, he examined differences in management procedures by ownership type. Second, he compared input choices.[34]

As discussed above, trustees of nonproprietary organizations may be constrained in the use of profit-sharing as "carrots" for high-level managerial performance and, may impose more-explicit rules as a result. Clarkson presented evidence from secondary sources indicating that, not only did for-profit hospitals have less-explicit bylaws, but also they were less likely to have (1) formal budgets approved by a governing board, (2) an American Hospital Association (AHA) chart of accounts, (3) written sets of staff regulations, (4) regularly scheduled staff meetings, (5) standing committees on the staff, (6) restrictions on staff physicians' surgical privileges, and (7) restrictions on nonstaff members practicing in the hospital.

Clarkson found that administrative staff spent more of their time

---

34. Clarkson, "Some Implications of Property Rights."

on night duty in for-profit hospitals. This was interpreted as evidence that management of nonproprietary hospitals enjoyed higher nonpecuniary benefits, since day work is generally preferable to working the night shift.

Clarkson hypothesized that nonproprietary hospital managers will use market information less frequently than will their counterparts in proprietary organizations. He reported that nonproprietary hospitals were most likely to use explicit nonprice rationing mechanisms for allocating beds among nonemergency patients. He gave some examples of these approaches but presented no evidence that any hospital allocated beds on the basis of a competitive bid.

It is difficult to evaluate a prospective manager's capability before hiring. Clarkson found nonproprietary hospitals more likely to employ a graduate of a hospital administration program, presumably an imperfect proxy for quality. He did not describe the criteria that for-profit firms used to select their managers.

Management interested in cost minimization would pay employees competitive wages based on their individual performances and would eschew automatic wage adjustments. Clarkson found nonproprietary hospitals, both private and public, much more likely to grant such increases.

Based on the assumption that managers of nonproprietary hospitals are less likely to share in hospital profits, one would expect that they devote less effort to collecting unpaid bills from patients. Clarkson found some evidence from a small sample of southern California hospitals that the nonproprietaries were less likely to pursue unpaid bills.

A second part of Clarkson's study dealt with variability of input selection. Once wage rates are known, allocatively efficient hospitals should employ similar labor mixes. Clarkson found greater variability for the nonproprietaries, which he interpreted as evidence of their allocative inefficiency.

Clarkson succeeded in advancing some very interesting ideas, but unfortunately most of his inferences are subject to alternative interpretations. First, his comparisons predate the investor-owned chain hospital. Many of the for-profit hospitals were owned and operated by a single physician or a small group of physicians. It should come as no surprise that hospital bylaws were not formalized; these were closely held corporations, and many were not even incorporated. If the physician owner-manager was in the hospital by day, it should come as no surprise that he employed administrative help for night duty. In some cases, the physician himself served as the administrator; therefore, there was no administrator at the hospital with a degree in hospital administration. Second, the hypothesis that managers of nonproprietary organizations have less reason to be concerned about profitability was plausible but, without direct evidence on the methods of manager compensation, the tests proffered must be considered weak at best. Third, a major reason that input mix varies among hospitals is that case mix varies. Unfortunately, Clarkson asserted that input mix should not be very sensitive to case mix variation and hence did not adjust for case mix differences. If the variation in case mix were greater for nonproprietary hospitals, one would expect to find more substantial input mix differences. Finally, as discussed more fully below, Clackson's evidence on unpaid bills contradicts more recent evidence based on a national sample. Also, hospitals may deliberately fail to collect some unpaid bills as an act of charity. Hence, such inaction is not necessarily indicative of inefficiency.

Lindsay (1976, 1980). In C. M. Lindsay's model, the government sponsor of a public enterprise places a value on certain attributes of the firm's output.[35] Whether or not the sponsor can evaluate profitability is largely irrelevant in Lindsay's view. If the government sponsor had wanted the firm to maximize profit, it would not have created the public enterprise in the first place. The enterprise's managers recognize the attributes the sponsor values and orient their businesses accordingly. Attributes invisible to the sponsor are not produced or produced only incidentally to something the sponsor values. Quality tends to be invisible to the sponsor and therefore is not emphasized by the public enterprise.

The test of the model provided a nexus to efficiency. Lindsay compared mean per diem cost in Veterans Administration (VA) hospitals with that of proprietary hospitals and found the latter to be appreciably higher. Staff-to-patient ratios were also found to be much lower in VA than in for-profit hospitals. This is plausible, Lindsay explained, because Congress would not reward the VA for offering patients more than a life-maintaining quality level. While cost per diem was lower

35. Cotton M. Lindsay, "A Theory of Government Enterprise," *Journal of Political Economy* 84, no. 5 (October 1976):1061–77.

in the VA hospitals, this saving was partly offset by longer mean lengths of stay in such institutions. Recognizing that many readers would argue that such comparisons are meaningless because the VA treats a "unique" case mix, Lindsay also contrasted lengths of stay in state and local short-term general hospitals with proprietary hospitals and found stays in the former to be about one to two days longer. Lindsay maintained that the longer stays for the public hospitals were consistent with his theory of government enterprise, because Congress values, or at least can monitor, quantity that takes the form of more patient days.

The 1980 study by Lindsay and coauthors compared lengths of stay in U.S. proprietary hospitals with those of the British National Health Service (NHS) by three-digit diagnosis category.[36] Without exception, stays in NHS hospitals were higher, more than twice as high for some diagnoses.

Ideally, Lindsay (and others) would have distinguished differences in cost per quality-adjusted patient day and in the number of patient days adjusted for quality. The lower per diem expense for the VA may have reflected lower quality, but perhaps government enterprise was indeed more efficient in this instance. The study did not contain even one measure of quality. Some aspects of quality are undoubtedly invisible to Congress, for example, the smile on the nurse's face when she wishes the patient "good night." Other aspects, such as the poor condition of the physical plant and lengthy waits in outpatient departments, would be highly visible to even the most casual visitor and most certainly to the media. Perhaps Congress has knowingly permitted a low amenity level to persist at some VA hospitals because it is unwilling to underwrite a higher quality level.

That stays tend to be longer in public hospitals probably has more to do with patients' time prices than with property rights. The poor, who are served by public hospitals in this country, and the median patient of the NHS, who when of employment age is more likely to have pay or employment status linked to the amount of sick leave taken than is his or her counterpart in the United States, are probably willing to trade some time for money. The longer stays in public hospitals need not reflect a misreading of such patients' demand curves.

---

36. Cotton M. Lindsay et al., *National Health Issues: The British Experience* (Nutley, N.J.: Hoffman-LaRouche, 1980).

Lewin, Derzon, and Margulies (1981).   Lewin and coauthors compared 53 matched pairs of for-profit and voluntary hospitals having 50 to 412 beds.[37] Each for-profit hospital had been owned by a chain for at least three years. Criteria for matching were size, location (same state and metropolitan area), and a common group of services. The two types of hospitals selected had almost the same average daily census, number of beds, occupancy rate, number of admissions, Medicare days as a percentage of total days, Medicaid days as a percentage of total days, and inpatient revenue as a percentage of total revenue.

The authors found that the for-profits had higher charges—8 percent higher routine (room and board) and 36 percent higher ancillary charges per inpatient day. These hospitals had mean routine and ancillary charges per admission in excess of their not-for-profit competitors by 4 percent and 26 percent, respectively. Medicare allowable costs, including Medicare's return on equity payment, which only profit-seeking hospitals are eligible to receive, were 13 percent higher in for-profits per inpatient day and 8 percent higher per admission. Net patient service revenue (defined as gross patient revenue less contractual adjustments obtained by some insurers, bad debts, and charity care) less taxes paid per adjusted patient day (an adjustment to convert outpatient visits into inpatient equivalents) was 12 percent higher for profit-seeking hospitals.

Overall, total operating cost per adjusted patient day and total inpatient cost per inpatient day were both about 8 percent higher in for-profit hospitals. However, inpatient cost per admission was about the same, since stays were shorter in the for-profit hospitals. An analysis of inpatient cost components revealed that the voluntary hospitals had lower ancillary service expenses (including radiology, laboratory, and pharmacy expenses) and lower administrative expenses, while the for-profits spent proportionately less on space and routine nursing care.

Not surprising in view of the above results, markups were higher in for-profit hospitals than in the voluntaries, and more so for routine care than for ancillary services. Total net income after income tax as a percentage of total net revenue was 3.7 percent in the for-profits and 1.3 percent in the not-for-profits. Net income after tax per ad-

37. Lawrence S. Lewin, Robert A. Derzon, and Rhea Margulies, "Investor-Owneds and Nonprofits Differ in Economic Performance," *Hospitals* 55, no. 13 (July 1, 1981):52–58.

justed day was, on average, $9.14 for the profit-seeking hospitals and $3.36 for the not-for-profits. The authors inferred from their empirical analysis that the not-for-profits may have been underpricing their services, especially for routine care.

Lewin and coauthors exercised far more care in drawing samples from a population of comparable hospitals than did most of the earlier researchers. Their study offers two potential lessons. One deals with relative efficiency and the other with pricing.

The two ownership types proved to be about equal in terms of cost per case, but there was a sizable difference in price per case. For purposes of making judgments about relative efficiency, neither the cost nor the charge measure is perfect. Irrespective of ownership, the theoretically correct measure of cost for making efficiency comparisons—economic cost—includes a competitive return to owner equity. Thus, the cost estimates reported by Lewin and coauthors provide a lower-bound estimate of economic cost. If hospitals of all ownership types had the same debt-to-equity ratio, accounting cost would equal economic cost up to a factor of proportionality. But proprietary hospitals have higher ratios on average.

The charge measures may over- or understate economic cost. They would overstate such cost if hospitals have the power to set price to earn more than a competitive return on equity. Such measures would understate economic cost for three reasons. First, charge data do not reflect hospital revenue from nonpatient sources, gifts and grants in particular. The Lewin et al. study did not adjust for differences in such revenue, which on average is higher for nonproprietary hospitals. Second, a private not-for-profit hospital may pay its community dividend in the form of free care. The value of such care would not be reflected in an estimate of mean charges computed as net patient revenue divided by patient days or admissions. By contrast, the dividend a for-profit hospital pays its shareholders comes out of the hospital's after-tax profit; this dividend is reflected in the hospital's net revenues. This criticism would have greater force if voluntary hospitals provided much more "free care" than their for-profit counterparts, but they do not.[38] Third, as Lewin and his colleagues suggested, some hospitals may price their services below the level needed to recover full economic cost.

38. Sloan, Valvona, and Mullner, "Identifying the Issues."

Sloan and Vraciu (1983).   Frank Sloan and Robert Vraciu compared for-profit and voluntary hospitals having less than 400 beds using financial data Florida hospitals were required to submit to that state's Hospital Cost Containment Board.[39] To compare efficiency, the authors developed two measures. The first was "net operating funds," defined as operating revenue (net of contractual adjustments and non-paid accounts) minus corporate income taxes. They could not subtract property taxes from operating revenue because such data were not available on an individual hospital basis. The second measure was total margin, the after-tax difference between total revenue and total expense. They included nonoperating revenue, part of which was income from gifts and grants, in total revenue. The nonoperating revenue measure did not capture all charitable giving since voluntary hospitals are permitted to pass restricted donations and income from restricted funds directly onto the balance sheet without showing such income on the income statement. Since the Cost Containment Board obtained only income statements, the authors could not consider "balance sheet only" charitable income.

The authors found that net operating funds per adjusted admission were identical for voluntary and for-profit chain hospitals in their Florida sample in 1980 ($1,978 each), whereas all for-profit hospitals, free-standing and chain, had slightly higher net operating funds per case ($2,009). The voluntaries had slightly lower net operating funds per adjusted patient day: $271 for not-for-profit, $276 for proprietary chains, and $279 for proprietaries overall. Based on these comparisons, Sloan and Vraciu concluded that the net operating cost to the community was virtually the same for voluntary and for-profit chain hospitals, and that the chain proprietaries were less costly than their free-standing counterparts. They found that the after-tax total margin was a little higher for the nonprofits: 5.6 percent, compared to 5.4 percent for the proprietary chains and 4.8 percent for proprietaries overall.

A controversial aspect of the Sloan-Vraciu study has been the authors' tax adjustment. Arnold Relman, editor of the *New England Journal of Medicine* and perhaps the most vocal opponent of the for-profit hospital movement, argued, "Whatever benefits those taxes might have produced were distributed throughout the economy and were not

39. Frank A. Sloan and Robert A. Vraciu, "Investor-Owned and Not-for-Profit Hospitals: Addressing Some Issues," *Health Affairs* 2, no. 1 (Spring 1983):25–37.

confined to health care or to those who paid the charges. Therefore, regardless of whether the community in some sense benefited from the taxes, it seems clear that the higher charges in the investor-owned chain hospitals increased the cost of health care, without a commensurate return to the health sector.[40] This type of argument would apply to all types of business taxes. If anything, Sloan and Vraciu and others are to be faulted for not taking account of all types of taxes.

Pattison and Katz (1983).   Pattison and Katz analyzed 1980 financial data that California hospitals were required to submit to the California Health Facilities Commission.[41] To compare like hospitals, the authors classified them into one of twelve peer groups. The peer groups were formed from a cluster analysis, with hospital size, location, teaching status, and service mix complexity constituting the clustering variables. Comparisons were limited to peer groups 4 and 5, which had relatively high for-profit representation. Mean bed size for the two groups was 140. Hospitals in all three ownership categories were represented in the comparisons.

The authors presented too many measures of hospital performance to review here; this discussion focuses only on the measures also used in other studies. As in the other studies reported above, the authors found that the for-profit hospitals had higher inpatient charges per admission and particularly per patient day. Patients at for-profit hospitals had more ancillary-intensive stays, as indicated by the percentage of the total bill for such services. Investor-owned chains were about 2 percent higher in terms of operating expenses per admission than were the voluntary hospitals. Free-standing proprietaries were 2 percent lower on this measure than were the voluntaries, all of which were free-standing. Public hospitals had the lowest operating cost per case. The for-profit hospitals tended to have higher, rather than lower, administrative costs, which seems inconsistent with the argument that profit-seeking hospitals reduce "slack."

Unfortunately, no data on income taxes were presented. Hence, a direct comparison between the Sloan-Vraciu and the Pattison-Katz re-

40. Arnold S. Relman, "Editorial: Investor-Owned Hospitals and Health-Care Costs," *New England Journal of Medicine* 309, no. 6 (August 11, 1983):370–72. Quotation is from p. 371.

41. Robert V. Pattison and Hallie M. Katz, "Investor-Owned and Not-for-Profit Hospitals," *New England Journal of Medicine* 309, no. 6 (August 11, 1983):347–53.

sults is not possible. Even without the tax adjustment, however, the differences were quite small.

There was no consistency among hospital types in relative after-tax profitability in the Pattison-Katz study. On net income per case after tax—a measure that included nonoperating revenue—voluntary hospitals ranked the highest, followed by chain for-profits, public hospitals, and independent for-profits, in descending order. However, voluntaries and independent for-profit hospitals had the highest net income to total assets. On net income to owners' equity, the for-profits were about twice as profitable as the voluntaries and three times more profitable than the public hospitals, again because the debt-to-equity ratio tends to be higher for proprietary hospitals. Also, an important part of the equity of public hospitals may not appear on their balance sheets.

Regression-based Studies

Some of the above studies presented comparisons among "matched samples" as a method for holding nonownership factors constant. Matched comparisons are necessarily limited, in that sample sizes become unacceptably small if more than a few criteria are used for matching. Regression analysis allows one to take many more factors into account. The following studies considered a number of explanatory variables in evaluating efficiency differences among hospitals.

Bays (1979).   Bays estimated a cost equation with the total cost per case as the dependent variable, using a sample of eighteen for-profit and twenty-eight private not-for-profit California hospitals observed in 1971 and 1972.[42] In contrast to almost all other hospital cost studies, Bays's dependent variable included estimated physicians' charges associated with the hospital stay as well as hospital cost. In addition to hospital ownership, he included a case mix variable, bed size, the percentage of hospital admissions that were "self-pay," and a measure of case flow, the number of cases treated per year per bed.

The coefficient on the binary variable on for-profit status, though positive, was insignificant at conventional levels. However, the coef-

---

42. Carson W. Bays, "Cost Comparisons of Forprofit and Nonprofit Hospitals," *Social Science and Medicine* 13C, no. 4 (December 1979):219–25.

ficient on an interaction term with respect to for-profit ownership and chain status was negative and statistically significant at the 1 percent level. Bays also estimated separate regressions on for-profit and voluntary hospital samples. Some structural differences in the cost equations between the two types of hospitals were detected, but such stratification was of limited value given the small sample size.

Becker and Sloan (1985).   Becker and Sloan combined data from two national hospital surveys, the Reimbursement Survey and the Annual Survey of Hospitals, both conducted by the American Hospital Association in 1979.[43] Combining the two surveys made 1,645 hospitals available for analysis.

The dependent variables were total hospital cost per adjusted patient day and per adjusted admission, patient revenue divided by total cost, and total revenue (patient plus nonpatient) divided by total cost. Total cost was accounting cost as it appeared on hospital income statements. The revenue measures excluded contractual adjustments and unpaid bills. As specified, the parameter estimates from the cost and profit equations could be added to yield equations for revenue per adjusted patient day and per adjusted admission. The authors discussed the role of taxes in interpreting their results, but did not adjust the data for tax payments prior to estimating their cost and profit equations.

A distinction was made, based on ownership status and affiliation with a chain, among nine different hospital types. Three categories of chain status were considered: independent, "recent," and "longstanding." The study distinguished among chains based on length of affiliation. A hospital may have been acquired because it was a poor performer, and some time may have been required before an improvement in efficiency could have been realized. Data was limited, so the dividing line between recent and longstanding was four years for proprietary and six years for private nonprofit and government chains. Hospitals that were contract managed but not owned by an outside group were classified as independent.

In addition to ownership, the authors included a number of explanatory "control" variables: teaching status, case mix (the Resource

---

43. Edmund R. Becker and Frank A. Sloan, "Hospital Ownership and Performance," *Economic Inquiry* 23, no. 1 (January 1985):21–36.

Need Index developed by the Commission on Professional and Hospital Activities), the mix of hospital patients by third-party payer, bed size, a binary variable for hospital age, per capita income of patients in the hospital's market area (to account for amenity differences), a measure of hospital wages, and region dummies.

Becker and Sloan found that independent for-profits were more expensive than other independent hospital ownership types in terms of cost per adjusted patient day, but they were the least costly, gauged on cost per adjusted admission, although the difference between independent for-profits and voluntaries was not significant at conventional levels. Independent public hospitals were almost identical to private nonprofits on both cost measures. The results were less favorable to proprietary hospitals affiliated with chains. Their cost per adjusted patient day was more than 10 percent higher than it was for independent voluntaries. On total cost per adjusted admission, newly affiliated proprietary chain hospitals were 12 percent higher than independent voluntaries; chain proprietaries with a longer affiliation were 6 percent higher on cost per case, but the coefficient on the binary variable for this group was insignificant.

The profit regression showed no difference in profitability between voluntary and for-profit hospitals—holding the other factors in the regression constant—but the public hospitals were less profitable. Neither these nor the cost results lent empirical support for standard property rights theory. The estimated ownership parameters were somewhat sensitive to equation specification, which gives some reason for concern that some of the comparisons from the less well controlled studies might be misleading.

Wilson and Jadlow (1982).   Wilson and Jadlow assessed the relative efficiency of hospitals of the three ownership types in the provision of nuclear medicine services.[44] Linear programming was used to estimate a frontier production function. Inefficiency could then be evaluated in terms of a given hospital's divergence from hospitals at or

44. George W. Wilson and Joseph M. Jadlow, "Competition, Profit Incentives, and Technical Efficiency in the Provision of Nuclear Medicine Services," *Bell Journal of Economics* 13, no. 2 (Autumn 1982):472–82.

near the frontier. Using an "efficiency divergence index" as the dependent variable, Wilson-Jadlow estimated equations with an index of competitive intensity and binary variables for public and for-profit ownership as independent variables. They found that government hospitals were less efficient and for-profit hospitals more efficient than the omitted reference group, private not-for-profits.

The Wilson-Jadlow study has the advantage of focusing on one department, thus reducing the likelihood of output heterogeneity, which is often a problem in hospital cost studies. Also, nuclear medicine output was adjusted for variations in service mix among nuclear medicine departments in the sample.

Wilson and Jadlow included very few explanatory variables in the efficiency equations, which may be a source of serious omitted-variables bias. For example, very few departments in for-profit hospitals have teaching programs. A leap of faith is required to generalize from one small hospital department to the hospital as a whole; additional confirmation from other departments would be desirable.

Sloan and Steinwald (1980a, 1980b).   Sloan and Steinwald presented regressions with earnings per full-time hospital employee as the dependent variable (1980a).[45] The authors found no difference in pay levels by ownership type. Their second study (1980b) specified and estimated an input employment model with six dependent variables: professional nurse (RN) employment per bed, licensed practical nurse (LPN) employment per bed, other employees per bed, net plant assets per bed, expenditures on current nonlabor inputs per bed (including hospital supplies, utility expense, interest, and annual depreciation), and number of beds.[46] They reported that proprietary hospitals had lower expenditures on RN and other employee use, and higher expenditures on current nonlabor inputs, than either voluntary or government hospitals. The proprietary hospitals had comparatively low labor expense, but this saving was fully offset by higher expense on the nonlabor side.

---

45. Frank A. Sloan and Bruce Steinwald, *Insurance, Regulation, and Hospital Costs* (Lexington, Mass.: Heath-Lexington Books, 1980).

46. Frank A. Sloan and Bruce Steinwald, *Hospital Labor Markets: Analysis of Wages and Work Force Competition* (Lexington, Mass.: Heath-Lexington Books, 1980).

Overall Assessment of Findings on Hospital Efficiency

In summary, empirical research to date suggests that for-profit and voluntary hospitals are quite similar in terms of accounting cost. For-profits may be slightly higher in price. Pay levels appear to be comparable, but for-profit hospital production tends to be less labor intensive. Public hospitals differ much more from the two types of private hospitals than the two private types do from each other. Since many public hospitals appear to offer lower-amenity care, observed differences in the efficiency measures are difficult to interpret.

Does the empirical evidence suggest that one ownership type is more efficient than the others? To make proper comparisons, it is necessary to take the following precautions.

First, cost should be measured as economic rather than as accounting cost. This means that a competitive return on equity should be included, irrespective of ownership type.[47] If a return on equity is not counted, hospitals with high debt-to-equity ratios will show higher capital cost and probably higher total cost. Rents or quasi-rents should not be counted.

Second, there should be an adjustment for differences in accounting practices that differ systematically by ownership type. For example, since they are subject to the corporate tax, for-profit hospitals have an incentive to use accelerated depreciation methods. For this reason alone, proprietary chain hospitals, which tend to be newer on average,[48] would tend to report higher cost. Care should be exercised in allocating home office costs to individual hospitals.

Third, there should be an attempt to avoid or correct for selectivity bias. For instance, hospitals recently acquired by chains may have been candidates for acquisition because they were mismanaged. It may take years for the chain organization to markedly improve the efficiency of such hospitals.

Fourth, tax payments should be removed from cost. Ideally, the only taxes that should be included in cost are those representing pay-

47. Douglas A. Conrad, "Returns on Equity to Not-for-Profit Hospitals: Theory and Implementation," *Health Services Research* 19, no. 1 (April 1984):41–63.

48. Center for Health Economics Research and Health Policy Center, Vanderbilt University, *Medicare-Medicaid Payment Policies and Capital Formation*, Final report to the U.S. Health Care Financing Administration, December 20, 1985.

ments for an input used in the production of hospital care. For example, if the city provides refuse collection and levies taxes to finance this service, this tax is a legitimate cost of producing hospital care and should be counted. A public good such as national defense may benefit the hospital (should the hospital retain its own militia?), but this input is more remotely related to the production of hospital care. As a practical matter, such hair-splitting is not necessary since all hospitals benefit from refuse collection and national defense, but only for-profit hospitals pay taxes.

Fifth, some weight should be given to "voluntary" taxes. What if a hospital taxes itself voluntarily by providing services for which price falls short of marginal cost or engages in teaching and unsponsored research? If society placed no value on these "good acts," they could be considered a form of slack, yielding pleasure to administrators, medical staff, trustees, and hospital employees, but no one else. But if they are valued by society at large (and some of the above undoubtedly are), they should be considered when efficiency comparisons are made. Three related questions should be posed: Which good acts were provided, and in what amounts? Who were the beneficiaries? And how much is society willing to pay for this amount of activity to benefit the groups identified?

Sixth, determinants of cost variation other than ownership should be held constant. Hospitals vary in case mix, quality (broadly conceived), and location. Since some of the other factors are correlated with ownership, crude comparisons are surely biased. Hospital studies conducted to date have attempted to hold these other factors constant to varying degrees.

None of the studies reviewed in this section incorporated all six adjustments, but some adjusted more than others. A deficiency of some of the descriptive studies is the failure to hold pertinent performance determinants other than ownership type constant. This problem is particularly severe in the earlier descriptive studies, such as Clarkson and Lindsay's. Some of the more recent descriptive studies, such as Lewin et al., Pattison and Katz, and Sloan and Vraciu, were largely successful attempts to hold other factors constant by dividing the sample into more homogenous hospital groups for the purpose of making comparisons. Thus, for example, small not-for-profit hospitals were compared with their small for-profit counterparts. Sloan and Vraciu came closest to measuring economic cost, and the authors were correct in removing taxes from cost. Becker and Sloan, who used cost-dependent variables in their regressions, were probably the most successful in controlling the influence of other factors and in dealing with the selectivity problem.

Considering results from all of the studies, it appears that efficiency differences between private not-for-profit and for-profit hospitals are small, at most. A verdict on public hospitals is not possible because they produce a very different product.

Contradictory Evidence on Efficiency
from the Nursing Home Industry

Nursing homes are similar to hospitals in a number of respects. The three ownership forms are found in both industries, although market shares of each differ between the two. Both employ large numbers of nursing personnel. There are many similarities (as well as some important differences) in payment methods.

Several empirical studies of efficiency by ownership type have been conducted on the nursing home industry.[49] These studies reached several consistent conclusions. First, cost per diem is appreciably lower in proprietary than in nonproprietary homes. Second, proprietary homes pay their employees less. Third, there is an interaction between cost per diem and wages, on the one hand, and the method that Medicaid, the dominant third-party payer in the nursing home industry, uses to pay nursing homes. In particular, proprietary homes appear to be most efficient when they face exogenous product prices. Conversely, the differences by ownership are much smaller when Medicaid pays on the basis of cost without imposing ceilings on the amount paid per unit of output. The authors stress this finding because it implies that

---

49. Christine E. Bishop, "Nursing Home Cost Studies and Reimbursement Issues," *Health Care Financing Review* 1, no. 4 (Spring 1980):47–64; Howard Birnbaum et al., *Public Pricing of Nursing Home Care* (Cambridge, Mass.: Abt Books, 1981); George J. Borjas, H. E. Frech III, and Paul B. Ginsburg, "Property Rights and Wages: The Case of Nursing Homes," *Journal of Human Resources,* 8, no. 2 (Spring 1983):231–46; Margaret B. Sulvetta and John Holahan, "Cost and Case-Mix Differences in Hospital-based and Free-standing Skilled Nursing Facilities," mimeograph (Washington, D.C.: Urban Institute, April 1984); H. E. Frech III and Paul B. Ginsburg, "The Cost of Nursing Home Care in the United States: Government Financing, Ownership, and Efficiency," in Jacques Van der Gaag and Mark Perlman, eds., *Health, Economics, and Health Economics* (Amsterdam: North Holland, 1981), chap. 5, pp. 67–81.

meaningful efficiency differences only emerge when firms in the industry have a real reason to be cost minimizers.

Two reasons may be advanced for the difference in results for the two industries. First, studies for one or the other may be deficient methodologically. This is unlikely; the studies seem to be of comparable quality. Second, there may be differences in incentives. In 1982, 12 percent of hospital revenue was derived from uninsured sources. The corresponding figure for nursing homes was 44 percent.[50] Also, self-pay hospital patients pay a lower percentage of hospital charges, on average, than do patients with insurance.[51] Although a comparable estimate is unavailable for nursing homes, it is doubtful that self-pay nursing home patients pay less than the dominant payer in that industry, Medicaid. Thus, nursing homes are interested in attracting the self-pay patient and do so by offering a low, quality-adjusted price. Price competition is much less important in the hospital industry. Certainly, most hospitals do not compete for the uninsured hospital patient.

EMPIRICAL EVIDENCE ON OTHER DIMENSIONS OF HOSPITAL PERFORMANCE

It is important to investigate dimensions other than "efficiency" in this review for at least two reasons. For one, advocates of nonprofit ownership of hospitals argue that the rationale for this ownership form is not performance gauged in terms of efficiency, but rather in terms of the "good acts" they perform. Presumably for this reason, state legislatures have granted these hospitals favorable treatment. Second, if not-for-profit hospitals do in fact perform more good acts, efficiency comparisons that do not take these acts into account will be biased. The direction of the bias is not as straightforward as might appear at first glance. If nonprofits provide more free care, their receipts per unit of output would appear relatively low; thus some would mistakenly conclude that such hospitals are more efficient. However, if such hospitals accept unusually complex cases for treatment or engage in teaching and unsponsored research, and if empirical analysis

---

50. Gibson, Waldo, and Levit, "National Health Expenditures, 1982."

51. Paul B. Ginsburg and Frank A. Sloan, "Hospital Cost Shifting," *New England Journal of Medicine* 310, no. 14 (April 5, 1984):893–98.

fails to take adequate account of these differences, for-profit hospitals may appear comparatively more efficient than they really are.

"Free" Care

Sloan, Valvona, and Mullner conducted a detailed analysis of the amounts of bad-debt and charity care community hospitals in the United States provided during 1978–83.[52] "Charity care" was defined as care rendered to patients whom the hospital judged unable to pay, and "bad debt care" as the value of care delivered to patients judged by the hospital to be able to pay but who did not. The value of such care was computed in terms of the hospital's own prices.

The authors calculated bad debt-charity care as a percentage of hospital charges by ownership location. They found that in metropolitan areas in 1982, these percentages were 3.7 for voluntaries, 8.6 for public, and 3.0 for profit-seeking hospitals; whereas in nonmetropolitan areas, corresponding percentages were 4.0, 5.3, and 4.2 respectively for the three ownership types. Thus, if anything, for-profit hospitals outside cities rendered more of such care in relation to charges than did their voluntary counterparts, and almost as much as did state and local government hospitals. In metropolitan areas, for-profit hospitals ranked third, but not far behind voluntaries. In fact, judging from other data presented in this paper, the two metropolitan hospital types would have been closer if the comparison had been limited to nonteaching hospitals.

Pattison and Katz presented estimates of charity care as a percentage of net patient revenue (gross revenue less contractual adjustment and bad debt-charity care).[53] For the two groups of hospitals on which their article was based, charity care as a percentage of net revenue was 0.4 percent for voluntaries and public hospitals and 0 percent for the for-profits. Apparently, none of these hospitals was particularly generous to indigent patients. Sloan and Vraciu found that voluntary and for-profit hospitals in their Florida sample both provided the same amount for bad debt and charity care per day in 1980, namely $16.[54]

52. Sloan, Valvona, and Mullner, "Identifying the Issues."
53. Pattison and Katz, "Investor-Owned and Not-for-Profit Hospitals."
54. Sloan and Vraciu, "Investor-Owned and Not-for-Profit Hospitals."

Although hospitals receive payment from Medicare and Medicaid, there are frequent complaints about the discount these programs obtain.[55] In fact, they do obtain a much higher discount on average than do private payers.[56] However, payments by Medicare and Medicaid as a percentage of total payments to hospitals appear to be remarkably similar by ownership type. Becker and Sloan found that, for hospitals in their national 1979 sample, state and local government hospitals derived 11 percent of their revenue from Medicaid;[57] both voluntary and for-profit hospitals derived 7 percent of their revenue from this source. All three hospital types obtained a third of their revenue from Medicare. Pattison and Katz reported that California hospitals in their study derived 13 percent of their revenue from Medi-Cal; for national chain and independent for-profit hospitals, the Medi-Cal shares were 11 and 14 percent, respectively.[58] Voluntary and public hospitals obtained 12 and 18 percent of their revenue, respectively, from Medi-Cal. For-profit hospitals were almost identical to voluntaries and public hospitals in terms of Medicare receipts as a percentage of revenue; independent for-profits received slightly less. Sloan and Vraciu reported that Medicare and Medicaid patient days were 55 percent of total acute patient days for voluntary hospitals in their Florida sample. The corresponding percentage for profit-seeking hospitals was 54 percent.[59]

Case Mix and Service Mix

It has often been alleged that for-profit hospitals engage in "cream skimming" by accepting those patients with the highest price/cost margins for treatment. Unfortunately, there is little empirical evidence on case mix differences by ownership type. Ownership-specific information by service mix is available, however.

Using a small sample of California hospitals observed during 1971 and 1972, Bays found that the for-profits admitted significantly more

55. Health Insurance Association of America, *Hospital Cost Shifting: The Hidden Tax* (Washington, D.C.: HIAA, 1982).
56. Ginsburg and Sloan, "Hospital Cost Shifting."
57. Becker and Sloan, "Hospital Ownership and Performance."
58. Pattison and Katz, "Investor-Owned and Not-for-Profit Hospitals."
59. Sloan and Vraciu, "Investor-Owned and Not-for-Profit Hospitals."

patients with infectious diseases, respiratory diseases, diseases of the skin, fractures, and trauma than did the voluntaries in his sample.[60] They admitted fewer cases involving neoplasms, central nervous system, maternity, and those categorized as "special service." Data on price/cost margins were not available to Bays, and so he could not conclude that for-profits accept either more or less profitable cases. However, based on results of regression analysis on hospital profitability by Sloan and coauthors, it appears likely that the maternity and trauma cases were comparatively unprofitable.[61] There is no way of making similar judgments about the other case types.

Sloan and Vraciu compared voluntary, for-profit, and chain for-profit hospitals in Florida in 1980 on the basis of the percentage of these hospitals that had particular types of facilities and services.[62] They found that voluntary and for-profit hospitals with fewer than 400 beds were equally likely to have an outpatient department and about the same in terms of radiology, laboratory, and pharmacy offerings. The private not-for-profits were more likely to offer "profitable" services such as open heart surgery, cardiac catheterization, and CT scanning, but were also more likely to have a premature nursery—an unprofitable service because so many of the cases are uncompensated.[63] Essentially the same patterns between facility/service availability and ownership applied nationally in 1982.[64]

So far this review has been limited to short-term general hospitals. A comparison by Schlesinger and Dorwart of psychiatric hospitals by ownership type in some ways contradicts the above findings for general hospitals.[65] As in the above studies, the authors found that for-profit and private not-for-profit facilities were equally likely to screen out nonpaying patients; government-run facilities were more likely to accept such patients. However, the authors found from their own review of the literature that for-profit hospitals were less likely than the

60. Carson W. Bays, "Case-Mix Differences between Nonprofit and For-Profit Hospitals," *Inquiry*, 14, no. 1 (March 1977):17–21.

61. Sloan, Valvona, and Mullner, "Identifying the Issues."

62. Sloan and Vraciu, "Investor-Owned and Not-for-Profit Hospitals."

63. James M. Perrin, "High Technology and Uncompensated Hospital Care," in Sloan, Blumstein, and Perrin, eds., *Uncompensated Hospital Care*, pp. 54–71.

64. American Hospital Association, *Hospital Statistics, 1983*.

65. Mark Schlesinger and Robert Dorwart, "Ownership and Mental-Health Services: A Reappraisal of the Shift toward Privately-Owned Facilities," *New England Journal of Medicine* 311, no. 15 (October 11, 1984):959–65.

other two types to provide some services that are inadequately reimbursed by conventional sources of financing: emergency psychiatric services provided by telephone, home care for psychiatric patients, and suicide prevention. A problem with Schlesinger and Dorwart's comparisons is that they reported on only a few services. A proper analysis of service offerings requires an examination of the full array of services provided by hospitals.

Medical Education

A major difference between for-profit hospitals and the other ownership types is that the former engage in medical education only very rarely. Although this difference is of some interest, it is doubtful that any of the comparisons presented in the previous section are misleading because of failure to consider the role of medical education. Many of the studies excluded teaching hospitals; a few included teaching as part of the explanatory variables.

In 1982, only 14 percent of community hospitals were affiliated with medical schools.[66] Such hospitals are thus in distinct minority. Nevertheless, given the absence of for-profit teaching hospitals, it is useful to consider why profit-seeking hospitals do not provide medical education.

For-profit hospitals would presumably be unwilling to provide an activity for which marginal cost exceeded marginal revenue, where marginal revenue includes direct compensation from foregone resident earnings as well as added revenue from patient care because of higher quality perceived by consumers. The fact that hardly any for-profit hospitals provide medical education suggests that marginal cost must generally exceed marginal revenue, properly calculated.

Some other empirical evidence suggests, however, that hospital care may be no more or perhaps only a little more costly in teaching settings,[67] and that residents bear most if not all of the cost of training themselves.[68] Thus, it is not so clear why for-profit hospitals have not

66. American Hospital Association, *Hospital Statistics*, 1983.

67. Frank A. Sloan, Roger D. Feldman, and Bruce Steinwald, "Effects of Teaching on Hospital Costs," *Journal of Health Economics* 2, no. 1 (March 1983):1–28; James R. Hosek and Adele R. Palmer, "Teaching and Hospital Costs: The Case of Radiology," *Journal of Health Economics* 2, no. 1 (March 1983):29–46.

68. William D. Marder and Douglas E. Hough, "Medical Residency as Investment in Human Capital," *Journal of Human Resources* 18, no. 1 (Winter 1983):49–64.

been involved in medical training to date. Perhaps the recent affiliation of two large hospital chains, Hospital Corporation of America
and Humana, with teaching programs reflects a newly found recognition that teaching is not as costly on a case mix–adjusted basis as
was once thought. It is also possible that profit-seeking medical schools
and hospitals (when they combine teaching and patient care) have
faced entry barriers since the Flexner Report in 1910 gave such institutions very low marks.[69]

CONCLUSIONS

On the whole, property rights theory does not fit the hospital industry
very well. The empirical evidence reveals little or no difference in
efficiency by ownership type. Certainly, the differences that are observed could be due entirely to quality and amenity variation by ownership type. Variation in quality-amenities is difficult to quantify in
objective terms. It is virtually impossible to gauge it with an acceptable degree of precision from secondary data sources.

The hospital industry is large by any standard, and evidence of
small differences in costs cannot easily be disregarded. It is very
doubtful that further analysis of hospital data up through the early
1980s would reveal efficiency differences that have not emerged in
previous studies. Nevertheless, the empirical findings from hospitals
should not be taken as evidence that property rights theory is "wrong."

The doctors on the voluntary hospital's medical staff may be the
residual claimants, and they would then have a financial stake in keeping
such hospitals efficient. Inefficient hospitals are candidates for acquisition. This mechanism for weeding out inefficient firms is not
present in other sectors in which public and private nonprofit firms
are found, such as public libraries and fire stations.

Because of the pervasiveness of cost pass-through, third-party payment, hospitals may not have faced a meaningful incentive to be
efficient. Money has been made in the industry by manipulating reimbursement rules rather than by cutting costs. And if this last explanation has merit, for-profit hospitals have only begun to have a reason
to prove themselves as efficient producers. Only recently have pro-

---

69. Abraham Flexner, *Medical Education in the United States and Canada,* Bulletin No.
4, The Carnegie Foundation for the Advancement of Teaching (Boston: D. B. Updike, 1910).

spective payment plans, health maintenance organizations (HMOs), and preferred provider organizations gained sufficient market shares to represent a meaningful influence on hospital behavior. There is some limited evidence that the average cost per case is lower in Kaiser hospitals, a private not-for-profit HMO, than in other private not-for-profit private hospitals with which they have been compared.[70] Under the new hospital payment systems that are emerging, only the fittest will survive, irrespective of ownership form.

It is clear from evidence presented in this review that the applicability of property rights theory depends to a considerable extent on special features of the industry being examined. *For-profit* does not necessarily mean "most efficient" in every industry in which such firms compete with others organized on a not-for-profit basis.

To the extent that new pressures from the payment side are now becoming evident, it is indeed an appropriate time to reconsider the rationale of hospital ownership forms other than for-profit. Competition may eliminate the inefficiency, but it may also weed out those hospitals that are costly because they provide many "good acts." Since society presumably values at least some of these acts, there is reason for concern. Furthermore, some third-party payers have already decided not to pay for the hospital care of the nonpaying patients, and some, such as Medicare, are now deciding whether to pay for graduate medical education.

It is beyond the scope of this study to determine societal willingness to pay for such hospital outputs as uncompensated care and medical education. However, several points can be made that are pertinent to the policy discussion of who should pay and what the social responsibilities are of various ownership types.

First, the evidence is quite clear that private hospitals, for-profit or not-for-profit, on the whole do not provide much "free care" or medical education. To date, tax-exempt status has usually been available to hospitals that want it. Thus, to the extent that a profit-seeking hospital would provide too few of such outputs, a subsidy in the form of tax-free status is a very inefficient way to go about achieving these social objectives. At a minimum, such status should be linked to pro-

---

70. See Harold S. Luft, *Health Maintenance Organizations: Dimensions of Performance* (New York: Wiley-Interscience, 1981), for a summary of this evidence, especially pp. 141–43.

vision of a minimum amount of "good acts." Property rights theory would predict that the only ones who would disagree with this conclusion are those who have a claim on the savings from not paying taxes. This is a refutable hypothesis that might be tested by surveying physicians, hospital administrators, hospital trade association officials, and taxpayers. The fact that the only hospitals to provide much care to uninsured patients are the public hospitals that receive an explicit subsidy for providing such output is some evidence that the income effect of a tax exemption on good acts is not enough.

Second, to the extent that some nonprofit hospitals have willingly cross-subsidized unprofitable outputs, the new competitive forces emerging in the hospital industry will put an end to this. Thus, if the public does indeed value such outputs, it must determine its willingness to pay, and then develop explicit tax and expenditure mechanisms to accomplish such an objective. A major deficiency of the current implicit tax subsidy is that society does not have to determine its willingness to pay but rather leaves such decisions to the bosses at the hospital. Whether or not these bosses are good at determining societal wants is perhaps an empirical question, but many informed observers are doubtful. Health care providers often contend that the public may select a much lower quality level of services, research, and education, and then be sorry when it sees the actual consequences. There is some merit to their point of view.

Third, "voluntarism" is again a popular concept in the 1980s. The rationale for voluntary activity is threefold. First, there is a wedge between taxes paid and public expenditures received. The government bureaucracy takes a slice of the tax dollar. The slice required for administration by voluntary agencies may be smaller. Second, people may be more willing to give if they are not compelled to do so. Third, expenditures made by voluntary agencies do not appear in public budgets. As a result, the public sector looks (and is) smaller. The merits of the first two points should be decided on the basis of the empirical evidence, which unfortunately is not available. The third may provide good fodder for political campaigns, but not much else.

In view of the rapid changes now occurring in the hospital industry, researchers have a virtually unprecedented opportunity to conduct useful studies of hospitals—studies that have a high likelihood of enhancing our understanding of the link between ownership and performance in the hospital field.

The conditions in which a hospital is likely to be acquired have not been fully specified, and measurement of this phenomenon has been limited to a few case studies. Only when the factors leading to acquisition have been documented will it be possible to deal meaningfully with potential selectivity bias in cost comparisions. Policymakers would want to know whether, for example, hospitals were acquired because they provided too much "free care" or because of mismanagement.

A closely related issue concerns efficiency improvements made after a hospital is acquired. Do various efficiency indicators show improvements with each post-acquisition year? Does the time path differ according to the ownership of the hospital before acquisition? To understand cost changes better, it would be advisable to examine data that hospitals must provide to a regulatory authority or payer (such as Medicare Cost Reports) rather than data that hospitals provide voluntarily (such as the AHA's Annual Survey of Hospitals). Policymakers will want to know if there is a meaningful reduction in free care, unsponsored research, and education where a public or private not-for-profit hospital is acquired by a for-profit hospital.

Often when a for-profit chain acquires a hospital of one of the other ownership types, a community-run foundation is established with proceeds of the sale. The foundation then has funds with which to purchase care for the poor, education, or any other type of service of potential benefit to citizens of the community. This kind of transaction is a property-rights proponent's dream. The hospital is operated by a profit-seeking firm while funds are available for explicit subsidies of externality-producing activities. Opponents argue that the for-profit hospital will just exploit its monopoly power by raising prices, lowering the real value of the foundation's real assets. This outcome is unlikely if there is competition among hospitals. Rather than debate what *might* occur, however, researchers should take an actual look.

Finally, it will be useful to see whether the relative performance of for-profit hospitals *really* improves in the new environment in which hospitals face prospectively determined prices. Will they finally demonstrate appreciable operating efficiencies? Or will they take advantage of the new incentives to "cream-skim?" Empirical evidence on these very important questions will have a large audience.

PART III

GOVERNMENT HEALTH INSURANCE

4

MEDIGAP INSURANCE: FRIEND OR FOE IN REDUCING MEDICARE DEFICITS?

Amy K. Taylor, Pamela Farley Short, and Constance M. Horgan

THE MEDICARE FINANCING PROBLEM

Medicare, the federal health insurance program serving principally the elderly but also younger persons who are either disabled or have end-stage renal disease, faces serious fiscal problems. Medicare consists of two parts, financed by separate trust funds with different sources of revenue. Revenues for part A, the Hospital Insurance (HI) portion, which helps participants pay for inpatient hospital care and posthospital skilled nursing facility care, are obtained primarily from the Social Security payroll tax. In contrast, revenues for part B, the Supplementary Medical Insurance (SMI) component, which assists beneficiaries to pay chiefly for physician services and outpatient hospital services, come from premiums paid by (or on behalf of) participants and from general revenues. Both parts of the Medicare program face financial difficulties because the growth in benefit payments that has occurred in recent years—and is anticipated to continue into the future under current financing policies—has been much more rapid than

Note: An earlier version of this paper was presented at the Annual Meeting of the American Public Health Association, November 13, 1984.

The views in this paper are those of the authors and no official endorsement by the National Center for Health Services Research and Health Care Technology Assessment is intended or should be inferred.

145

the growth in revenues from premiums, payroll taxes, and general revenues. Some of this rapid growth is due to the aging of the population, but most of the growth is due to rising medical care costs.[1]

Although the hospital prospective payment provisions of the Social Security Amendments of 1983 and the cutbacks of the Tax Equity and Fiscal Responsibility Act (TEFRA) of 1982 have reduced the long-range deficit in the HI trust fund, it is still projected to be exhausted within a decade.[2] Since transfers from general revenues assure the solvency of the SMI trust fund, concerns regarding its financial situation arise because the general revenues going to the SMI trust fund are projected to grow at a much higher rate than the overall growth in general revenues. Despite enactment of TEFRA, which guarantees that premium payments will be set to cover 25 percent of SMI program costs until July 1985—thus reversing the trend of a decreasing share of costs being covered by premium payments—SMI costs still consume a growing share of the federal budget. Because of the rapid growth in costs for both parts of the Medicare program, and the extent to which general revenues have become a major source of financing, the Medicare Board of Trustees has recommended that Congress take further action to curtail the rapid growth in the cost of the HI program and the rapid growth in the SMI program.[3]

Proposals for dealing with the financial problems of the Medicare program are likely to rely on one or any combination of four general approaches: (1) controlling payments to the provider, (2) raising premium payments by the beneficiary, (3) raising taxes on the younger population (increasing payroll taxes or allocating a larger proportion of general revenues to Medicare), and (4) requiring additional cost-sharing by the beneficiary.[4] The recently introduced hospital prospective payment system based on diagnosis-related groups (DRGs) is an example of the first type of approach. The second and third

1. Paul Ginsburg and Marilyn Moon, "An Introduction to the Medicare Financing Problem," *Conference on the Future of Medicare,* Committee on Ways and Means, U.S. House of Representatives (Washington, D.C.: Government Printing Office, 1983).

2. Marilyn Moon, "Changing the Structure of Medicare Benefits: Issues and Options," Congressional Budget Office (Washington, D.C.: CBO, 1983).

3. Summary of the 1984 Annual Reports of the Medicare Board of Trustees (Washington, D.C.: Government Printing Office, 1984).

4. William Hsiao and Nancy Kelly, "Restructuring Medicare Benefits," *Conference on the Future of Medicare,* Committee on Ways and Means, U.S. House of Representatives (Washington, D.C.: Government Printing Office, 1983).

approaches have been used to increase revenues throughout the existence of Medicare. The last approach has also been used in the past and would restrict benefits by requiring greater cost-sharing by the beneficiary. Like an increase in Medicare premiums, such a change in benefits would place some of the burden for reducing Medicare's deficits on the beneficiaries rather than on providers or younger taxpayers.

SOLUTIONS INVOLVING THE BENEFICIARY

This paper examines the approaches that focus on the beneficiary rather than on the provider or the taxpayer. Specifically, the implications of the cost-sharing option as a means of reducing federal outlays on Medicare is examined and contrasted with an approach that would increase premium payments as a means of increasing Medicare revenues.[5]

Increased cost-sharing requirements could take several forms. Larger deductibles, coinsurance, or copayments could be required; presently included services could be excluded; or lower limits could be placed on the allowable charge for bills from physicians who do not accept Medicare assignment, leaving the beneficiary to pay the rest. These types of cost-sharing techniques would reduce Medicare outlays (1) directly, by shifting them from the federal government to the beneficiary or others paying on behalf of the beneficiary, and (2) indirectly, by discouraging use of covered services. Cost-sharing is currently required for both HI and SMI, and increased cost-sharing could be structured to shift off budget outlays for both parts of the Medicare program.

The impact on the beneficiary of increased cost-sharing would of course depend on the specific type of arrangement implemented; however, since cost-sharing is linked to utilization, its burden would fall most heavily on those beneficiaries who are sicker. Given patterns of medical utilization, increased cost-sharing would therefore tend to fall relatively more heavily on the older and poorer elderly.[6] Although increased cost-sharing would reduce Medicare outlays, not all of the

5. For an in-depth discussion of the implications of increased cost-sharing under Medicare, see Moon, "Changing the Structure of Medicare Benefits."
6. Ibid.

shifted costs would be paid directly by the beneficiary, because extensive supplementation of Medicare is provided by other sources, such as private insurance and Medicaid. Almost 66 percent of the elderly have both Medicare and private supplementary insurance, whereas 11 percent have Medicare plus Medicaid, 20 percent have Medicare only, and the remaining 3.8 percent are either uninsured or have other kinds of coverage. Thus, over 20 percent of the elderly would be directly at risk of paying additional cost-sharing requirements completely out-of-pocket. Additionally, those with private supplementary insurance would pay higher costs through higher insurance premiums. Because so many of the elderly have insurance supplementary to Medicare, the indirect effect of reduced utilization induced by higher cost-sharing is mitigated. Thus, the existence of supplementary coverage allows expenditures to be shifted from the Medicare budget without exposing most of the elderly to the risk of high out-of-pocket expenses; however, this shift may subvert the beneficial effect of curbing utilization.

In assessing the impact of increased cost-sharing, it should also be recalled that Medicare already requires substantial cost-sharing by beneficiaries. Some services, most notably custodial nursing home care and prescription drug and dental services, are specifically excluded. In 1978 only 44 percent of total health care expenditures of the elderly were paid by Medicare, although Medicare did pay for 75 percent of hospital services and 56 percent of physician services.[7] The burden of out-of-pocket expenses is already high for some Medicare beneficiaries, especially those without Medicaid or supplementary private insurance.[8]

Although increasing the SMI premium could be considered a form of increased cost-sharing, its impact would be very different from cost-sharing that is implicitly linked to the use of services. The direct effect of raising the SMI premium would be to increase revenues by raising costs evenly across all beneficiaries who participate in SMI. It would not have the indirect effect of curbing utilization. Moreover,

7. Charles Fisher, "Differences by Age Groups in Health Care Spending," *Health Care Financing Review* 1, no. 4 (Spring 1980).
8. Gail Cafferata and Mark Meiners, "Public and Private Insurance and the Medicare Population's Out-of-Pocket Expenditures: Does Medigap Make a Difference?" (Paper presented at the American Public Health Association Annual Meeting, Anaheim, California, November 1984).

raising the SMI premium would only assist in solving the SMI financing problem. Currently, premiums are not employed for HI; but, if premiums were to be addressed, the impact would be the same as for SMI. Raising premiums would affect all beneficiaries evenly, although it would represent a greater burden for lower-income Medicare participants.

SUPPLEMENTATION

The extent of supplementation to Medicare is a key factor in the relative similarity between increasing cost-sharing requirements and raising premium payments as means of solving the Medicare financing problem. If all Medicare beneficiaries purchased supplementary insurance to cover the cost-sharing requirements of Medicare, the end result would be similar to covering the expenditures under Medicare and financing through Medicare rather than private premiums. However, not all Medicare participants have supplementation through private insurance or Medicaid, and the breadth and depth of coverage under private plans can vary considerably.

Supplementary insurance, sometimes known as Medigap insurance, is offered by private insurers to cover the gaps in Medicare coverage caused by cost-sharing requirements.[9] The implications of Medicare beneficiaries' buying Medigap policies are assuming greater importance for the Medicare trust funds, since a growing proportion of the elderly now purchase this type of coverage or have other, employment-related private insurance. In 1967, 46 percent of Medicare beneficiaries had supplementary insurance,[10] and by 1977, 67 percent of the elderly were covered by both Medicare and private insurance.

In 1977 about two-thirds of the privately insured Medicare beneficiaries had nongroup coverage that was obtained directly from insurers, and the remaining one-third had group coverage that was largely employment related. Group policies, some of them obtained by work-

9. For a more detailed description of the private health insurance coverage of elderly Medicare beneficiaries, see Gail Cafferata, "Private Health Insurance Coverage of the Medicare Population," *National Health Care Expenditures Study, Data Preview 18*, DHHS Publication No. (PHS) 84–3362 (Washington, D.C.: U.S. Department of Health and Human Services, National Center for Health Services Research, 1984).

10. Marjorie Mueller, "Private Health Insurance in 1970," *Social Security Bulletin* 35 (February 1972).

ing spouses, tend to be more comprehensive than nongroup policies. The total annual premium for group policies is consequently more than twice that for nongroup policies covering Medicare beneficiaries. In 1977, this amounted to $383 per insured beneficiary for group plans, compared to $189 for nongroup policies. Since employers paid more than 60 percent of the premium costs of group plans, the out-of-pocket premium expenses for persons with group plans were slightly less than those for persons with nongroup plans.[11]

The extent and type of Medigap coverage is clearly an important consideration in determining the impact of any changes in Medicare cost-sharing provisions. Although Medigap can be considered a friend of the Medicare trust funds because it pays for the expenditures that Medicare is able to shift off budget through cost-sharing, it can at the same time be considered a foe because it induces additional utilization of health care services as the beneficiary effectively faces reduced cost-sharing.[12] The specific objective of the remainder of this paper is to describe the increase in Medicare expenditures attributable to the effective elimination of cost-sharing by Medigap policies. The next section presents a simultaneous equations model of the role of supplemental health insurance in determining Medicare expenditures and reimbursement levels. The final section uses parameter estimates from that model and others to calculate the effects of restructuring Medicare benefits.

OVERVIEW OF THE MODEL

Using an econometric model of expenditures and insurance within the Medicare system, this study explores the reasons for, and implications of, supplemental insurance for Medicare recipients. The equations presented here describe the variations in seven important variables for Medicare recipients: the purchase of nongroup supplemental insurance, the hospital admission rate, total expenses for hospital care, the decision to see a doctor, ambulatory physician expenditures, whether the Medicare deductible was exceeded, and total Medicare reimbursement in dollars. The predetermined variables in the model include

11. Cafferata, "Private Health Insurance Coverage of the Medicare Population."
12. Charles Link, Stephen Long, and Russell Settle, "Cost Sharing, Supplementary Insurance and Health Services Utilization Among the Medicare Elderly," *Health Care Financing Review* 2 (Fall 1980).

sociodemographic characteristics (age, income, race, sex, education, employment), region of the country and size of the city, characteristics of the local health care system (hospital beds per 100,000 population, doctors per 100,000 population, average hospital costs in the county, mean supplemental health insurance premiums, Medicare's prevailing fee for a follow-up office visit), perceived health status and disability days, and third-party coverage (Medicaid and employment-related group insurance).

Of the 67 percent of the population 65 years and older covered by both Medicare and private insurance in 1977, about one-third had group coverage, mostly obtained through present or past employment. This insurance can be considered exogenous to the model developed here because these policies are determined independently of the benefits of the Medicare system. Similarly, Medicaid, which covered 10.6 percent of Medicare recipients, can also be viewed as exogenous. However, those elderly who are covered by neither Medicaid nor private group insurance have to decide whether to purchase nongroup insurance to supplement their Medicare coverage. The factors that influence this decision and the implications of all three types of supplementary coverage are estimated as part of the econometric model.

The decision to purchase insurance and the levels of expenditure that are in part a function of insurance coverage can be viewed as a simultaneous equations system in which both latent variables and their realized qualitative variables figure in the model.

The general form of this model is

(4.1)　　　　　　　　$Y_1^* = a_1 X_1 + u_1$

(4.2)　　　　　　　　$Y_2 = b_2 Y_1 + a_2 X_2 + u_2$

where

$$Y_1 = 1 \quad \text{if} \quad Y_1^* > 0$$

otherwise

$$Y_1 = 0$$

In this case, Y_1 equals 1 if an individual has nongroup supplemental insurance; otherwise Y_1 equals 0. The Xs are vectors comprised of the appropriate combinations of the independent variables listed above.

Y_2 represents three pairs of equations, which describe: (1) the probability of a hospital admission and hospital expenditures, conditional on use; (2) the probability of a doctor visit and expenditures for physicians' services, conditional on at least one visit; and (3) the probability of Medicare reimbursement for medical care, and the magnitude of these payments for beneficiaries with reimbursement greater than zero. In each of these sets, the first equation is estimated using a linear probability model.[13] The expenditure equations are logarithmic to correct for the skewed distribution of medical care expenditures.[14]

If the decision to purchase insurance is influenced by unobserved factors reflected in u_2 that contribute to higher expenditures, then u_1 is not independent of u_2 and an instrumental variable technique is required for an unbiased estimate of b_2. In other words, if the decision to purchase insurance is related to a person's anticipated expenditures, then differences in expenditures that are observed between nongroup enrollees and those without supplemental coverage may be due to self-selection rather than to the insurance itself. However, if u_1 and u_2 are independent, use of an instrument is less efficient than use of Y_1 itself. By estimating equation (4.1) to obtain an instrument for Y_1 that is independent of u_2,[15] we employed Hausman's test of simultaneity bias to determine the appropriate estimation procedure.[16] We could not reject the hypothesis that the estimate of an ordinary least-squares regression is unbiased, and consequently use the actual value of Y_1 rather than an instrument in the second set of equations.

The data used for this analysis were taken from the National Medical Care Expenditure Survey (NMCES). NMCES was conducted in 1977 to assess health-related utilization, costs, and sources of payment for the United States from a multistage national probability sam-

13. A linear probability model was used for estimation for several reasons. The probability of having at least one doctor visit was 80 percent, and of having a hospital stay, 20 percent. A linear probability model works well in this range for a linear approximation. See Takeshi Amemiya, "Qualitative Response Models: A Survey," *Journal of Economic Literature* 19, no. 4 (December 1981):1483–1536. Probit equations were also run, and the results did not differ. The linear probability model is presented here for ease of interpretation.

14. For an interpretation of the coefficients of dummy variables in an equation where the dependent variable is expressed in logarithms, see Robert Halvorsen and Raymond Palmquist, "The Interpretation of Dummy Variables in Semilogarithmic Equations," *American Economic Review* 70, no. 3 (June 1980):474–75.

15. James Heckman, "Dummy Endogenous Variables in a Simultaneous Equation System," *Econometrica* 46, no. 6 (July 1978):931–59.

16. Jerry Hausman, "Specification Tests in Econometrics," *Econometrica* 46, no. 6 (November 1978).

ple of 13,500 households (40,000 persons). The survey also provides extensive information on the benefit provisions, premiums, and financing of the health insurance held by the noninstitutionalized civilian population of the United States.

EMPIRICAL RESULTS

The first equation in this model helps us to understand the factors that influence the decision about whether to purchase nongroup supplementary insurance (and also to test for the endogeneity of insurance in the utilization equations). What types of persons are more likely than others to purchase nongroup supplemental coverage? The probability of having this type of insurance is likely to be influenced by sociodemographic factors (including income), health status, region of the country and urbanization, premium levels, medical care prices, and predicted routine use of care. The results of estimating this equation are shown in Table 4–1.

As expected, low-, middle-, and high-income individuals are more likely to purchase supplemental insurance than are the poor or near poor. The probability of having insurance is 22 percent higher for whites than nonwhites. Individuals in the South and West were less likely than those in the North-central (the omitted category) to supplement their Medicare coverage, while living in an urban area had no significant effect. Males were also less likely to have coverage than were females, perhaps reflecting the fact that many men are eligible to use Veterans Administration facilities. The probability of having supplemental coverage is much lower for those in fair or poor health than for others. Although this group might be expected to want more health insurance than those in better health, it may be that they are less able to get coverage or that only less desirable coverage is available to them. Another important influence appears to be education, with those having at least a high school education being more likely to buy supplemental insurance.

The next set of equations examines the influence of insurance and other factors on hospital admissions and expenditures for hospital services. Hospital admissions tend to increase with age, and nearly 20 percent of the elderly had at least one hospital event in 1977. It is expected that among those over age 65, the oldest will have even higher admission rates than others. For the population as a whole,

Table 4–1.   Determinants of Nongroup Supplemental Coverage (Dependent variable = 1 if individual had nongroup supplemental insurance; Otherwise = 0).

Independent Variable	Coefficient	Standard Error
Constant	.675***	.085
Age[a]		
70–74	−.001	.027
75+	−.029	.025
Income[b]		
Low	.060**	.029
Middle	.093***	.029
High	.075**	.033
White	.234***	.025
Male	−.066***	.023
Education		
12 years+	.117***	.022
Perceived health status[c]		
Good	−.006	.024
Fair	−.068**	.027
Poor	−.127***	.043
Married	−.012	.023
Region[d]		
Northeast	−.013	.030
South	−.097***	.027
West	−.118***	.033
SMSA	.004	.023
Follow-up fee	−.0002**	.00008
Mean premiums	.0002	.0002

SOURCE: U.S. Department of Health and Human Services, National Center for Health Services Research, *National Medical Care Expenditure Study, 1977,* DHHS Publication No. (PHS) 81–3280, (Washington, D.C.: DHHS, 1981), available from National Technical Information Service, Springfield, VA 22161.

[a]omitted category is 65–69 years
[b]omitted category is poor and near poor
[c]omitted category is excellent
[d]omitted category is North-central
*significant at .10 level
**significant at .05 level
***significant at .01 level

income is negatively correlated with the percentage of people with a hospital event.[17] However, since Medicare is a universal program with nearly complete hospital coverage, it is not known what the impact of income would be in this case. The presence of supplementary in-

17. Amy Taylor, "Inpatient Hospital Services: Use, Expenditures and Sources of Payment," *National Health Care Expenditures Study, Data Preview 15,* DHHS Publication No.

surance and Medicaid might also influence the decision to enter the hospital. Health status is another important determinant of hospital admissions. It is entered in the equation in two ways, as self-perceived health status and as the number of disability days out of the hospital. Where hospital beds are more abundant, doctors might be more likely to hospitalize patients.[18] The availability of physicians per capita is also included, along with average hospital costs per day in the county.

The estimated hospital admissions equations are shown in Table 4–2. The presence of supplementary insurance and Medicaid did not seem to influence hospital admissions, perhaps because of the comprehensive hospital coverage under Medicare. Once the one-day deductible has been exceeded, hospital patients face no additional charges for hospital services for up to 60 days, whether they have additional coverage or not. As expected, being over age 75 significantly increases the probability of being admitted to the hospital. Income has no effect on admissions when health status and insurance coverage are held constant. Males on Medicare had a higher likelihood of a hospital admission than did females. Both measures of health status had a major impact on the hospital admission rate. For those in fair or poor health, the probability of a hospital event was 4–6 percent higher than for those in excellent health; in addition, the likelihood of a hospital admission was 30 percent less for those with no disability days outside the hospital than for those with one to seven days, while those with more than thirty days were 10 percent more likely to have gone to the hospital. The average cost of hospital care had a very small, negative effect on the admission rate.

Hospital expenditures are the product of average cost per day times length of stay, and so are likely to be influenced by these two determinants. Table 4–2 shows the results of estimating the hospital expenditures equation. Having a group supplemental insurance plan increased expenditures by more than 30 percent, although nongroup plans and Medicaid did not have similar effects. Although age and perceived health status had no effect on total hospital expenditures, the number of disability days outside the hospital was a significant

---

(PHS) 83–3360 (Washington, D.C.: U.S. Department of Health and Human Services, National Center for Health Services Research, 1984).

18. Martin Feldstein, "An Econometric Model of the Medicare System," *The Quarterly Journal of Economics* 85, no. 1 (February 1971).

Table 4–2. Hospital Admissions and Expenditures.

| | Hospital Admission (1 = yes) | | Hospital Expenditures (Log $) | |
	Coefficient	Standard Error	Coefficient	Standard Error
Constant	.281***	.043	7.519***	1.161
Insurance[a]				
Nongroup plan	.025	.017	.028	.131
Group plan	.029	.020	.273*	.154
Medicaid	.015	.023	−.008	.155
Age[b]				
70–74	−.002	.017	.085	.134
75+	.052***	.016	.178	.116
Income[c]				
Low	.003	.019	−.331**	.134
Middle	−.013	.018	−.306	.137
High	.009	.021	−.053	.157
White	−.011	.016	−.107	.116
Male	.067***	.013	.129	.099
Education				
12 years+	−.019	.014	.274**	.109
Perceived health status[d]				
Good	.019	.016	.006	.132
Fair	.041**	.018	−.168	.137
Poor	.062**	.028	−.096	.176
Disability days[e]†			.146**	.027
None	−.300***	.018		
7–30	−.027	.022		
30+	.104***	.021		
Region[f]				
Northeast	.001	.020	.182	.142
South	−.018	.018	−.093	.132
West	−.019	.020	−.264*	.158
SMSA	.013	.017	.070	.139
Doctors per 100,000†	−.00003	.00009	.213*	.111
Hospital beds per 100,000†	.00003	.00003	−.136**	.063
Average cost per patient day in county†	−.0003**	.0001	−.150	.654

Source: *National Medical Care Expenditure Study, 1977.*

[a]omitted category is no supplemental coverage
[b]omitted category is 65–69 years
[c]omitted category is poor and near poor
[d]omitted category is excellent
[e]omitted category is 1–6 days
[f]omitted category is North-central
*significant at .10 level
**significant at .05 level
***significant at .01 level
†The variables are expressed in logarithms in the expenditure equations.

determinant of hospital expenditures, with an elasticity of 0.14. Income was also an important influence; expenditures for lower- and middle-income individuals were 26 to 28 percent lower than for the poor or near poor. Expenditures also tended to be lower in the western region of the country. Those with at least a high school education had much higher hospital expenses than others. Another significant influence on expenditures was the number of doctors per capita, which indicates that doctors are complements to hospital services for this group of patients. On the other hand, in areas where there are relatively more hospital beds, total hospital expenditures tended to be lower.

Coverage under Medicare part B for physicians' services includes both a yearly deductible and coinsurance. Supplemental insurance and Medicaid fill these gaps in coverage to varying extents. Both group and nongroup insurance as well as Medicaid increased by up to 13 percent the probability of having a doctor visit (Table 4–3). Whites were more likely to have a doctor visit than others, as were people who lived in the South. Health status had the expected effect on the probability of seeing a doctor during the year, with those in fair or poor health being 10 to 12 percent more likely to visit a doctor than those in excellent health. The probability of a doctor visit was 5 percent higher for those with seven or more disability days than for those with one to six days, and 16 percent lower for those with no disability.

Supplemental insurance coverage also significantly increased expenditures for physicians' services, once the decision had been made to see a doctor. Having group or nongroup coverage led to expenditures 26 to 39 percent higher than having Medicare only. Middle- and high-income individuals also tended to have larger expenditures than others, perhaps reflecting a choice of more expensive physicians. The most important determinant of expenditures, however, was the price of a physician office visit, as measured by Medicare allowed fees for a follow-up visit to a general practitioner, with an elasticity of 0.85; this is not surprising, since expenditures equal the product of price times quantity. However, since it is less than 1.0, this implies a price-elasticity of demand greater than zero. Being in less than excellent health also led to higher expenditures, as did more disability days. Living in the West also significantly increased expenditures for ambulatory visits (by 30 percent), as did living in an urban area (by 10 percent).

Table 4–3.   Doctor Visits and Expenditures.

Independent Variables	Doctor Visit (1 = yes)		Expenditures for Physician Office Visits (Log $)	
	Coefficient	Standard Error	Coefficient	Standard Error
Constant	.553***	.060	−2.383**	1.135
Insurance[a]				
Nongroup plan	.135***	.018	.333***	.061
Group plan	.114***	.021	.234***	.070
Medicaid	.062***	.024	.109	.081
Age[b]				
70–74	.002	.017	.028	.057
75+	−.012	.016	.053	.054
Income[c]				
Low	.003	.020	.045	.066
Middle	.003	.019	.108*	.065
High	.024	.022	.116	.074
White	.116***	.017	−.072	.059
Male	−.018	.014	.030	.047
Education				
12 years+	−.007	.015	.070	.050
Perceived health status[d]				
Good	.063***	.016	.219***	.056
Fair	.119***	.019	.133**	.063
Poor	.101***	.029	.361***	.095
Disability days[e]†			.204***	.013
None	−.158***	.020		
7–30	.051**	.023		
30+	.049**	.023		
Region[d]				
Northeast	.032	.021	−.010	.070
South	.057***	.018	.083	.063
West	.027	.022	.260***	.074
SMSA	.003	.017	.102*	.059
Doctors per 100,000†	−.00002	.0001	.066	.055
Hospital beds per 100,000†	−.00002	.00003	−.010	.024
Follow-up fee†	.00005	.00005	.848***	.176

SOURCE: *National Medical Care Expenditure Study, 1977.*

[a]omitted category is no supplemental coverage
[b]omitted category is 65–69 years
[c]omitted category is poor and near poor
[d]omitted category is excellent
[e]omitted category is 1–6 days
[f]omitted category is North-central
*significant at .10 level
**significant at .05 level
***significant at .01 level
†The variables are expressed in logarithms in the expenditure equations.

The two final equations examine the determinants of exceeding the Medicare deductible and the impact of various factors on Medicare reimbursements. While the previous equations helped explain the underlying behavior of Medicare recipients with respect to their use of, and expenditures for, medical care, these can be considered reduced-form equations that show the net effect of exogenous variables on government payments for part B of the Medicare system.

The estimated equation (Table 4-4) shows that health-related variables are important determinants of whether or not individuals exceeded the Medicare deductible of $60 in 1977. The probability of having any Medicare reimbursements was substantially higher for those 70 years of age and older, for those in less than excellent health, and for those with more than seven disability days. On the other hand, those with no disability days had a 20 percent smaller chance of exceeding their deductible. Location was also an important factor; persons living in the West or in urban areas were more likely to exceed their deductible than those living elsewhere. Males, too, had a slightly higher chance of having ambulatory medical services reimbursed by Medicare. Finally, supplemental health insurance, both group and nongroup, significantly increased—by 10 to 13 percent—the likelihood of exceeding the deductible.

Table 4-4 also shows the determinants of Medicare reimbursements once the deductible has been met. It is interesting to note that having nongroup supplemental coverage increases government outlays for Medicare by about $30 for each person who exceeds the deductible. Surprisingly, neither group health insurance nor Medicaid had a similar effect. The Medicare allowed fee for a follow-up office visit had a significant positive impact; for each dollar the fee goes up, it appears that Medicare reimbursements will increase by $11 over a year. Good and poor health, as opposed to excellent, also led to higher reimbursement levels ($37 to $46), as did more disability days. Another important factor is region of the country, with those living in the West having Medicare reimbursements more than $50 higher than those in the North-central region. Males also had slightly higher reimbursement levels ($17) than did females. Finally, Medicare paid $26 more for those with at least a high school education, perhaps because this group would be more likely to see specialists rather than general practitioners.

Table 4–4. Probability of Exceeding Medicare Deductible and Medicare Reimbursement Levels.

Independent Variables	Exceed Deductible (1 = yes)		Medicare Reimbursement Ambulatory	
	Coefficient	Standard Error	Coefficient	Standard Error
Constant	.250**	.073	−52.508	46.688
Insurance[a]				
Nongroup plan	.131***	.022	30.888**	14.694
Group plan	.096***	.025	8.107	17.064
Medicaid	.044	.029	14.260	18.849
Age[b]				
70–74	.094***	.021	3.224	14.018
75+	.094***	.020	−2.704	13.090
Income[c]				
Low	−.017	.024	7.730	15.710
Middle	−.006	.024	−14.257	15.597
High	−.004	.027	14.995	17.868
White	.027	.021	−15.456	13.505
Male	.028*	.017	19.027*	13.585
Education				
12 years+	−.014	.019	25.912**	11.816
Perceived health status[d]				
Good	.042**	.020	37.230***	13.585
Fair	.093***	.023	10.462	14.846
Poor	.089**	.035	45.917**	21.128
Disability days[e]			.297***	.075
None	−.213***	.023		
7–30	.048*	.028		
30+	.151***	.027		
Region[f]				
Northeast	.039	.026	1.003	16.529
South	.019	.023	−2.828	15.096
West	.090***	.027	51.499***	17.176
SMSA	.036*	.021	15.267	13.917
Doctors per 100,000	.0002*	.0001	.064	.078
Hospital beds per 100,000	−.0003	.0004	−.025	.026
Follow-up fee	−.0001	.0001	.116**	.044

SOURCE: *National Medical Care Expenditure Study, 1977.*

[a]omitted category is no supplemental coverage
[b]omitted category is 65–69 years
[c]omitted category is poor and near poor
[d]omitted category is excellent
[e]omitted category is 1–6 days
[f]omitted category is North-central
*significant at .10 level
**significant at .05 level
***significant at .01 level

THE EFFECT OF RESTRUCTURING MEDICARE BENEFITS

The estimates from the model just presented describe the effects of supplemental insurance within the Medicare system as it is currently structured. The last section of this paper turns to the question of how the presence of supplemental insurance influences the effects on the system of changing benefits for Medicare recipients. More specifically, we look at a hypothetical cost-sharing option and examine the implications of increased cost-sharing for both the elderly and for government outlays, given the presence of Medigap coverage. We also compare this hypothetical policy with that of changing premiums for part B or introducing premiums for part A of Medicare.

As we noted earlier, an alternative to restructuring Medicare's benefits is to raise the part B premium or to introduce a premium for part A hospital benefits as a way of shifting onto beneficiaries some of the burden of reducing the program's projected deficits. The latter approach has the virtue of spreading the burden evenly, rather than unequally in proportion to utilization, and it can be modified rather easily to allow those with lower incomes to pay less. However, all beneficiaries, including those who use few services, would be affected by a certain increase in their monthly outlays in lieu of cost-sharing in the uncertain event of needing care.

The relative appeal of restructuring Medicare benefits, compared to the alternative, is dependent on the reaction of Medicare beneficiaries to the change in benefits in two ways. First, as the econometric analysis in the preceding section demonstrates, Medicare's present cost-sharing requirements encourage a lower level of use and total expenditures among beneficiaries who are subject to them, saving the program its substantial share of the reduction in expenditures. Depending on the sensitivity of total expenditures to cost-sharing, an increase in cost-sharing will effect further savings. Second, the magnitude of these savings depends crucially on the number of beneficiaries who are subject to cost-sharing, and in particular on how the tendency to purchase private supplementary insurance might respond to a change in the amount and type of expenditures covered by Medicare. Currently, only about a fifth of elderly beneficiaries are without supplementary coverage from either private sources or Medicaid and fully subject to Medicare's cost-sharing. Whether beneficiaries would buy more or less private insurance, so that cost-sharing would have its effect on a smaller or larger number, is an open question. On the one hand, a reduction in the expenditures covered by Medicare would increase the risk of out-of-pocket expenditures, making supplementary insurance more attractive. On the other hand, as the expenses covered by supplementary insurance increased, so too would the premiums, making the insurance less attractive.

Because nearly all of the elderly are covered by Medicare, and because Medicare's current cost-sharing provisions are identical for all beneficiaries, it is impossible to observe the effect of hospital cost-sharing provisions on the use and expenditures of the elderly outside the range of the present system. The results of the preceding section suggest that present cost-sharing provisions have little or no effect on hospital use, but there is no empirical evidence since 1965 that can be used to predict the potential effect of higher levels of cost-sharing. Nor is it possible to observe the effect of alternative Medicare cost-sharing provisions on the supplementary private insurance purchases of beneficiaries, since Medicare cost-sharing is identical for everyone and has remained essentially unchanged over time.

Yet enough information is available to place boundaries on the range of responses that might reasonably be expected from a restructuring of Medicare's benefits. First, for about 40 percent of elderly Medicare beneficiaries, the fact that they have supplementary coverage is unlikely to change: 25 percent have group insurance through their current and former employers and 17 percent are covered by Medicaid. This leaves only 60 percent who are at risk of paying the cost-sharing and who would have to decide whether or not to purchase supplementary insurance.

It is also unlikely that a catastrophic-illness limit on a person's cost-sharing under Medicare's present provisions would, as is sometimes suggested, encourage a significant number of beneficiaries to give up their private insurance. Medicare's lack of catastrophic-illness protection is apparently not the primary reason for buying supplementary insurance, since only 14 percent of persons with nongroup hospital policies in 1977 were fully covered if they exceeded Medicare's 150-day hospital maximum, while 43 percent were only partially covered and 30 percent were not fully covered for the copayments after 90 days.[19]

19. Cafferata, "Private Health Insurance Coverage of the Medicare Population."

Finally, given the present tailoring of nongroup supplementary policies to the cost-sharing requirements of the present system, it is likely that many would continue to cover whatever was excluded from Medicare benefits. For example, in 1977 most Medigap plans specifically covered the $124 Medicare hospital deductible, the $31 and $62 copayments, and the $60 deductible and 20 percent of Medicare allowable charges not covered by part B, while excluding coverage for expenses like prescription drugs, which are also excluded by Medicare.

While it is impossible to observe the elderly supplementing any benefits except those now offered by Medicare, Marquis and Phelps have analyzed the response of the nonelderly families in the Rand Health Insurance Experiment to hypothetical offers of supplementary insurance to different base plans.[20] In addition to the difference in age of the buyers, the Rand experiment involved a concept of supplementary insurance different from that currently observed with Medicare, allowing purchasers only to "buy down" their catastrophic-illness limit on cost-sharing rather than "buy up" to increasing amounts of first-dollar coverage. In this context, they found that the probability of purchasing a supplementary plan (which would lower the out-of-pocket limit by two-thirds) decreased from 69 percent with a base plan having 25 percent coinsurance to 57–59 percent with base plans having 50 percent coinsurance or more, a decline of 15 to 20 percent in the purchase of supplementary plans as premiums rose to cover additional expenses excluded by the base plan.

Suppose a new part A hospital copayment were instituted in the Medicare program, equal to 10 percent of the first-day deductible, for days 2 to 60, which are now fully covered, and that the part B coinsurance were raised from 20 to 25 percent. For hospital care, this is a change from essentially free care (except for the deductible) to 10 percent coinsurance. The Marquis-Phelps experiment suggests that the number of beneficiaries purchasing supplementary plans might decline by as much as 20 percent, probably an outside guess as to the number of additional enrollees whose behavior in seeking medical care would be altered.

However, the Marquis-Phelps analysis also underlines the apparently strong inclination toward first-dollar coverage rather than coverage

---

20. Susan Marquis and Charles Phelps, "Demand for Supplementary Insurance" (Paper presented at the American Economic Association Annual Meeting, New York, New York, 1982).

near the Rand Health Insurance Experiment's catastrophic-illness limits. At the 15 to 30 percent loading fees that might be expected of nongroup insurance, the probability of fully supplementing base plans ranging from 25 to 95 percent coinsurance was, respectively, 54 to 49 percent. In other words, about half the families preferred no cost-sharing at all. This phenomenon, although it contradicts the theory of expected utility maximization, has been widely observed elsewhere.[21] It is also evident in the supplementary insurance presently purchased by Medicare beneficiaries, who are willing to add the additional cost of the insurance company's loading fee to the cost-sharing associated with the deductibles rather than pay the costs out-of-pocket. That hospital copayments would significantly reduce the front-end protection of Medicare beneficiaries without supplementary insurance is therefore likely to be a significant consideration in the decision to insure, and one that might well lead to an increase in supplementary coverage. The preferences that Marquis and Phelps observed among younger persons might also be quite different among elderly persons on fixed incomes, who face a greater likelihood of large medical expenses.

As a result, the range of possibilities also includes a shift toward more rather than less supplementary insurance, and toward a reduction in the number of Medicare beneficiaries subject to any newly imposed cost-sharing provisions. Supplementary insurance that covered the additional expenses excluded by Medicare would necessarily cost more, however, and our analysis of the preceding section indicates that income is already a constraint on insurance purchases. Since a quarter of the potential buyers of nongroup insurance are poor (as are 32 percent of nonpurchasers) and only a third of potential buyers do not presently buy a plan, it seems unlikely that the proportion without coverage would drop to less than 20 percent.

Under these various scenarios, including an increase, a decrease, or no change in the number of beneficiaries with supplementary insurance, we have estimated the effects in 1977 of introducing a 10 percent hospital copayment and an increase to 25 percent physician coinsurance on Medicare outlays and out-of-pocket expenditures for

---

21. See, for example, Howard Kunreuther et al., *Disaster Insurance Protection: Public Policy Lessons* (New York: Wiley, 1978); Daniel Kahneman and Amos Tversky, "Prospect Theory: An Analysis of Decision under Risk," *Econometrica* 47, no. 7 (1979):263–92.

medical care.[22] These estimates are restricted to the elderly, noninstitutionalized Medicare population. The figures assume a change to an annual part A deductible, no change in the part B deductible, and no Medicare limit on out-of-pocket expenses. Marilyn Moon offers a comprehensive and thoughtful analysis of a much wider range of benefit options, including cost-sharing limits, and considers the effect on heavy users as well as on the average enrollee.[23] However, although she discusses the possibility of behavioral responses in utilization and supplementary insurance purchases, she does not attempt to quantify them as we do here.

The calculations assume that private insurance will continue to ensure the same level of out-of-pocket expenditures as it does under the present Medicare system, so that reductions in Medicare reimbursements are entirely offset by the supplementary coverage. The average reduction in Medicare payments is consequently matched by an increase in the average benefits paid by private insurance plus a loading fee (assumed to be 20 percent for nongroup and 10 percent for group insurance). Group enrollees, however, pay only 37 percent of their premiums under the present system. Although they might be required to pay the full additional cost to their employer's plan of Medicare's change in benefits, the increase in their private benefits might also be spread over the actuarial experience of the younger members of the group. A continuing 37 percent share is assumed.

Findings from the Rand Health Insurance Experiment—again for the nonelderly population—indicate that 25 percent coinsurance lowered the rate of hospital admissions from 13.3 percent when care was free to 10.4 percent, a 22 percent reduction.[24] The introduction of 10 percent coinsurance in Medicare is consequently assumed to produce a 10 percent reduction in admissions for those without supplementary insurance, but to have no additional effect on Medicare payments for hospitalized patients under DRGs.

The estimates of the preceding section indicate that coverage of the

---

22. Table A4–1 shows the effect of this policy change on the detailed components of total expenditures, including expenditures for hospital care and ambulatory physician visits, Medicare reimbursements, out-of-pocket payments, and private insurance premiums.

23. Moon, "Changing the Structure of Medicare Benefits."

24. Joseph Newhouse; Willard Manning et al., "Some Interim Results from a Controlled Trial of Cost Sharing in Health Insurance," *New England Journal of Medicine* 305 (December 17, 1981):1501–7.

part B deductible and 20 percent of Medicare allowable charges by the typical nongroup plan currently raises the probability of a physician visit by 13.5 percentage points and the average subsequent expenditure by 39 percent. If that is the effect of the difference in cost-sharing between those with nongroup plans and those facing the present Medicare requirements, then an additional 5 percent coinsurance might effect a further reduction in expenditures per user on the order of 10 percent. We assume that the probability of use would not be further affected by an increase in the coinsurance above the deductible. Finally, the calculations make the simplifying assumption that a representative cross-section of persons with nongroup coverage would give up their plans and vice versa, so that the utilization of those who change their insurance status would be the group average prior to switching.

The 1977 NMCES estimate of Medicare outlays for the hospital and ambulatory physician services of the noninstitutionalized elderly population is about $11 billion, 89 percent of which is for hospital care.[25] The introduction of 10 percent hospital coinsurance therefore accounts for a large component of any savings from the assumed benefit changes.

Estimates of the effect of increased Medicare cost-sharing are shown in Table 4–5. Consider first the scenario that assumes no change in nongroup enrollment. If there were also no change in utilization behavior, the direct savings from the shifting of hospital and physician expenses onto enrollees in the form of cost-sharing would be $37 per person, or $805 million overall. A $37 increase in Medicare premiums would have an identical effect on Medicare outlays. However, because of their already lower utilization of hospital and physician services, this increase in Medicare premiums would exceed what those without supplementary coverage would pay on average with more cost-sharing ($30). Those with above-average utilization would, of course, pay more under the cost-sharing approach. The private premiums of nongroup enrollees would increase by more than the comparable increase in Medicare premiums because of their higher-than-average utilization and the additional loading fee. Group enrollees would pay only about a third as much in private premiums as a $37 increase in Medicare premiums, while $50 per Medicaid enrollee would be shifted

---

25. See Appendix Table A4–1.

Table 4–5.   Effect of Increased Medicare Cost-Sharing on Medicare Budget and Out-of-Pocket Expenditures.

Scenario	Total Change in Medicare Payments ($ million)	Budgetary Equivalent (Increase in Medicare Premiums)	Increase in Out-of-Pocket Expenses,[a] Including Private Premiums ($ per person)			
			Medicare Only	Non-group	Group	Medicaid[b]
No change in supplementation; no utilization effect	805	37	30	46	14	50
No change in supplementation, with utilization effect	1022	47	25	46	14	50
Decrease in supplementation[c]	1197	55	25	46	14	50
Increase in supplementation[d]	892	41	25	46	14	50
Persons (000)			4,465	9,087	5,526	2,677

SOURCE: *National Medical Care Expenditure Survey, 1977.*

Note: The assumed cost-sharing is 10 percent of the one-day annual hospital deductible for days 2–60 and 25 percent physician coinsurance.

[a]Only medical expenses for hospital and ambulatory physician care are included.

[b]Additional expenditures covered by Medicaid rather than Medicare are shown, not out-of-pocket expenditures.

[c]Assuming that 20 percent of those with nongroup plans—8.4 percent of the Medicare population—were to give up their supplementary insurance.

[d]Assuming that the proportion of those who purchase supplementary insurance would rise from 67 percent to 80 percent of Medicare recipients.

off the Medicare budget to be shared with state governments. The cost-sharing approach thus works to the greater advantage of the federal government, given that a significant number of elderly Medicaid enrollees are heavy users of medical services by definition of the "medically needy" eligibility criteria.

A 10 percent reduction in hospital admissions and physician expenditures in response to cost-sharing by those who face these payments—the present one-fifth of enrollees without supplementary coverage—would produce an additional savings of $10 per person, up to $1.022 billion in total. The equivalent increase in Medicare premiums would consequently be $47 per person. On average, the introduction of increased cost-sharing would be more financially advantageous than a comparable premium increase to all parties except state governments. The increased private premiums of nongroup as well as group enrollees and the average out-of-pocket expenses of those without supplementary coverage would be less than $47. These monetary savings would come at the cost, however, of a further reduction in the services used by those covered by Medicare alone, who already make fewer physician visits than their more fully insured counterparts. The resulting increase in out-of-pocket payments for this group would be $25, with a reduction in utilization. The increase in out-of-pocket payments for other groups would be the same as if we assumed no utilization effect, since the increase in their private insurance coverage would mean no change in cost-sharing for those with supplemental insurance.

The premiums for nongroup insurance, as indicated, would increase by $46 (plus the cost of additional benefits for inpatient physician services). If 8.4 percent of the Medicare population—20 percent of those with nongroup plans—were to give up their insurance as a result, Medicare's savings could be as much as $1.197 billion. To have a comparable effect on outlays, a $55 increase in Medicare premiums would be required. These additional savings come from the reduction in utilization of the 1.8 million beneficiaries who would forego their supplemental coverage and consequently be faced with the old cost-sharing provisions as well as the new. The average out-of-pocket expenses of this group would increase by more than $100 for hospital and ambulatory physician services—despite the cutback in utilization—plus the cost-sharing associated with inpatient physician services and other expenses now covered by their private insurance. In turn, they would save the $185 premium for supplementary insurance. With respect to the distribution of expenditures between the federal and state governments under Medicaid, a $55 increase in premiums would be required to achieve the same savings to the federal government as the $50 reduction in Medicare benefits.

If the proportion of potential buyers who chose to purchase supplementary coverage rose to 80 percent from the current 67 percent, Medicare's savings would drop to $892 million, or $41 per capita. Reflecting our finding that supplemental coverage has a significant effect on ambulatory physician expenditures by enrollees that adds to Medicare's outlays, the increase in Medicare's part B outlays for new nongroup enrollees would more than offset its savings on their hospital care. At the same time, the part A savings would be substantially less than if the new nongroup enrollees were subject to the 10 percent cost-sharing. Thus, the increase in supplementary insurance dilutes the budgetary effect of the change in benefit provisions. In this scenario, those presently enrolled in nongroup plans would face an increase of about $46 in outlays, while the comparable increase in Medicare premiums is $41. The out-of-pocket expenditures for hospital and outpatient physician care of those newly enrolling in supplementary insurance would decrease by $73, with their new private insurance benefits somewhat offset by the predicted increase in their amount of physician care. They would also have to pay $231 in premiums for the insurance coverage.

CONCLUSION

We have seen that supplemental insurance not only affects the outlays of the current Medicare program, it also influences the impact of proposed changes in Medicare benefits. Considering the scenarios presented here, the federal government would have saved $800 million to $1.2 billion in 1977 from the contemplated change in Medicare's benefit provisions. This would have been equivalent to an increase in Medicare premiums in the range of $37 to $55 per person per year in terms of its effect on Medicare outlays. The average out-of-pocket expenditures of those without supplementary coverage would have increased by about $27, with the possibility of much higher than average cost-sharing payments, and the amount of their health care would have been reduced by about 10 percent. Group enrollees would fare better under a change in benefits than under a universal increase in Medicare premiums, assuming that employers or younger group members would continue to share in the added cost of their premiums. Unless private supplementary insurance decreases substantially, the burden on states is slightly lower if a premium is imposed than if cost-sharing is increased. Cost-sharing would allow the federal government to shift more outlays from the Medicare program to Medicaid, saving federal revenues at the expense of state governments. Those presently enrolled in nongroup plans might pay the same, more, or less with cost-sharing than with an equivalent increase in Medicare premiums, depending on the behavioral response of beneficiaries with respect to utilization and supplementation. Rather than increase Medicare premiums by $37 to $55, the decision to change Medicare's benefit provisions would thus save group enrollees $23 to $41, non-group enrollees as much as $9 per person, and the federal government the states' share of up to $13 per Medicaid enrollee. To be balanced against the potential benefits to these parties is the added burden on state governments and on Medicare enrollees who are presently without supplementary coverage. Those Medicare beneficiaries who chose either to buy or give up their supplementary coverage might be worse or better off as well.

APPENDIX

Table A4–1. Medicare Outlays and Savings Under New Cost-Sharing Provisions.

	Total[a]	Medicare[a] Only	Non-group Insurance	Group Insurance	Medicaid
Baseline 1977					
Persons (000)	21,755	4,465	9,087	5,526	2,677
Percent of beneficiaries	100.0	20.5	41.8	25.4	12.3
Average per person					
Premiums	N/A	N/A	$185	$142	N/A
Hospital					
Total expense	623	557	543	680	889
Medicare expense	443	443	415	469	487
Out-of-pocket expense	26	51	22	15	19
Users (%)	19.8	17.3	20.4	18.1	25.7
Ambulatory physician					
Total expense	157	109	166	170	181
Medicare expense	56	38	65	52	64
Out-of-pocket expense	61	52	71	67	24
Users (%)	80.0	68.6	84.4	81.7	80.2
Total Medicare payments					
(millions)[b]	10,856	2,148	4,362	2,879	1,475
Hospital	9,637	1,978	3,771	2,592	1,304
Physician	1,218	170	591	287	171

Scenario One: No change in nongroup enrollment

	Total		Medicare Only		Non-group Insurance		Group Insurance		Medicaid
Average change									
per person									
Premiums	N/A				N/A		+46	+14	N/A
Hospital									
Total expense	−11	(0)			−44	(0)	0	0	0
Medicare expense	−42	(−33)			−69	(−27)	−34	−31	−46

171

Table A4–1.   (continued)

	Total[a]	Medicare[a] Only	Non-group Insurance	Group Insurance		Medicaid
Out-of-pocket expense	+5	(+6)	+24	(+27)	0	0	0
Users (%)	−0.4	(0)	−1.7	(0)	0	0	0
Ambulatory physician							
Total expense	−3	(0)	−11	(0)	0	0	0
Medicare expense	−5	(−4)	−12	(−3)	−4	−3	−4
Out-of-pocket expense	+1	(+1)	+1	(+3)	0	0	0
Users (%)	0	(0)	0	(0)	0	0	0
Total change in Medicare payments (millions)[b]	−1,022	(−805)	−362	(−134)	−345	−188	−134
Hospital	−914	(−718)	−308	(−121)	−309	−171	−123
Physician	−109	(−87)	−54	(−13)	−36	−17	−11

	Total	Medicare only	Changing Insurance	Nongroup Insurance	Group Insurance	Medicaid
Scenario Two: Decrease in population with supplementary insurance						
Persons (000)	21,755	4,465	1,817	7,270	5,526	2,677
Percent of beneficiaries	100.0	20.5	8.4	33.4	25.4	12.3
Average change per person						
Premiums	N/A	N/A	−185	+46	+14	N/A
Hospital						
Total expense	−13	−44	−42	0	0	0
Medicare expense	−45	−69	−72	−34	−31	−46
Out-of-pocket expense	+9	+24	+53	0	0	0
Users (%)	−0.5	−1.7	−2.0	0	0	0
Ambulatory physician						
Total expense	−8	−11	−72	0	0	0
Medicare expense	−10	−12	−56	−4	−3	−4
Out-of-pocket expense	+4	+1	+50	0	0	0
Users (%)	−1.1	0	−13.5	0	0	0
Total change in Medicare payments (millions)[b]	−1,197	−362	−233	−276	−188	−134
Hospital	−979	−308	−131	−247	−171	−123
Physician	−218	−54	−102	−29	−17	−11
Scenario Three: Increase in population with supplementary insurance						
Persons (000)	21,755	2,710	1,755	9,087	5,526	2,677
Percent of beneficiaries	100.0	12.5	8.1	41.8	25.4	12.3
Average per person						
Premiums	N/A	N/A	+231	+46	+14	N/A
Hospital						
Total expense	−6	−44	0	0	0	0
Medicare expense	−39	−69	−27	−34	−31	−46
Out-of-pocket expense	+1	+24	−21	0	0	0

Table A4–1.   (continued)

	Total[a]	Medicare[a] Only	Non-group Insurance	Group Insurance	Medicaid
Users (%)	−0.2	−1.7	0	0	0	0
Ambulatory physician						
Total expense	+4	−11	+72	0	0	0
Medicare expense	−2	−12	+34	−4	−3	−4
Out-of-pocket expense	−4	+1	−52	0	0	0
Users (%)	+1.1	0	+13.5	0	0	0
Total change in Medicare (millions)[b]	−892	−220	+12	−345	−188	−134
Hospital	−848	−187	−47	−309	−171	−123
Physician	−44	−33	+60	−36	−17	−11

SOURCE: *National Medical Care Expenditure Study, 1977.*

[a]Figures in parentheses indicate estimates assuming no change in utilization.
[b]Components do not add up to total because of rounding.

SELECTED BIBLIOGRAPHY

Amemiya, Takeshi. "Qualitative Response Models: A Survey." *Journal of Economic Literature* 19, no. 4 (December 1981):1483–1536.

Bonham, G. S., and L. S. Corder. *National Medical Care Expenditures Study (NMCES) Household Interview Instruments: Instruments and Procedures 1,* DHHS Publication No. (PHS) 81–3280. Washington, D.C.: U.S. Department of Health and Human Services, National Center for Health Services Research, 1981.

Cafferata, Gail. "Private Health Insurance Coverage of the Medicare Population." In *National Health Care Expenditures Study, Data Preview 18,* DHHS Publication No. (PHS) 84–3362. Washington, D.C.: U.S. Department of Health and Human Services, National Center for Health Services Research, 1984.

Cafferata, Gail, and Mark Meiners. "Public and Private Insurance and the Medicare Population's Out-of-Pocket Expenditures: Does Medigap Make a Difference?" Paper presented at the American Public Health Association Annual Meeting, Anaheim, California, November 1984.

Feldstein, Martin. "An Econometric Model of the Medicare System." *The Quarterly Journal of Economics* 85, no. 1 (February 1971).

Fisher, Charles. "Differences by Age Groups in Health Care Spending." *Health Care Financing Review* 1, no. 4 (Spring 1980).

Ginsburg, Paul, and Marilyn Moon. "An Introduction to the Medicare Financing Problem." In Committee on Ways and Means, U.S. House of Representatives, *Conference on the Future of Medicare.* Washington, D.C.: Government Printing Office, 1983.

Halvorsen, Robert, and Raymond Palmquist. "The Interpretation of Dummy Variables in Semilogarithmic Equations." *American Economic Review* 70, no. 3 (June 1980):474–75.

Hausman, Jerry. "Specification Tests in Econometrics." *Econometrica* 46, no. 6 (November 1978).

Heckman, James. "Dummy Endogenous Variables in a Simultaneous Equation System." *Econometrica* 46, no. 6 (July 1978):931–59.

Hsiao, William. "Public versus Private Administration of Health Insurance: A Study in Relative Economic Efficiency." *Inquiry* 15 (December 1978):379.

Hsiao, William, and Nancy Kelly. "Restructuring Medicare Benefits." In Committee on Ways and Means, U.S. House of Representatives, *Conference on the Future of Medicare*. Washington, D.C.: Government Printing Office, 1983.

Kahneman, Daniel, and Amos Tversky, "Prospect Theory: An Analysis of Decision under Risk." *Econometrica* 47, no. 7 (1979):263–92.

Kunreuther, Howard, R. Ginsberg, L. Miller, P. Sagi, P. Slovic, B. Borken, and N. Katz. *Disaster Insurance Protection: Public Policy Lessons*. New York: Wiley, 1978.

Link, Charles, Stephen Long, and Russell Settle. "Cost Sharing, Supplementary Insurance and Health Services Utilization Among the Medicare Elderly." *Health Care Financing Review* 2 (Fall 1980).

Long, Stephen, Russell Settle, and Charles R. Link. "Who Bears the Burden of Medicare Cost Sharing?" *Inquiry* 19 (Fall 1982):222–34.

Long, Stephen, and Russell Settle. "Medicare Cost Sharing and Supplementary Health Insurance: Selected Research Findings." Paper presented at American Public Health Association Meetings, Montreal, Canada, November 1982.

Marquis, Susan, and Charles Phelps. "Demand for Supplementary Insurance." Paper presented at the American Economic Association Annual Meeting, New York, 1982.

Moon, Marilyn. "Changing the Structure of Medicare Benefits: Issues and Options." Washington, D.C.: Congressional Budget Office, 1983.

Mueller, Marjorie. "Private Health Insurance in 1970." *Social Security Bulletin* 35 (February 1972).

Scitovsky, Ann, and Nelda Snyder. "Effect of Coinsurance on Use of Physician Services," *Social Security Bulletin* 35 (1972):3–19.

Summary of the 1984 Annual Reports of the Medicare Board of Trustees. Washington, D.C.: Government Printing Office, 1984.

Taylor, Amy. "Inpatient Hospital Services: Use, Expenditures and Sources of Payment." In *National Health Care Expenditure Study, Data Preview 15*, DHHS Publication No. (PHS) 83–3360. Washington, D.C.: U.S.

Department of Health and Human Services, National Center for Health Services Research, 1984.

U.S. Senate, Special Committee on Aging. *Medicare and the Health Costs of Older Americans: The Extent and Effects of Cost Sharing.* S. Prt. 98–116. Washington, D.C.: Government Printing Office, 1984.

Waldo, Daniel, and Helen C. Lazenby. "Demographic Characteristics and Health Care Use and Expenditures by the Aged in the United States: 1977–1984." *Health Care Financing Review* 6, no. 1 (Fall 1984):1–29.

5

PUBLIC INSURANCE PROGRAMS: MEDICARE AND MEDICAID

Paul B. Ginsburg

INTRODUCTION

More than twenty years have passed since the inception of the Medicare and Medicaid programs. While these public programs, which finance medical services for the elderly and the poor, have thus far not turned out to be the initial steps toward national health insurance that some had predicted, they nevertheless have had a profound influence on the medical care system. They may become even more influential in the near future as the major reforms recently enacted reach their full impact.

The influence of Medicare and Medicaid on the health system is often summarized in terms of numbers of persons covered and dollars paid out to purchase medical services. Medicare provides health insurance for approximately 30 million persons—27 million who are eligible on the basis of age and 3 million who are eligible on the basis of disability. In 1985, 23 million persons were expected to receive Medicaid benefits.[1] Combined federal, state, and local outlays for the two programs were projected to total $113 billion. Medicare and Medicaid patients account for roughly half of the revenues received by community hospitals.

1. This included about 4 million persons also enrolled in Medicare.

The nature of this influence is changing dramatically. Until recently, these programs attempted to purchase services in as unobtrusive a manner as possible, for eligible persons. Eligibles could choose virtually any provider of services who would be paid, for the most part, in a manner similar to that used by private insurers. Thus, hospitals were paid on the basis of incurred costs—the mechanism used by many Blue Cross plans—and, except for Medicaid programs in some states, physicians were paid on the basis of "customary, prevailing, and reasonable" charges.[2] It is not surprising, at least in hindsight, that increasing the proportion of the population with insurance, with only limited restrictions on the amount reimbursed, would result in an acceleration of the rate of increase in costs.

In recent years, however, as reforms have been implemented to control these programs' outlays, the influence of Medicare and Medicaid have gone in different directions. Medicare's prospective payment system for hospitals appears to have helped trigger a dramatic slowdown in the rate of growth in hospital costs. Both programs now make it attractive for covered individuals to enroll in health maintenance organizations (HMOs), which is likely to increase the competitive pressure on fee-for-service providers.

Additional change in these programs is expected over the next ten years. The previously abstract question raised by economists—what proportion of resources society should devote to health services—will be faced by these programs because they are financed with taxes. While the general population has not yet been inspired to think in terms of the trade-off between health services and other goods and services, it has focused on the trade-off between spending in these programs and higher taxes. Indeed, the results of decisions to constrain spending in the Medicare and Medicaid programs may influence the proportion of resources devoted to health services for the rest of the population as well.

This chapter begins with a section on the origins of these public insurance programs, followed by a description of their rapid growth from their inception to approximately 1980. The third section de-

2. In 1975, Medicare departed somewhat from this practice by limiting the rate of increase in "prevailing" screens to an index of physicians' practice expenses. Medicaid programs that did not follow Medicare methods paid physicians on the basis of a fee schedule, with the average fee often substantially lower than that paid by private insurers or Medicare.

scribes the major reforms enacted during the early 1980s and analyzes their likely impact over the long term. The next section is devoted to a review of a number of broad policy options for the next series of major reforms. These include broadening the hospital PPS, changing the programs' benefit structures, further encouraging the use of private health plans by beneficiaries, and encouraging the use of preferred provider arrangements. Underlying these options are the broadest issues, such as the role of government in the health care system, whether a "two-tiered" health care system is inevitable, and whether different forms of rationing are inevitable.

ORIGINS OF MEDICARE AND MEDICAID

The enactment of Medicare and Medicaid in 1965 was the culmination of a lengthy debate on the role of the federal government in the financing of health services. This section reviews that debate briefly and describes the basic features of the two programs that were so heavily influenced by that debate.

The Debate

Interest in having the federal government play a role in the financing of medical services goes back to at least the 1930s.[3] Throughout the period that culminated with the passage of Medicare and Medicaid in 1965, the merits of two opposing models were debated. Under a universal coverage model, the federal government would provide health insurance to all on a compulsory basis, financed by taxes on earnings. The alternative limited government's role to the provision of assistance to the needy. This "gap-filling" approach often emphasized program administration by state governments, with financial assistance from the federal government to the states.

Prior to 1965, most federal legislation affecting health care financing followed the latter approach. A particularly important milestone was the 1950 Amendments to the Social Security Act, which authorized matching grants to the states for direct payments to pro-

---

3. This section draws on the excellent summary in Kathleen N. Lohr and M. Susan Marquis, *Medicare and Medicaid: Past, Present, and Future*, N-2088-HHS/RC (Santa Monica, Calif.: Rand Corporation, May 1984).

viders of medical care ("vendor payments") for treatment of those on public assistance. Previously, federal matching funds could be used for medical care, but only to calculate the monthly cash payment to recipients of public assistance. That is, a state could include the average monthly cost of medical care for a family in calculating a monthly cash assistance benefit, but it could not provide a health insurance benefit. Given the uneven and unpredictable nature of a single family's medical care expenses, such an approach did not provide much access to medical care for the poor.

In 1960, the Kerr-Mills Act expanded federal matching payments to the states for vendor payments and permitted states to include the "medically needy"—elderly, blind, and disabled persons with low incomes who are not on public assistance. During this period, proponents of universal health insurance focused their efforts on coverage for the elderly. Since the elderly had lower incomes, less private health insurance, and higher medical expenses than did the rest of the population, focus on this group might head off arguments that national health insurance would help too many persons who were well off. To avoid opposition from the formidable American Medical Association (AMA), these proposals were limited to payment of hospital bills. Despite these limitations on the scope of the proposals, passage of such legislation did not come about until after the landslide election of Lyndon Johnson in 1964.

Health insurance was at the top of the legislative agenda in 1965, however, with three major proposals put forth. The Johnson administration proposed hospital insurance for the aged, financed by payroll taxes. Republicans offered a proposal for subsidized voluntary insurance for the aged. This proposal, which included coverage for physicians' services, would be financed through general revenues. The AMA opposed both plans, but countered with a plan of its own to expand the Kerr-Mills program of matching grants to the states for vendor payments for the needy.

As chairman of the House Ways and Means Committee, Wilbur Mills crafted a compromise that encompassed all three approaches. It included a compulsory health insurance program for the elderly financed through payroll taxes (Medicare part A), a voluntary insurance program for physicians' services subsidized through general revenues (Medicare part B), and an expanded means-tested program administered by the states (Medicaid). This structure has not been altered to date.

Medicare Part A

Medicare's Hospital Insurance (HI) program is closely linked with the Social Security program.[4] Eligibility is based on entitlement to Social Security or Railroad Retirement benefits. All persons aged 65 and over with such an entitlement are eligible for Medicare. In 1972, those under 65 who had been entitled to Social Security or Railroad Retirement disability benefits for twenty-four months and those with end-stage renal disease were added to the program. Persons aged 65 and over who are not eligible can enroll through the payment of a premium that reflects per capita costs.

HI covers the costs of ninety days of hospitalization for each spell of illness after the payment of a deductible ($400 in 1985). The sixty-first through ninetieth days are subject to a daily copayment equal to one-quarter of the deductible amount. In addition, each beneficiary has a lifetime reserve of sixty days that are subject to a daily copayment of one-half the deductible amount.

HI covers the costs of up to 100 days of care after hospitalization in a skilled nursing facility, with all but the first twenty days subject to a copayment of one-eighth of the hospital deductible amount. For a homebound individual, unlimited home health visits by health workers are covered without copayment. A hospice benefit is provided for those with a life expectancy of less than six months.

Reimbursement has undergone significant changes in the past few years. Historically, hospitals, skilled nursing facilities, and home health agencies have been reimbursed on a "reasonable cost" basis. "Reasonable" has generally meant all costs associated with the care of Medicare patients. Beginning in fiscal year 1984, virtually all Medicare reimbursements to hospitals have been made on the basis of a prospective payment per discharge (this system is described later). Skilled nursing facility reimbursements are now limited to 112 percent of costs in a comparison group of facilities, and home health payments are limited to the 75th percentile of average agency costs per visit.[5] Providers are not permitted to collect from beneficiaries the difference between charges and what Medicare reimburses.[6]

4. Only the highlights are covered here. The reader seeking additional detail should refer to the annual supplements of the *Social Security Bulletin*.

5. A limit is established for each type of service. Each agency's limit is then based on the weighted average of these limits, with the weights based on the agency's service mix.

6. Providers do collect the required deductibles and copayments, however.

HI is financed by a trust fund. The income of the HI Trust Fund consists of payroll tax receipts, premiums from those not otherwise eligible, and interest earned on trust fund balances. Outlays are limited to balances in the trust fund.

Insurance companies (mostly Blue Cross plans) process claims under the program and audit providers' cost reports. These intermediaries are reimbursed for their services on a cost basis, though binding ceilings have constrained resources available for these functions in recent years.

Medicare Part B

Medicare's Supplementary Medical Insurance (SMI) program is not linked to Social Security; thus, persons aged 65 and over who do not have the required participation in Social Security are nevertheless eligible.[7] Benefits include physician services (whether inpatient or outpatient), outpatient hospital services, outpatient laboratory and radiology services, and home health services. All benefits are subject to a $75 annual deductible and 20 percent coinsurance.[8] No limits exist on either the amount of services covered or the beneficiary's liability for coinsurance.

Physicians are reimbursed for their charges, which are subject to screens for "reasonableness." A charge for a service is limited to the lower of the physician's customary charge, defined as the 50th percentile of the physician's charges for the service in the previous year, and the area prevailing charge, defined as the 75th percentile of area physicians' customary charges for the procedure in the previous year. Since the mid-1970s, increases in prevailing charges have been limited by an index of practice expenses. Physician reimbursements were frozen from July 1, 1984, through September 30, 1985. Hospital outpatient departments are reimbursed on a reasonable cost basis.

Unlike hospitals, physicians are permitted to charge the patient more than the amount deemed reasonable by Medicare. A physician can either accept assignment and receive from Medicare reimbursement of the reasonable charge less applicable deductibles and coinsurance, or not accept assignment and bill the patient, who in turn files a claim

---

7. Persons eligible for part A on the basis of disability or end-stage renal disease are also eligible for part B.

8. These are waived for home health services.

with Medicare. In 1983, 83 percent of approved claims had their charges reduced by these screens for reasonableness. The average reduction was 23 percent. Fifty-four percent of claims in that year were assigned. In 1984, the concept of a participating physician was initiated. Participating physicians agree in advance to accept assignments on all cases and are included in a directory of such physicians.

SMI is also financed through a trust fund, but this trust fund is able to draw from general revenues as needed. Originally, monthly premiums financed 50 percent of outlays for SMI. In 1972, however, percentage increases in premiums were limited to increases in Social Security cash benefits. By the early 1980s, the proportion financed by premiums had fallen to approximately 25 percent. The practice of having premiums underwrite a constant percentage of SMI outlays was restored at that point. As for HI, insurance companies perform the claims processing. Most of the part B "carriers" are Blue Shield plans.

Medicaid

Medicaid programs are state-run programs to finance health services for the needy. They must conform to federal requirements; in turn they receive federal matching grants to underwrite their cost. In the areas of eligibility and benefits, federal legislation has established categories of persons and types of services that must be included as well as categories that are optional.

Medicaid programs must cover persons receiving benefits under the Aid to Families with Dependent Children (AFDC) program, and most persons receiving benefits under the Supplemental Security Income (SSI) program.[9] Persons whose coverage is optional under federal law tend to be low-income persons who do not receive cash assistance but have the same demographic characteristics as those covered by AFDC or SSI. For example, states can elect to cover children in low-income families with two parents, even though the presence of two parents generally precludes cash assistance. Legislation enacted in 1984, however, requires states to cover all low-income children born after October 1, 1983, up to age five. Another important optional group consists of persons who qualify for cash assistance but do not actually receive it. Finally, states can extend coverage to the medically needy—

9. Some states have been permitted to use more restrictive income standards than SSI.

persons meeting all of the categorical requirements for Medicaid eligibility and whose income, after deducting medical expenses, is less than the state's "medically needy" income standard.

Mandatory Medicaid benefits include hospital and physician services, diagnostic services, family planning consultation, care in skilled nursing facilities, and screening and treatment of children for various illnesses and impairments. The most important optional services include nursing home care in intermediate care facilities, prescription drugs, and dental care. Medicaid nursing home benefits are much more important than their Medicare equivalents, since they are not restricted to persons recuperating from an acute illness. Approximately 43 percent of Medicaid outlays in 1983 went for nursing home care. In contrast, coverage of home health services is more restrictive in Medicaid than in Medicare. States must seek a waiver to provide home health services, and assure the Health Care Financing Administration (HCFA) that the addition of the benefit will not increase outlays. Most states pay the SMI premiums for eligible Medicaid recipients as well as deductibles and coinsurance for both parts of Medicare. For these dually eligible persons, Medicaid acts as a supplemental insurance policy.

While only very limited cost-sharing by beneficiaries is permitted under Medicaid, states are permitted to restrict the amount of services per beneficiary. Some states restrict hospital care to twenty-one days per year and limit the number of covered physician visits.

States have extensive discretion concerning methods of payment to providers. While states originally had to pay hospitals according to Medicare principles, they can now use any method so long as payments are "reasonable and adequate." States can pay physicians according to Medicare principles or on the basis of a fee schedule. All providers must accept Medicaid's reimbursement as payment in full. As a consequence, and because of the very low rates of physician payment in some states, large numbers of physicians refuse to treat Medicaid patients.[10]

Rates for matching federal grants to the states are based on a for-

10. A recent survey by John Holahan found that seven states—New York, New Jersey, Pennsylvania, Maryland, Florida, Rhode Island, and Connecticut—reimbursed specialists at rates less than 50 percent of Medicare rates in those respective states. See John Holahan, "Paying for Physician Services in State Medicaid Programs," *Health Care Financing Review* (Spring 1984):99–110.

mula that results in higher rates for states with lower per capita income. Regardless of the formula, however, 50 percent is the lowest rate. In 1985, 77.63 percent was the highest rate. During the 1982–1984 period, matching rates were reduced, but they have since been restored.

1966–1980: RAPID GROWTH

The first fifteen years of Medicare and Medicaid were a period of rapid growth in spending. Not only did the original programs prove much more expensive than had been anticipated, but a major expansion of Medicare was enacted in 1972. Further expansions might well have been enacted if not for the cost problems that could not be resolved.

Growth in Outlays

Almost from the beginning, outlays for Medicare and Medicaid exceeded initial projections (see Tables 5–1 and 5–2). As early as 1967, Congress was faced with a projected depletion in the Hospital Insurance Trust Fund. It chose to increase revenues rather than attempt to control costs.[11] The federal government had deliberately chosen to reimburse providers in a generous manner when Medicare was enacted, both to win their political support and to ensure access to services by beneficiaries, and it was not about to change that policy so soon.

Instead, cost-control concerns were focused on the entire health care system. In 1967, a National Conference on Medical Costs was convened to discuss the problem of rising costs. According to one astute observer: "The conference conclusions were conspicuous in their failure to suggest restraint on the rates of Medicare payment as a possibility for action. Rather, the point was made over and over that a better organized health care system was required—a suggestion that is more easily made than implemented."[12]

In Medicare, rapid cost increases were, for the most part, a reflection of developments in the health care system. Rates of use of services by Medicare beneficiaries had increased as a result of Medicare coverage, but not to a degree inconsistent with actuarial fore-

11. Irwin Wolkstein, "Medicare's Financial Status: How Did We Get Here?" *Milbank Memorial Fund Quarterly: Health and Society* (Spring 1984):183–206.
12. Ibid., p. 185.

Table 5–1.   Medicare Outlays, Fiscal Years 1967–1984.

Fiscal Year	Part A		Part B		Total	
	$ Millions	Percent Increase Over Prior Year	$ Millions	Percent Increase Over Prior Year	$ Millions	Percent Increase Over Prior Year
1967	2,597	—	799	—	3,396	—
1968	3,815	46.9	1,532	91.7	5,347	57.4
1969	4.758	24.7	1,840	20.1	6,598	23.4
1970	4,953	4.1	2,196	19.3	7,149	8.4
1971	5,592	12.9	2,283	4.0	7,875	10.2
1972	6,276	12.2	2,544	11.4	8,820	12.0
1973	6,842	9.0	2,637	3.7	9,479	7.5
1974	8,065	17.9	3,283	24.5	11,348	19.7
1975	10,612	31.6	4,170	27.0	14,782	30.3
1976[a]	12,579	18.5	5,200	24.7	17.779	20.3
1977	15,207	20.9	6,342	22.0	21,549	21.2
1978	17,862	17.5	7,350	15.9	25,211	17.0
1979	20,343	13.9	8,805	19.8	29,148	15.6
1980	24,287	19.4	10,746	22.1	35,034	20.2
1981	29,248	20.4	13,240	23.2	42,488	21.3
1982	34,864	19.2	15,559	17.5	50,423	18.7
1983	38,551	10.6	18,317	17.7	56,868	12.8
1984	42,295	9.7	20,374	11.2	62,669	10.2

SOURCE: 1983 Annual Report of the Board of Trustees: Federal Hospital Insurance Trust Fund and Supplementary Medical Insurance Trust Fund, as reported in U.S. House of Representatives, Committee on Ways and Means, *Background Material and Data on Programs within the Jurisdiction of the Committee on Ways and Means*, WMCP: 99–2 (Washington, D.C.: Government Printing Office, 1985), pp. 138–39.

[a]In the transition quarter from July to October 1976 (when the beginning of the federal fiscal year was changed), outlays were $4,805 million. These outlays do not appear in the table.

casts. Survey data indicate that days in short-stay hospitals per hundred Social Security beneficiaries aged 65 and over increased by 25 percent between 1965 and 1967. There were no significant differences in rates of physician visits, however.[13]

Trends over the 1970–1981 period show these developments clearly. The number of Medicare enrollees grew at an average annual rate of 3.1 percent, a figure that includes the addition of disabled enrollees beginning July 1, 1973. Hospital discharges per enrollee increased at

13. Regina Loewenstein, "Early Effects of Medicare on the Health Care of the Aged," *Social Security Bulletin* (April 1971):3–20.

Table 5–2.   History of Medicaid Program Costs.

Fiscal Year	Total $ Millions	Total % Increase	Federal $ Millions	Federal % Increase	State $ Millions	State % Increase
1966[a]	1,658	—	789	—	869	—
1967[a]	2,368	42.9	1,209	53.2	1,159	33.5
1968[a]	3,659	55.6	1,837	51.9	1,849	59.5
1969[a]	4,166	13.0	2,276	23.9	1,890	2.2
1970[a]	4,852	16.5	2,617	15.0	2,235	18.3
1971	6,176	27.3	3,374	28.9	2,802	25.3
1972[b]	8,434	36.6	4,361	29.2	4,074	45.4
1973	9,111	8.0	4,998	14.6	4,113	1.0
1974	10,229	12.3	5,833	16.7	4,396	6.9
1975	12,637	23.5	7,060	21.0	5,578	26.9
1976	14,644	15.9	8,312	17.7	6,332	13.5
TQ[c]	4,106	NA	2,354	NA	1,752	NA
1977	17,103	16.8[a]	9,713	16.9[d]	7,389	16.7[d]
1978	18,949	10.8	10,680	10.0	8,269	11.9
1979	21,755	14.8	12,267	14.9	9,489	14.8
1980	25,781	18.5	14,550	18.6	11,231	18.4
1981	30,377	17.8	17,074	17.3	13,303	18.4
1982	32,446	6.8	17,514	2.6	14,931	12.2
1983	34,956	7.7	18,985	8.4	15,971	7.0
1984 (current law estimate)	37,631	7.7	20,094	5.8	17,537	9.8

SOURCE: Budget of the U.S. Government, fiscal years 1969–85, and conversations with officials of the Health Care Financing Administration, as reported in U.S. House of Representatives, Committee on Ways and Means, *Background Material and Data on Programs within the Jurisdiction of the Committee on Ways and Means*, WMCP: 99–2 (Washington, D.C.: Government Printing Office, 1985), pp. 138–39.

Note: Totals may not add, due to rounding.

[a]Includes related programs not identified separately, though for each successive year a larger portion of the total represents Medicaid expenditures. As of January 1, 1970, federal matching was only available under Medicaid.

[b]Intermediate care facilities were transferred from the cash assistance programs to Medicaid effective January 1, 1972; data for prior periods do not include these costs.

[c]Transitional quarter (beginning of federal fiscal year moved from July 1 to October 1).

[d]Represents increase over fiscal year 1976, i.e., five calendar quarters.

an average rate of 1.7 percent per year. But charges per discharge increased at an annual rate of 11.2 percent, exceeding general inflation (as measured by the Consumer Price Index) by 2.9 percentage points per year. This increase in resources per discharge came in spite of a decline of 2.2 percent per year in average length of stay.

To a large extent, these trends had been in place before Medicare, but had not been noticed by many. While precise data for resource use by the aged are not available prior to Medicare, data on short-term general hospitals from the American Hospital Association's Annual Survey can be used to track resource use generally. From 1950 to 1965, real expenditures per discharge increased at an average annual rate of 5.0 percent per year, compared to 5.9 percent per year for 1965 to 1980.[14] This last figure also reflects the sharp change that occurred at the beginning of Medicare in the proportion of patients over age 65.

In Medicaid, which experienced a more rapid increase in outlays during its initial years, growth in the number of eligibles was the principal factor. For the population eligible for Medicaid on the basis of eligibility for AFDC, outlays increased at a 36.6 percent annual rate during the 1967–1972 period. More than two-thirds of this growth is attributable to increased numbers of eligible persons.[15]

Eligibility for Medicaid increased for a number of reasons, most of which were not related to Medicaid policies. First, many states increased their need standards for AFDC, enabling more families to qualify for cash assistance. The initiation of work incentive programs also increased the number of AFDC recipients by permitting higher payments at higher income levels. Also, the administration of AFDC was liberalized. Second, the number of female-headed households—those categorically eligible for AFDC—increased, reflecting important demographic trends that have continued to this day. Third, many organizations mounted public information programs to increase participation in AFDC. Finally, the number of Medicaid eligibles was increased by additional states initiating Medicaid programs during that period.

Expenditures per user increased at an annual rate of only 4.5 percent for the AFDC population—a rate comparable to general inflation during that period. This figure is in marked contrast to increased real spending per enrollee in Medicare. Two explanations come to mind. First, Medicaid data record only the number of users of reimbursed services, not the number eligible. In the Medicaid population eligible

14. Neither of these trends has had outpatient visits removed from them, since estimates of outpatient visits are not available for years prior to 1965. However, removing outpatient costs for the 1965–1980 period raises the trend by only 0.4 percentage points.

15. John Holahan, *Financing Health Care to the Poor* (Lexington, Mass.: Lexington Books, 1975), pp. 28–29.

through AFDC, the number of users per eligible increased at a 5.3 percent annual rate.[16] While many writers have characterized this phenomenon as an increase in participation rates reflecting more information about the availability of program benefits, a portion of the increase could reflect growing rates of service use.

Second, the slow increase in expenditures per user may reflect the effects of early policies by states, such as more stringent reimbursement policies, to reduce the costs of the program. States were shocked at how costly Medicaid was to them and began early to look for ways to control program costs.

After the initial period of extreme growth in Medicaid, increases slowed. The number of eligibles continued to rise until 1976, though at a much slower pace, and then leveled off. The number of aged eligibles declined, probably a result of the substantial real increases in Social Security benefits in the early 1970s.

Expansions

Despite the rapid growth in outlays, a major expansion in Medicare was enacted in 1972. All those receiving Social Security Disability Insurance payments for twenty-four months were covered under Medicare. In addition, most persons with end-stage renal disease were granted Medicare eligibility.

Both expansions of the program were costly. Together they accounted for $7.6 billion in 1984. In that year, 2.9 million disabled persons had coverage under part A, and 2.7 million under part B. The average annual benefit per disabled person enrolled in both programs was $2,737, compared to $1,998 per aged enrollee.

The end-stage renal disease program cost $2.1 billion in 1984 (included in the $7.6 billion figure above). The program's success in encouraging the construction of facilities and in extending lives has contributed to its high costs today. In 1984, there were 87,000 beneficiaries, compared to 16,000 in 1974.

The Social Security Amendments of 1972 also increased the use of general revenues to finance SMI. As noted above, the amendments severed the link between premium increases and increases in the program's outlays. They also authorized a limited expansion of Medicaid

16. Ibid.

by allowing states to make all those receiving benefits from the then-new SSI program eligible for Medicaid. However, states could elect to continue with more restrictive eligibility standards.

Cost Containment

Beginning in 1972, the federal government took steps to control its costs in the Medicare and Medicaid programs on a number of fronts. Legislation focused both on the programs themselves and on the health care system in general, but in hindsight, what was enacted had only small effects.

Program-Specific Policies.   The Social Security Amendments of 1972 included numerous provisions to contain program costs, especially in Medicare. The amendments authorized the Professional Standards Review Organization (PSRO) program, which used peer review to control costs and increase quality. Perhaps because the administration implemented the program with an emphasis on quality of care rather than cost containment, evaluations of the program showed that savings from the reduction in utilization were comparable in magnitude to the costs of running the program.[17]

The 1972 amendments sought to endorse state-level efforts at health planning by not reimbursing capital costs for hospital facilities disapproved by state planning agencies. At that time, roughly half the states had recently enacted Certificate of Need (CON) programs, which reviewed major capital expenditures as a condition of licensure. The provision was essentially symbolic, indicating federal support of state-level attempts to contain costs through project review. The penalties were far less stringent than those already applied by the state programs. In 1974, the National Health Planning and Resource Development Act required states to adopt CON programs.

More significant changes were made in reimbursement policy. Section 223 of the amendments authorized the Secretary of Health, Education and Welfare to establish limits on costs recognized as rea-

17. Evaluations by the Health Care Financing Administration and the Congressional Budget Office each estimated a reduction in hospital days of about 2 percent, but disagreed on whether the savings from this reduction was larger than the costs of review. In either case, the net impact was very small. See Congressional Budget Office, *The Effects of PSROs on Health Care Costs: Current Findings and Future Evaluations* (Washington, D.C.: Government Printing Office, June 1979).

sonable. Under this authority, the administration developed limits on routine (hospital and nursing services) costs per patient day. While these limits were progressively tightened, the aggregate reimbursement reduction was never that large. In 1981, reimbursements were reduced by only 0.6 percent.[18] Nevertheless, the Section 223 limits were an important first step toward the prospective payment system enacted in 1983.

A general tightening of policies regarding allowable costs may have been more important than the Section 223 limits as far as dollars saved. While it is difficult to put a number on the effects of such policies, in Medicare, nonrecoverable charges as a percentage of billed charges increased from 14 percent in 1975 to 23 percent in 1981.[19] Since most Medicaid programs used Medicare principles of reimbursement, these steps reduced Medicaid outlays as well.

Limitations on physician reimbursement also proved to be of quantitative importance. Recall that physician reimbursements are limited to the lowest of three charges: the actual charge, the customary charge, and the prevailing charge. The 1972 amendments limited the increase in prevailing charges to an index of physicians' practice expenses. By means of this index, the cost of the physician's own time is proxied by changes in earnings throughout the economy. Application of this economic index is the major factor behind the increase in the percentage of charges reduced—from 66 percent in 1974 to 83 percent in 1983—and behind the increase in the average reduction in charges— from 13 percent in 1974 to 23 percent in 1983. As was the case for hospital reimbursement, many Medicaid programs followed Medicare reimbursement rules, so these policies reduced Medicaid outlays as well.

A number of Medicaid programs were more aggressive than Medicare was in using reimbursement policies to contain the rise in outlays. Some sought, and received permission, to pay hospitals on a prospective basis. New York adopted particularly stringent prospective rates for Medicaid during its budgetary crisis in the mid-

18. Unpublished data, Health Care Financing Administration.
19. The figures were provided by Helen Lazenby of the Health Care Financing Administration. Discussions with hospital financial experts corroborate a distinct tightening in the administration of the cost-reimbursement system. However, other factors may also have contributed to the increasing proportion of nonrecoverable charges. Hospitals may have increased markups to privately insured patients, probably as a reaction to the understatement of capital costs by conventional accounting rules during a period of high inflation.

1970s. While some states limited their prospective payment policies to Medicaid, others applied them to private payers, and a few received authority to apply them to Medicare as well. The experience of states with systems that applied to payers other than Medicaid was important to the enactment of a Medicare prospective payment system (PPS) in 1983.

Some states did not follow Medicare policies for the payment of physicians' charges. The alternatives were not as innovative as those for the payment of hospitals, however, and consisted mainly of fee schedules, with fees far below levels charged private patients. In response to budget pressures, many states froze their fees schedules, while charges increased rapidly.

Health Care System Policies.   Federal attempts to control the rising costs of Medicare and Medicaid policies through reform of the health system were less successful. Through the National Health Planning and Resource Development Act of 1974, the federal government required states to set up CON programs, a process to review major capital expenditures. As indicated above, roughly half of the states had already been performing such reviews, though many of these states had to change aspects of the review process to conform to federal requirements. Research on the CON programs has not been encouraging concerning the programs' record of cost containment.[20]

Federal policies toward the health work force probably increased Medicare and Medicaid costs. In the early 1960s, the federal government began a program of support for medical education designed to increase the number of trained physicians. By all accounts, the program was highly successful in increasing the supply of physicians. While this contributed to an achievement of some objectives, such as increased access to physician services in rural areas,[21] it also increased expenditures for physician services. Economists have debated for some time whether physicians can create demand for their own services.[22]

---

20. For a review of this literature and background on federal health planning legislation, see Congressional Budget Office, *Health Planning: Issues for Reauthorization* (Washington, D.C.: Government Printing Office, March 1982).

21. W. B. Schwartz et al., "The Changing Geographic Distribution of Board-certified Physicians," *The New England Journal of Medicine* 303 (1980):1032–38.

22. See, for example, the debate between Reinhardt and Sloan in Federal Trade Commission, *Competition in the Health Care Sector: Past, Present, and Future* (Washington, D.C.: Government Printing Office, March 1978).

But even with a classical model of the physician services market, an exogenous increase in the number of physicians is likely to increase expenditures, as the quantity increase overwhelms the price reduction.[23]

The Economic Stabilization Program, the economywide wage and price controls in effect from 1971 to 1974, provided a brief experience with reimbursement limitations affecting all payers. Hospital prices were subject to the limitations, though with very limited effect until a special set of pricing rules tailored to the unique methods of paying for hospital services could be formulated. While price controls did reduce hospital revenues, their impact on costs appeared slight, principally because of the avowedly temporary nature of the controls.[24] Consideration was given to maintaining the hospital controls as a permanent system, but no action was taken.

In 1977, the Carter administration proposed a series of all-payer revenue controls on hospitals. Known as "hospital cost containment," the initiative followed the methods developed during the Economic Stabilization Program and were quite similar to those that would have taken effect in 1974 had the controls on the hospital industry been extended. Projected reductions in Medicare and Medicaid outlays were a very important argument by the Carter administration in support of its proposal.

After three years of legislative battles, the initiative was defeated. While some observers feel that the time had been right for such an initiative and that its defeat was a combination of mismanagement by the administration and outstanding effort on the part of the American Hospital Association, such a favorable period did not last long, since deregulation became the theme for both parties at the end of the 1970s. Had hospital cost containment passed, it might well have been repealed a few years later.

23. This interpretation does not come from conventional microeconomic models, since in this case demand and supply are too inelastic for an exogenous increase in supply to increase expenditures. However, if one incorporates some nonprice variables in the model, such as waiting time and distance, such predictions can be made. Sloan and Schwartz have reviewed the literature and use a 0.4 expenditure elasticity—that is, for every 10 percent increase in physician supply, expenditures increase by 4 percent. See Frank A. Sloan and William B. Schwartz, "More Doctors: What Will They Cost?" *Journal of American Medical Association* 249 (February 11, 1983):766–69.

24. Paul B. Ginsburg, "Impact of the Economic Stabilization Program on Hospital Costs: An Analysis with Aggregate Data," in Michael Zubkoff, Ira Raskin, and Ruth Hanft, eds., *Hospital Cost Containment: Selected Notes for Future Policy* (New York: Prodist, 1978) pp. 293–323.

1981–1984: MAJOR REFORMS

During the 1981–1984 period, a series of enormously important reforms in Medicare and Medicaid were enacted. While the large federal budget deficits that began in fiscal year 1982 were the primary motivation, the policies share a consistency of theme. The debate between program-specific reform versus health system reform was resolved decisively in favor of the former. The federal government, although now clearly in favor of a more market-oriented health system, would promote the necessary reforms only through revision to Medicare and Medicaid policies; private purchasers would have to take their own steps to contain costs, with minimal interference from the federal government.

Four major pieces of legislation affecting Medicare and Medicaid were enacted during this period: (1) the Omnibus Budget Reconciliation Act of 1981 (OBRA), (2) the Tax Equity and Fiscal Responsibility Act of 1982 (TEFRA), (3) the Social Security Amendments of 1983, and (4) the Deficit Reduction Act of 1984 (DEFRA).

The provisions affecting Medicare and Medicaid are so numerous that space precludes even a brief mention of many. Instead of breadth, this paper will aim for depth, and will limit discussion to the following four areas of reform, which are likely to have the greatest importance over the long term:

1. Medicare prospective payment of hospitals,
2. Increased state discretion in Medicaid, especially regarding recipients' freedom of choice of provider,
3. Medicare payment of HMOs and other alternative delivery systems on a capitation basis,
4. Medicare participating physicians.

Medicare Prospective Payment of Hospitals

Medicare prospective payment was enacted in two stages. The first stage was the addition of a series of reimbursement limits to the cost-based system that was a part of TEFRA.

TEFRA Limits.   One of the reimbursement limits was an extension of the Section 223 limits described above. The TEFRA limits applied to both routine and ancillary (e.g., lab tests, X-rays, operating room) costs, and were on a per discharge rather than a per diem basis. Each hospital's costs per discharge were adjusted for case mix and compared to adjusted costs in peer hospitals to establish a limit.[25]

The second reimbursement limit applied to rates of increase in costs per admission. Increases from each hospital's 1982 levels that exceeded specified percentages would not be recognized for reimbursement. Hospitals with cost increases below these limits would be eligible for bonuses equal to a portion of the difference.

The TEFRA limits had elements of the two possible approaches to prospective payment. The first group of limits set payment rates (or, in this case, limits on cost reimbursements) by making comparisons across hospitals. The second group of limits was based on increases from each hospital's actual costs during a base period. Each approach has its strong and weak points, and there is a great deal of wisdom in combining them.

The TEFRA provisions were motivated not by the notion of giving hospitals incentives to slow cost increases, but rather by the need to reduce outlays drastically. Spurred by the requirements of the budget process, TEFRA reduced hospital payments by an unprecedented degree from what they would otherwise have been. According to calculations by the Congressional Budget Office, by fiscal year 1985 TEFRA reimbursement limits would reduce Medicare payments to hospitals by 9 percent.

Despite the origins of these provisions in the budget process, the notion of incentives was brought into Medicare reimbursement policy for the first time. The bonuses for low rates of increase in costs per admission were projected to increase outlays, since the cost of bonuses for low rates of increase that would have occurred anyway would probably have exceeded the savings to the program from the portion of induced cost reductions not paid as bonuses. To many the notion of Medicare paying a hospital more than its costs was quite radical.

Prospective Payment System (PPS).   TEFRA had a three-year sunset provision applying to the reimbursement limits on rates of increase in costs per admission, and a requirement that the Secretary of Health and Human Services report to Congress with a proposal for a per-

25. During a phase-in period, one-quarter of costs in excess of this limit were reimbursed.

manent Medicare PPS. Political historians are likely to write extensively about the speed with which implementation of the system was begun: Within five months of the passage of TEFRA, the Secretary placed before Congress a comprehensive proposal for prospective payment; less than four months afterward, the President signed legislation for a system along the lines of what had been proposed; and six months later, a phased implementation of the system began.

After a three-year transitional period, PPS uses a pure peer-comparison approach. A hospital's actual costs during a base period do not enter into the formula for its payment rate. Under PPS, patients are classified into one of 468 diagnosis related groups (DRGs). Each DRG is given a relative payment rate (called a weight) based on its cost relative to the other DRGs. Hospital payment rates for each DRG are modified according to local wage rates, whether the hospital is in an urban or rural area, and the number of interns and residents per bed.

While each hospital's actual 1982 costs affect its payment rate during the transition, even then hospitals are at complete risk for their costs. Except for certain distinct categories of costs not yet included in the system, such as capital costs and direct costs for graduate medical education, a hospital's current costs do not enter into the payment formula.[26] Thus, incentives to reduce costs are quite strong.

State Discretion in Medicaid

In 1981, the Reagan administration sought to cap federal grants to states for Medicaid and to give them more discretion with regard to decisions on eligibility, benefits, and reimbursement of providers. While Congress did not go along with capping grants—choosing other means to reduce grants to the states—it did endorse granting them additional flexibility in a number of areas.

One area of flexibility concerned hospital reimbursement. Prior to the passage of OBRA, Medicaid programs had to use Medicare reimbursement principles unless they applied for a special waiver. OBRA permitted states to use any reimbursement technique as long as payments to hospitals were "reasonable and adequate." To date, this au-

26. The legislation called for a proposal by the Secretary of Health and Human Services to incorporate reimbursement of capital costs into the PPS. While the legislation did not mention eventual inclusion of direct medical education, numerous legislative proposals have recently been introduced to put these reimbursements on a prospective basis.

thority has been used extensively. While some states have followed the lead of Medicare in paying on the basis of DRGs, others have implemented different types of prospective payment systems.

One aspect of the flexibility provisions that may have more long-run importance is the ability of states to seek waivers from requirements to allow beneficiaries to choose their providers. This provision permits Medicaid programs to pursue a number of interesting approaches to cost containment. It has been used in California to purchase hospital care on the basis of competitive bidding. Such bidding could not have been conducted if the program had not been able to prevent recipients from using hospitals that were not successful bidders.

The provisions allowing waiver of freedom of choice may also be important in allowing Medicaid programs greater use of alternative delivery systems. Under waiver, states have developed case management arrangements: Recipients in an area must choose from among a panel of primary care physicians participating in the program and obtain all nonemergency services from that physician, or upon referral from that physician.

Medicare Payment of HMOs and Competitive Medical Plans (CMPs)

Until recently, most Medicare reimbursement of HMOs was on a fee-for-service basis. HMOs using their own hospitals filed Medicare cost reports, and all of them billed the program for physician services. While the 1972 amendments had established a procedure for Medicare to pay HMOs on a capitation basis, virtually all HMOs considered the procedure so unattractive that they preferred to do the extra paperwork involved in fee-for-service reimbursement.

With HMOs being reimbursed on a fee-for-service basis, they were unable to offer Medicare beneficiaries an incentive to join. Savings from lower rates of hospital use went directly to Medicare, as fewer claims were made for hospital stays. Thus a much smaller share of the Medicare population than the general population was enrolled in HMOs. Most of the Medicare beneficiaries enrolled had "aged in," that is, had been enrolled through an employment-based health plan before reaching age 65 and then continued in the HMO as a Medicare beneficiary.

TEFRA set up a procedure for paying HMOs on a capitation basis that was more attractive to the HMOs. Briefly, under this plan Medicare pays the HMO a monthly amount that reflects what it reimburses fee-for-service providers for comparable beneficiaries—those of the same age and sex and in the same county of residence. Medicare pays 95 percent of the average adjusted per capita cost (AAPCC) to the HMO, which in turn must provide benefits at least as generous as those of the standard Medicare benefits package. HMOs are not permitted to earn a higher rate of profit on their Medicare capitation business than they do on their non-Medicare business. If costs plus normal profit are less than the Medicare payment, the difference must go to either increased benefits or reduced premiums.

While these provisions have just begun to be implemented, early indications are that a substantial number of Medicare beneficiaries will enroll. Many HMOs have sought to qualify for this type of reimbursement, and earlier demonstrations indicated significant popularity among the elderly.

An important aspect of the legislative provision is the broad definition of eligible organizations. In addition to HMOs (defined under Section 1301 of the Public Health Service Act), the law and regulations define a competitive medical plan (CMP) as one that provides medical services on a prepaid capitation basis. Physician services must be provided primarily through physicians who are either employees or partners of the organization or who have a contract with it. Encompassed in this definition are not only HMOs that are not federally qualified, but also a wide variety of other organizations, such as preferred provider organizations (PPOs), to the extent that they are at risk for medical care expenditures. A traditional insurance plan might qualify if it had a contractual relationship with a group of physicians. Thus, the broad definition of a CMP could make available to the Medicare population an important part of the range of private plans that are being experimented with today.

Medicare Participating Physicians

The Deficit Reduction Act of 1984 made an important change in the way Medicare reimburses physicians. It defined a participating physician as one who agrees in advance to accept assignment on all Medicare claims. Medicare publicizes which physicians have made this agreement so that beneficiaries seeking to reduce their out-of-pocket costs have a low-cost way of shopping for physicians.

In addition to the benefits of publicity, it is clear that Medicare will eventually reimburse participating physicians at a higher rate than they do the others. DEFRA permits only participating physicians to raise their charges during the period in which the fifteen-month freeze is in effect. While raising charges will not increase payments during the period of the freeze, it will permit a higher customary charge screen after the freeze is discontinued.

The "participating physician" concept is Medicare's first step toward using its market power to buy physician services for less. For hospital services, where providers have been unable to charge beneficiaries anything beyond the required deductible and copayment, Medicare has successfully paid less than have private insurers. But for physician services, where physicians have decided on a claim-by-claim basis whether to accept assignment and thus not charge beneficiaries more than the required deductible and coinsurance, Medicare has exercised little of its market power. By providing information to beneficiaries on physicians who will accept assignment, and establishing a payment differential between assigned and unassigned services, Medicare will be functioning more like a PPO. As long as beneficiaries make use of this information and increase the fraction of services that they obtain from participating physicians, Medicare is likely to be able to purchase physician services for less.

OUTLOOK UNDER CURRENT POLICIES

As a result of the reforms enacted during the 1981–1984 period, the costs of the Medicare and Medicaid programs will be substantially lower than they would otherwise have been. Nevertheless, federal and state outlays may increase at a more rapid rate than budgets permit. In addition, the unevenness of the incentives recently put in place could cause some undesirable distortions. This section discusses the basic forces behind the rising costs of these two programs, and how the recent reforms described above are likely to affect them.

Enrollment, service use, and real prices paid to providers are the basic forces that determine outlays in Medicare and Medicaid.[27] They are discussed, respectively, below.[27]

---

27. The analysis abstracts from general inflation since inflation also has a corresponding effect on the revenues to pay for these programs.

Enrollment

Enrollment has been, and is likely to continue to be, an important factor in cost increases in Medicare and Medicaid. In Medicare, enrollment is expected to increase by 1.9 percent per year through 1995.[28] While this is more rapid than the projected growth in the general population—0.8 percent per year—it is small compared to the expected effects of the baby boom generation's reaching the age of 65 beginning in 2010. But that is an issue beyond the scope of this paper.

The aging of the enrolled population, while also a factor, is of much less importance than the number of enrollees. Using age-specific rates of Medicare reimbursement, I have calculated that aging of the Medicare population will increase outlays by 0.2 percent per year. As Victor Fuchs has pointed out, such calculations probably overstate the role of aging, as they are heavily influenced by spending in the last year of life.[29]

Enrollment (or, more precisely, eligibility) is likely to increase Medicaid outlays but is more difficult to project. The size of the AFDC population will depend on state-level welfare policies, such as the level of the need standard; on demographic trends, such as the proportion of female-headed households; and on the economy. But 45 percent of Medicaid outlays in 1983 were for long-term care, so the rate of growth of the population aged 75 and over—the prime users of long-term care—will be an important determinant of the growth in outlays. This population is expected to increase at an average annual rate of 2.9 percent through 1995.

Reforms put in place during the 1980s will have only small effects on enrollment. Legislation made Medicare the secondary payer for those who are 65–69 and still employed, but this group is a very small minority of the Medicare population. The additional discretion given the states by OBRA may have encouraged some reductions in eligibility during the last recession, but states have been restoring them. Indeed, as the health care system becomes more competitive and institutions are less able to serve the uninsured poor through cross-subsidization, expanding coverage for the poor has taken on a higher

28. Office of the Actuary, Social Security Administration.
29. Victor R. Fuchs, " 'Though Much Is Taken': Reflections on Aging, Health, and Medical Care," *Milbank Memorial Fund Quarterly: Health and Society* 62 (Spring 1984):143–66.

priority. In 1984, DEFRA expanded Medicaid eligibility for children and pregnant women. Policy changes over the next few years are likely to extend eligibility for Medicaid even further.

Service Use

Rising rates of use of health services have been an important factor behind the growth in Medicare and Medicaid outlays. As discussed in the previous section, real hospital resources per Medicare enrollee increased at an average annual rate of 4.7 percent during the 1970–1981 period. Real increases in physicians' services have been more rapid—at least in Medicare. While visits per capita have been roughly constant over time, real spending per Medicare enrollee increased by 6.1 percent per year.[30] In Medicaid, by contrast, real spending per recipient did not increase. Medicaid's greater tightening of reimbursement limits probably contributed, but more opportunities to apply new technology to an elderly population may also have been a factor.[31]

Real increases in reimbursements for nursing home services in the Medicaid program were somewhat smaller. Reimbursements per patient day in skilled nursing facilities increased by 10.3 percent per year, only slightly higher than the 9.2 percent annual increase in the CPI over the period 1973–1980. For intermediate care facilities, however, reimbursements per patient day for 1975–1980 increased 12.9 percent per year, while the CPI for that period increased at an annual rate of 8.9 percent.

The legislation of the 1980s is likely to have a substantial impact on service use, but in an unbalanced way. Medicare's PPS is likely to slow substantially the rate of increase in services per admission. Budget analysts have been assuming that payment rates per admission will increase at only one percentage point more than the rate of general inflation each year—in contrast to the cost increases of 3 to 4 percentage points more than the rate of inflation experience during the 1970s. But the early data on cost trends since PPS was instituted have been so encouraging that the administration and both congres-

---

30. Reimbursements per SMI enrollee were deflated by the physician fee component of the CPI.

31. Most Medicaid physician payments are for young women and children. While many of the elderly are also eligible for Medicaid, the program is a secondary payer to Medicare—that is, it only pays for amounts not covered by Medicare.

sional budget committees have proposed a freeze in payment rates for fiscal year 1986.

While a slowdown in the rate of increase of resources per admission will be a step in the right direction, PPS does not include incentives to reduce the number of admissions per enrolled person. Indeed, with a fixed payment per admission, many had feared that PPS would induce an increased rate of admissions, since the payments would exceed hospitals' marginal costs of an additional admission.

To date, these fears have not been borne out, and indeed Medicare admissions have dropped dramatically. Over the two-year period from the first quarter of 1983 to the first quarter of 1985, admissions for persons aged 65 and over declined by about 6 percent. The long-term trend in admissions for this age group had been increases of 3 percent per year. Thus, admissions in the first quarter of 1985 were about 12 percent lower than they would have been if the long-term trend had continued.

Analysts do not yet understand the basis for this dramatic decline in admissions. One likely factor is the changes in employment-based health plans over the past few years. These plans have sharply increased the use of deductibles and coinsurance for hospital services and have instituted effective preadmission certification programs. Some allege that changes in physicians' practice patterns for persons with employment-based health plans have carried over to treatment of the Medicare population.

In addition, utilization review by the Medicare program may have become more effective with the advent of PPS, since resources spent monitoring length of stay can now be focused on the admission decision. Also, the peer review organizations (PROs) have been using a promising tool of preadmission certification for elective admissions. Indeed, coincident with the July 1, 1984, start date of many of the PROs, the decline in Medicare admissions (from the corresponding month of the previous year) appears to have accelerated.

A third possible explanation is that, for some surgical procedures, hospitals have an incentive to favor their outpatient departments over inpatient care. In contrast to inpatient reimbursements, which have been tightened substantially over the past few years, outpatient services are still reimbursed on the basis of costs. Thus, a hospital often is paid more for the ancillary services involved in a surgical procedure when it is performed in the outpatient department.

The problems with decreasing physician costs are somewhat more difficult. While Medicare and Medicaid have tightened reimbursement rates for physician services, broadening the payment unit has not been attempted.[32] The major reform in physician payment—participating Medicare physicians—is aimed at constraining prices without shifting as much of the burden to beneficiaries, but not at reducing service use. Thus, a continuation of increases in services per enrollee is expected.

In fact, however, the use of physicians' services, will most likely be reduced as a result of responses to the payment incentives that the PPS offers hospitals. For example, as length of stay declines, fewer hospital visits are made. In addition, more judicious use of x-rays and laboratory tests means a reduction in the need for the services of radiologists and pathologists. While data from SMI are not as current as those from HI, there are indications of a slowdown in the growth of physicians' services per enrollee.

In contrast to the hospital and physician payment policies discussed above, provisions permitting payment of HMOs and CMPs on a capitation basis have a better chance of controlling the rate of hospital admissions and the volume of physician services. The literature on HMOs suggests that such plans have been very successful at reducing the rate of hospital admissions.[33] HMOs might also be more successful than Medicare in slowing the growth in the volume of physician services through the use of incentives.

While difficult to project, Medicare beneficiaries' enrollment in HMOs is likely to increase substantially. Many HMOs and CMPs have already applied to Medicare to be paid on a capitation basis, and those gaining approval have been marketing to the Medicare population. The terms offered to beneficiaries are often attractive, with a substantial increase in the benefits commonly offered without the payment of additional premiums.

Nevertheless, substantial increases in HMO and CMP enrollment

32. The proposal to pay for inpatient physicians' services on a per case basis is discussed in the following section on policy options.

33. For a review of the literature, see Harold Luft, *Health Maintenance Organizations* (New York: Wiley, 1981). In addition, the reader should read the report on a randomized trial of HMO enrollment: W. G. Manning et al., "A Controlled Trial of the Effect of Prepaid Group Practice on Use of Services," *New England Journal of Medicine* 310 (June 7, 1984): 1505–10.

are unlikely to reduce Medicare outlays significantly. First, while the enrollment projections predict a substantial increase from current levels, the proportion of Medicare beneficiaries enrolled in 1990 will still be small. Second, and probably more important, most of the resource savings accomplished by the HMOs will go to the beneficiaries—not the program.

In order to provide incentives for health plans to participate and for beneficiaries to enroll in the plans, Medicare capitation payments are quite generous. Medicare pays 95 percent of what it estimates it would have paid in the fee-for-service sector. If a plan's costs are 80 percent of those in the fee-for-service sector, then Medicare gets only one-quarter of the savings. The possibility of biased selection further reduces the prospects for program savings. A study of some of the early demonstrations of this policy indicate that those who enrolled had lower rates of claims in prior years than did persons of the same age, sex, and location who did not enroll.[34]

The outlook for HMOs and CMPs reducing Medicaid outlays is somewhat more optimistic. First, Medicaid programs are in a position to capture a much larger share of the resource use reductions expected from capitated plans. These plans are attractive to many recipients because of the improved access to services offered. Second, Medicaid programs exercise a great deal more control over the enrollment process, so they are in a better position to avoid biased selection. Indeed, Medicaid programs often conduct the enrollment directly, and can take steps to protect against preferred risk selection by the HMOs.

FUTURE POLICY OPTIONS

A discussion of future policy options in Medicare and Medicaid will differ significantly at this time from typical discussions of policy options. The distinction stems from the great uncertainty over the outlook under current policies. A phenomenally important set of reforms has recently been put in place for these two programs and, while there are reasoned predictions concerning the general direction of the effects, there remains a great deal of uncertainty over how much these

34. Paul Eggers and Ronald Prihoda, "Pre-enrollment Reimbursement Patterns of Medicare Beneficiaries Enrolled in 'At-Risk' HMOs," *Health Care Financing Review* 4 (September 1982):55–74.

policy changes will accomplish. It is possible that refinements of recent policy changes will be all that is needed, but judgment must await a number of years of additional experience and some careful research.

During the interim, however, it is useful to review alternative policy reforms. A judgment as to whether there are attractive alternatives "on the shelf" will be important in focusing research and development efforts and in deciding the degree of effort that should go into refining existing policies.

As background to this discussion, it is useful to keep in mind that, with Medicare and Medicaid, the United States has come to grips with the issue of the proportion of resources that should go toward medical care. After fifteen years of rapid growth in outlays, major reforms have been enacted and are now in place.

Two important questions have not yet been faced, however. First, since we have taken a somewhat market-oriented approach to reform, the reality of our two-tiered system of medical care may become more visible. If Medicare and Medicaid eligibles concentrate their use of services in a subset of providers in response to incentives, will that be acceptable to society? Second, as we pursue cost containment, most assume that resources can be saved by eliminating services that make no contribution to health at the margin—"unnecessary" care. It is not clear how far we can cut back on services before resource savings require true trade-offs between health and other consumption. If and when we arrive at that point—assuming it is recognized—will we stop trying to economize? And if we continue, will we let the serious rationing be done by the marketplace, or through the political process?

This section will discuss the following broad policy options: (1) expansion of prospective payment, (2) increased cost-sharing and beneficiary premiums, (3) expansion of capitation, and (4) use of PPOs.

Expansion of Prospective Payment

Hospital prospective payment can be expanded in at least three different directions. First, the range of services included in the case payment can be increased to include inpatient physicians' services and/ or posthospitalization services such as care in skilled nursing facilities and home health services. Second, prospective payment could be expanded from a Medicare (and sometimes Medicaid) system to an all-payer system. Third, the use of competitive bids could be explored to replace the administered prices of the current system.

Range of Services. In the Social Security Amendments of 1983, Congress requested a report from the administration on the feasibility and desirability of including inpatient physicians' services in the PPS. The request stimulated a great deal of discussion. The attractiveness of the option is that it appears to be the only tool appropriate to non-capitated settings that gives physicians incentives to reduce the volume of services that they provide. But the option has a number of drawbacks.

First, some believe that the addition of direct physicians incentives to reduce services per case to the existing hospital incentives would be too much. They feel that threats to the quality of care would become too large, as would the degree of "gaming" activities such as coding patients into higher-paying DRGs. I doubt that these problems would be that serious, but the risks (and other uncertainties discussed below) lead one to prefer not to proceed with such a policy before conducting a demonstration of the concept.[35]

Second, DRGs may not be sufficiently homogeneous to make prospective payment to physicians feasible. The coefficient of variation of reasonable charges is very high in some DRGs (exceeding 1.0), and individual physicians may find the risks associated with this heterogeneity to be unacceptable. This problem could probably be resolved through a blend of fee-for-service payments in DRGs with high coefficients of variation.

Third, per case reimbursement of physicians would require a change in assignment policy. Under current policies, physicians have the choice of (1) accepting assignment on cases where the DRG payment exceeds the fee-for-service payment and (2) not accepting assignment but billing the patient on a fee-for-service basis. At minimum, physicians would have to be required to make an all-or-nothing assignment decision for all of their inpatient services, and physicians other than the attending would have to agree to bill only the attending phy-

---

35. The merits of this option and the design of a possible demonstration project are discussed in Paul B. Ginsburg et al., *Planning a Demonstration of Per-Case Reimbursement of Inpatient Physician Services under Medicare*, Report R–3378–HCFA (Santa Monica, Calif.: Rand Corporation, April 1986).

sician and not the patient for their services. Some contend that per case payment would work only under mandatory assignment. The changes in assignment policy required to make per case reimbursement a feasible option might have greater ramifactions than per case reimbursement itself, making this an example of "the tail wagging the dog."

Extending PPS to posthospital care is somewhat more compelling and subject to fewer problems. PPS, as it stands, distorts hospital decisions concerning the timing of discharge. Since skilled nursing facilities and home health services are still reimbursed on a fee-for-service basis while hospital care is reimbursed on a per case basis, hospitals can increase their net revenues through earlier discharge, whether it reduces overall costs or not.

The DRG payments that are made to hospitals could be increased to reflect the posthospital cost experience of patients in each DRG, and the hospital could be made financially responsible for patients' posthospital costs. That would remove the distortion in incentives. In addition, Medicare would benefit from hospitals' expertise as purchasers. It is likely that hospitals would develop better ways to purchase posthospital services (or provide them directly) than could Medicare. While it is likely that current amounts of posthospital services used per patient have a large coefficient of variation, the additional financial risk to hospitals would probably be small. The serious assignment problem encountered in per case payment of physicians does not arise here, as mandatory assignment has long applied to all of the services involved.

All-Payer Prospective Payment.   The debate over all-payer systems has changed radically of late. Proponents once argued that only all-payer systems would induce a hospital to contain costs, while opponents pointed out the difficulties inherent in regulating such a complex enterprise. The experience of PPS to date appears to indicate that Medicare prospective payment alone is sufficient to induce substantial cost containment. The widely feared cost-shifting has not taken place; indeed, the Medicare discount from billed charges has actually declined.

Ironically, while PPS applies only to one payer, it nevertheless faces many problems associated with regulation. Since it is an administered price system, it faces the problem of errors in relative prices.

These could make certain types of patients unattractive to hospitals and pose risks to independent hospitals with the "wrong" specialization. With its influence so pervasive, Medicare administrators are lobbied by those with an interest in a particular DRG; they are also beset by an important debate concerning national versus regional versus hospital-specific rates. PPS still has not accepted responsibility for its rates being "adequate," but such demands may come before the transition is complete.

Today the driving issue behind all-payer systems is not cost containment, but rather "equity" among payers and the financing of care to the uninsured indigent. Commercial insurers see themselves paying more than do Blue Cross plans, HMOs, and PPOs, which are receiving discounts from charges, and they are asking states to regulate payment differentials. Hospitals point out that they can no longer cross-subsidize care to the indigent and other services in the new competitive environment. All-payer systems can either reduce the degree of competition among hospitals by prohibiting most discounts, or place a surcharge on insurance premiums or hospital revenues to raise funds for grants to hospitals with a large burden of uncompensated care. The surcharge can be pursued without rate-setting, however.

With the success of PPS in containing costs, all-payer systems have lost a great deal of their attractiveness. They appear to have the potential to pose significant barriers to competition and do not offer clear benefits to make the risk worth taking.

Bidding.   While PPS has been successful to date, the fact that it is an administered price system poses a number of problems for the future. Mentioned above was the problem of errors in relative prices, for which there is no automatic corrective mechanism. In addition, hospitals cannot compete for Medicare patients on the basis of price. Under PPS, low-cost hospitals will be rewarded by a payment that exceeds their costs, but they will not be able to attract additional patients other than through actions—such as increasing amenity levels—that increase costs. With Medicare ultimately basing its payment rates on average costs, the inability of low-cost hospitals to attract more Medicare patients through the price mechanism will reduce some of the long-run potential of PPS to reduce costs.

Bidding has the potential to concentrate Medicare patients in the lower-cost hospitals, which is likely to save resources both directly and indirectly through stronger competitive pressures on hospitals to reduce their costs. Bidding has been used by California's Medicaid program, but I have not seen an evaluation of the results using sophisticated techniques.

The bidding option requires a great deal of development before it can be fully considered or even demonstrated. The use of bidding to purchase hospital care for patients with a wide variety of medical conditions raises several problems. Difficult issues must be resolved, such as whether patients would be allowed to pay more to use hospitals whose bid was too high. The issue of two-tiered medical care would have to be dealt with; for example, would only low-quality hospitals be available to Medicare enrollees? Nevertheless, development work on bidding mechanisms seems worthwhile.

Cost-Sharing and Premiums

The Medicare benefit structure has often been criticized as providing too much first-dollar coverage and too little catastrophic coverage. While the latter is certainly true, the former may not be—the $400 hospital deductible per spell of illness is substantial. But with a very high proportion of Medicare beneficiaries using either private supplemental coverage or Medicaid, the effective degree of cost-sharing is in fact very small.[36]

Many attempts to reform the Medicare benefit structure by increasing deductibles and coinsurance while improving catastrophic protection have failed. While economists think of cost-sharing as a device partially to offset the moral hazard problem in health insurance, many politicians see it as burdening those unfortunate enough to be ill. Indeed, the incentive effects of cost-sharing are feared rather than welcomed, the concern being that low-income persons served by Medicare and/or Medicaid will be forced to forgo needed care.

While increased cost-sharing is unlikely, asking the elderly to shoulder more of the burden of Medicare through additional premiums is a strong possibility. Already, TEFRA and subsequent legislation have halted the drift toward covering a smaller share of SMI

36. The most significant cost-sharing may be the amounts by which physicians' charges exceed Medicare's "reasonable" screens. Private supplemental policies tend not to cover such amounts. All claims for services covered under Medicaid must be assigned, even for those persons eligible for both Medicare and Medicaid, so there is no cost-sharing in those cases.

costs with premiums that began with the 1972 amendments. Many proposals in Congress call for having higher-income Medicare beneficiaries pay a much higher proportion of the costs of their SMI coverage.[37]

Indeed, greater cost-sharing for higher-income beneficiaries is a possibility, as long as a method could be found to limit the administrative burden. A premium rebate scheme like the one described by Zweifel in chapter 9 might accomplish this. While the maximum rebate would be uniform, premiums might vary by income.

An option that I have proposed would place a tax on premiums paid for private supplemental insurance ("Medigap").[38] Medigap insurance is implicitly subsidized by Medicare through the former's impact on use of services. If having supplemental coverage induces an additional hospitalization, Medicare will bear all but $400 of the cost. Since the costs that Medicare pays will not be reflected in the premium for the supplemental plan, the latter will be underpriced and too many people will purchase it. Since beneficiaries whose incomes are higher are more likely to purchase such supplemental coverage (see chapter 4), the distributional effects of this implicit subsidy should be a concern to many. An excise tax of approximately 35 percent on Medigap premiums would eliminate this distortion in incentives and increase Medicare trust fund balances through a combination of reduced outlays (from those no longer purchasing supplemental policies) and excise tax revenues.

Capitation Options

TEFRA's provision allowing Medicare to pay HMOs and CMPs on a capitation basis marked the first step in the direction of decentralizing cost-containment efforts. For those enrolling in such plans, efforts to control health care costs will be made by the HMO or CMP instead of directly by Medicare.

HMOs and CMPs have greater potential than does Medicare, along a number of dimensions, to contain costs without reducing access to

37. In July 1985, the House Ways and Means Subcommittee on Health recommended to the full Committee on Ways and Means a tax to finance SMI applicable to all part B enrollees with adjusted gross income in excess of $20,000 for individuals or $40,000 for couples. The subcommittee envisioned financing 25 percent of SMI outlays through the tax.

38. See Congressional Budget Office, *Containing Medical Care Costs through Market Forces* (Washington, D.C.: Government Printing Office, May 1982), pp. 54–55.

care. Control of the volume of hospital admissions is the most obvious and possibly the most important example. With PPS focusing on costs per admission, the only tool currently available to Medicare is utilization review by the PROs. On the other hand, HMOs and CMPs can (1) use informal incentives to physicians, (2) select physicians with conservative practice styles, and (3) engage in various utilization review activities. As indicated above, the research literature indicates impressive accomplishments in these areas. Control of the volume of physician services is another area where HMOs and CMPs might do better than Medicare.[39]

While Medicare vouchers have been debated frequently ever since they were proposed by Rep. Richard Gephardt and then-Rep. David Stockman, refinements to these TEFRA provisions may be the most fruitful road to greater use of cost-effective private health plans in Medicare. In many ways, the TEFRA arrangement achieves what vouchers are purported to do, but with easier administration. The major goal of a voucher is to allow those benefiting from a public subsidy to use the subsidy for services provided privately. This is accomplished by TEFRA, which allows beneficiaries to enroll in a qualifying HMO or CMP and benefit from all but 5 percentage points of any cost advantages the plan has over Medicare. Some people (though not I) would prefer a broader choice of qualifying plans, but that issue is different from the one involving a choice between the TEFRA approach and a voucher. The TEFRA definition could be broadened, and in any case vouchers must define what a qualifying plan is. TEFRA avoids the administrative problems involved in giving millions of beneficiaries pieces of paper to forward to qualifying health plans.

TEFRA could be improved in a number of areas, however. First, the restriction preventing health plans from earning a rate of profit in excess of the rate in their private business should be dropped. The experience to date seems to indicate substantial competition among plans, in which case the market can ensure that beneficiaries get the benefits of cost savings.

Second, the process of varying capitation payments according to the expected costliness of each beneficiary needs improvement. Within the Medicare population, age and sex explain very little of the vari-

39. For a more detailed discussion of this issue, see Paul B. Ginsburg and Glenn Hackbarth, "Alternative Delivery Systems and Medicare," *Health Affairs* 5 (Spring 1986):6–22.

ation in medical care costs. Information on prior use of services should be employed to reduce the risks of biased selection. That should give protection to individual plans as well as to the U.S. Treasury.

Third, at some time in the future, the level of Medicare payments should be revised so that the savings from HMOs and CMPs are translated into reduced outlays. This does not mean reducing the percentage of fee-for-service reimbursements from its current 95 percent level, however; that would reduce incentives for beneficiaries to use the most efficient financing arrangement. Instead, the standard Medicare contribution should be based on premiums charged by HMOs and CMPs, and those wishing to remain in the more expensive traditional Medicare should pay the difference. This change should not be made now, however, as it would be viewed as a major reduction in Medicare benefits. Nevertheless, if HMOs and CMPs pass a market test with Medicare beneficiaries and serve a substantial proportion of them in most areas, it would be appropriate to consider their premiums the cost of a standard health care financing package.

Preferred Provider Organizations

PPOs are gaining significant attention in employment-based health plans. The arrangements give policyholders incentives to concentrate their use of services among a select group of providers. The "preferred" providers may be those willing to provide services at a discount, those with lower prices to begin with and/or those believed to practice in a lower-cost style.

PPOs appear to have very limited potential in the Medicare or Medicaid programs. As far as getting lower prices from providers, the government programs already have gone quite far. In terms of hospital care, neither program will pay benefits for care in hospitals that will not accept the program's reimbursements as payment in full. Because the programs have such a large market share, few hospitals have turned down this "take it or leave it" offer.

As concerns physician services, Medicaid is very much like a PPO. Only a minority of physicians are willing to accept the program's reimbursements as payment in full, so Medicaid recipients are restricted to a panel of "preferred" physicians. With its participating physician concept, Medicare too is moving toward a preferred provider arrangement. Medicare's reimbursements are lower than regular charges, and the program guides the beneficiaries toward physicians willing to accept those rates as payment in full.

Selecting physicians on criteria other than low price would probably not be practical in either program. The criteria tend to be subjective, and public officials are not generally allowed such discretion. One can imagine the letters to members of Congress from physicians excluded because their practice styles were deemed moderately extravagent. PROs were set up to discipline providers whose practice styles deviate substantially from norms.

Of course, one could consider having private organizations make these judgments. But in order to maintain competition in that function, Medicare and Medicaid would need a way of monitoring success in cost containment. I doubt that there are practical ways of doing so on an ongoing basis other than through capitation payments—but then we would have a CMP, which is already a part of current policies.

SELECTED BIBLIOGRAPHY

Aiken, L. H., and K. D. Bays. "The Medicare Debate—Round One." *New England Journal of Medicine* 311 (1984):1196–1200.

Congressional Budget Office. *Changing the Structure of Medicare Benefits: Issues and Options*. Washington, D.C.: Government Printing Office, 1983.

———. *Containing Medical Care Costs through Market Forces*. Washington, D.C.: Government Printing Office, 1982.

———. *Medicaid: Choices for 1982 and Beyond*. Washington, D.C.: Government Printing Office, 1981.

Feder, J. M. *Medicare: The Politics of Federal Hospital Insurance*. Lexington, Mass.: Lexington Books, 1977.

"Financing Medicare: Explorations in Controlling Costs and Rising Revenues," Special issue, *Milbrank Memorial Fund Quarterly: Health and Society* 62 (1984): 143–355.

Ginsburg, P. B. and M. J. Curtis. "Prospects for Medicare's Hospital Insurance Trust Fund." *Health Affairs* 2 (1983): 102–12.

Holahan, J. *Financing Health Care to the Poor*. Lexington, Mass.: Lexington Books, 1975.

Lohr, K. N. and M. S. Marquis. *Medicare and Medicaid: Past, Present, and Future*, N–2088–HHS/RC. Santa Monica, Calif.: Rand Corporation, May 1984.

Meyer, J. A., ed. *Market Reforms in Health Care: Current Issues, New Directions, Strategic Decisions*. Washington, D.C.: American Enterprise Institute, 1983.

Office of Technology Assessment. *Diagnosis Related Groups (DRGs) and* the Medicare Program: Inplications for Medical Technology*. Washington, D.C.: Government Printing Office, 1983.

Rogers, D. E.; R. J. Blendon; and T. W. Maloney. "Who Needs Medicaid?" *New England Journal of Medicine* 307 (1982):13–18.

Sawyer, D., M. Ruther, A. Pagan-Berlucchi, and D. N. Muse. *The Medicare and Medicaid Data Book, 1983*. Baltimore, Md.: Health Care Financing Administration, 1983.

Social Security Administration. *Social Security Bulletin, Annual Statistical Supplement*. Washington, D.C.: Government Printing Office, annual.

Stevens, R., and R. Stevens. *Welfare Medicine in America: A Case Study of Medicaid*. New York: Free Press, 1974.

U.S. House of Representatives, Committee on Ways and Means. *Background Material and Data on Programs within the Jurisdiction of the Committee of Ways and Means*, WMCP:99–2. Washington, D.C.: Government Printing Office, 1985.

————. *Proceedings of the Conference on the Future of Medicare*, WMCP: 98–23. Washington, D.C.: Government Printing Office, 1984.

U.S. Senate, Special Committee on Aging. *Medicare and the Health Costs of Older Americans: The Extent and Effects of Cost Sharing*, S. Prt. 98–166. Washington, D.C.: Government Printing Office, 1984.

PART IV

PRIVATE HEALTH INSURANCE

6

THE QUESTIONABLE COST-CONTAINMENT RECORD OF COMMERCIAL HEALTH INSURERS

Clark C. Havighurst

INTRODUCTION: INSURANCE, MORAL HAZARD, AND EFFICIENCY

Repeated declarations that rising expenditures in health care are a serious national problem are not easy to reconcile with the favorable public attitude toward other "growth" industries. One reason for the general lack of enthusiasm over the health care industry's perennially increasing claims on the gross national product is, of course, that much of the burden of constantly rising costs falls on the public sector, playing havoc with government budgets. But the issue of health care costs is usually framed more broadly, to encompass private sector as well as public burdens. Since we normally presume that an industry grows because it is providing what people want, any questions raised concerning the increasing flow of private resources into health care must spring from a lack of confidence in the market mechanism that is at work. Specifically, observers question the market's allocation of resources to health care because they see major defects in private health insurance, the vehicle through which most privately financed health care is paid. The interposition of a third-party payer in transactions between providers and patients is widely said to constitute a market failure justifying concern that increased consumer spending on health care is not truly voluntary and therefore cannot be automatically equated with increased consumer welfare.

Although private health insurance undeniably contributes to increased societal spending on health services, that fact alone does not establish that resources are being seriously misallocated. One reason why people buy insurance is precisely to enable them to purchase services that they might not otherwise be able to afford in the event of a medical catastrophe; similarly, many consumers probably also buy insurance to avoid having to face painful economizing choices in obtaining medical treatment for themselves or a loved one. Health insurance has other, less welcome cost-raising effects, however. These fall under the heading of "moral hazard," the somewhat unfortunate term that economists use to describe the higher costs that result when normal economizing incentives are diluted by the opportunity to risk or spend another's funds. The moral hazard problem is inherent in insurance of all kinds and manifests itself in many ways, including outright fraud (such as arson), reduced precautions by insureds to avert the calamity insured against, wasteful spending on insured repairs, inefficiently high levels of quality or "gold-plating" in repair services, and reduced price-shopping by insureds. But even though moral hazard is an ever-present problem and introduces unwanted distortions in resource allocation, it does not by itself invalidate health insurance as an institution. The financial protection that such insurance provides may more than justify its higher costs.

In judging the health care market, it is important to recognize that there are two objectives at war with each other. Protection of individuals against unpredictable medical costs and efficiency in the allocation of resources to and within the health care sector are both desirable goals. Unfortunately, neither can be obtained without some sacrifice of the other. Because of this trade-off, some inefficiency is an inevitable and therefore tolerable part of the cost of reducing risks. This insight is important in making policy. As economist Paul Joskow has stated in discussing hospital costs, "The presence of moral hazard problems implies an inherent inefficiency in the hospital market. However, the system is inefficient only in relation to an abstract ideal, which is unlikely to be economically achievable. From a useful policy perspective, we can characterize the resulting allocation of resources as being inefficient only if we can identify institutional changes or government interventions that reduce the inefficiencies associated with moral hazard problems *without* incurring additional risk-bearing costs and transactions costs that exceed the implied savings."[1] Private insurance may thus be efficient even if it causes substantial apparent inefficiency in the market for health services.

In accordance with Joskow's observations, a major issue in judging the institution of private health insurance is whether insurers have done all that efficiency requires to counter the adverse effects of moral hazard. In theory, there are many things that insurers could do to ensure that only economically justified services are rendered at the expense of the insurance pool and that the prices paid for those services are competitive. In practice, as Joskow observes, many of the things that might be done may not be worth doing because they cost more than they save, or because they have other unwanted consequences. Nevertheless, the prevalent perception of waste and over-payment in the health care system is based in large part on the perception that insurers have been unduly passive in confronting their cost-containment task. Moreover, proponents of market reforms and increased competition in health care argue that insurers can be encouraged to perform this task more effectively. A leading topic of health policy debate is thus the past and future performance of the health insurance industry.

Structuring the issues in this debate—which is the aim of this chapter—is not an easy undertaking, because our understanding of the health insurance industry and its performance remains primitive. Ultimately, the questions are empirical ones, but many empirical studies to date have lacked a sound theoretical grounding, with the result that their conclusions and policy recommendations remain debatable. It is hoped that a careful exposition of hypotheses that might explain the industry's performance will give others a basis for more insightful empirical analysis.

The discussion presented here proceeds by first describing the apparent shortcomings of industry performance and then suggesting some possible explanations for it. Depending upon the empirical findings, possible conclusions are that (1) the market is doing very well in solving an extraordinarily difficult problem, (2) the market could do a

---

1. Paul Joskow, *Controlling Hospital Costs: The Role of Government Regulation,* MIT Press Series in Health and Public Policy (Cambridge: MIT Press, 1981), p. 22.

substantially better job if policy-makers would act to remove certain impediments to its operation, or (3) the obstacles to acceptable market performance are so great that a nonmarket solution should be tried. The analysis here, though incomplete, tends toward acceptance of, and action based upon, the second of these propositions.

This chapter's primary focus is on commercial health insurers, as distinct from both nonprofit Blue Cross and Blue Shield plans, which provide a roughly equivalent amount of coverage, and such alternative financing mechanisms as health maintenance organizations (HMOs). The reasons for treating the commercial carriers separately will be discussed later. Essentially, the commercial carriers have encountered quite different pressures and circumstances than have the others, in part because of their different historical relationship with health care providers. The issue to be examined is why their greater independence did not translate into more aggressive action to overcome the effects of moral hazard—that is, into effective control of health care costs.

THE PERFORMANCE THAT NEEDS TO BE EXPLAINED

Definitive assessment of the performance of the health insurance industry in controlling health care costs is not only beyond the scope of this chapter but also probably beyond the capacity of even the most skilled analysts. Although it is possible that the perceived shortcomings reflect only the difficulty of the cost-containment task and the unavoidable trade-off between risk-pooling and efficiency, there are some reasons for thinking that more could have been done and that substantial improvements in industry performance are possible if policy-makers attend to correcting incentives, removing legal constraints, and improving competitive conditions. The first section of this chapter suggests that industry performance has fallen short of what was feasible. The next section examines a variety of possible explanations for the suboptimal performance that is detected inconclusively here.

One way to begin an assessment of insurer cost-containment efforts is to compare what one sees in practice with what one speculates might have been done. Recognizing that the feasibility and acceptability of particular measures are hard to judge in the abstract, one may still imagine possible approaches to solving the moral hazard problem and, on the basis of what is conceived to be feasible, judge whether the health insurance industry has passed up promising strategies. Although this approach has obvious pitfalls, the following paragraphs setting forth measures that private insurers might have taken but seem never to have tried (until recently, in some cases) suggest that the innovative spirit has been lacking.

Selective Use of Cost-Sharing.   Cost-sharing has always been the commercial carriers' favorite approach to cost containment, but wherever it has been used it has almost always been imposed across the board and not on a diagnosis- or procedure-specific basis. With the exception of outpatient psychiatric care, which is frequently subject to a 50 percent copayment, specific treatments or procedures have seldom been made subject to cost-sharing that reflects their particular discretionary character or the variability of cost/benefit ratios from case to case. The trade-offs between risk-pooling and efficiency are such that the optimal terms and extent of insurance coverage will vary significantly from one risk to another, yet insurers have shown no awareness of this fact in failing to tailor coverage to fit particular risks.[2]

Benefit Cutoffs.   Insurers have seldom, if ever, placed special limitations on the duration of full coverage of hospitalization for particular diagnoses or procedures. Imposition of copayments for later days of a hospital stay—perhaps subject to exceptions for special circumstances—would give basic protection while also reflecting the rapidly declining marginal benefit of additional care. Great efficiency gains and only a small loss of financial protection would probably flow from shifting to the patient the determination, with professional advice, of whether additional, highly discretionary hospital care would be worth its cost.

Prior Authorization.   Although prior authorization of spending and

---

2. According to Martin Feldstein, "Economic theory suggests that optimal insurance coverage for an individual is a function of four things: the degree of risk, the individual's aversion to risk, the elasticity of demand for the insured services, and the administrative costs of the insurance plan." Martin Feldstein, "The Welfare Loss of Excess Health Insurance," *Journal of Political Economy* 81, no. 2 (1973):251. The new system for classifying services by diagnosis-related groups (DRGs) offers a potentially practical way for insurers to write policies with selective coverage. I am not aware of any private insurer that has used DRGs in specifying coverage, however. This would appear to be an interesting avenue for innovation in benefit design.

predetermination of benefits are finally beginning to be required, these strategies were long neglected. There are reports of significantly reduced utilization following such innovations even when no proposed treatment or hospitalization is turned down. Insurers once again appear to have passed up an opportunity to economize.

Contracting With Providers. Direct negotiation with providers over their prices and their willingness to submit to administrative checks on utilization has only recently been employed by commercial insurers as a cost-containment measure. Again, it is not obvious why what is workable today would not have been workable in the past.

Provider-Specific Coverage. Insurance carriers have recently begun to employ the preferred-provider concept, under which the services of certain providers are covered on a more favorable basis than those of others because they have agreed to accept a certain price or have submitted to administrative controls. This concept does not require provider agreement, however, and might have taken the form of benefit or premium variations based on an insured's prospective choice of a lower-cost hospital or physician group.[3] Such relatively simple innovations were long untried.

Insurer Financing of Out-of-Pocket Payments. Insurers might have paid providers in full and collected from patients any deductibles and copayments that they owed (perhaps through a wage checkoff arranged with the employer). They might also have offered to lend their insureds any funds needed to pay such out-of-pocket costs or to purchase noncovered services. Such practices, in addition to increasing the attractiveness of an insurer's subscribers to providers (perhaps warranting a discount), would have assured patients that credit would be available when it was needed, thus reducing their need for full insurance protection and making high deductibles and exclusions from coverage somewhat easier for them to accept.

The foregoing ideas for discharging insurers' cost-containment responsibilities (and others that could be mentioned[4]) appear to have enough merit to warrant raising questions about their widespread ne-

---

3. This idea was suggested prominently (to deaf ears) some time ago. See Joseph Newhouse and Vincent Taylor, "How Shall We Pay for Hospital Care?" *Public Interest* 23 (Spring 1971):78.

4. See Clark Havighurst and Glenn Hackbarth, "Private Cost Containment," *New England Journal of Medicine* 300, no. 23 (1979):1298; Clark Havighurst, "Health Insurers and Health-Care Costs: Can the Problem Be Part of the Solution?" *Health Communications and Informatics* 5, nos. 5–6 (1979):319; idem, "Professional Restraints on Innovation in Health Care Financing," *Duke Law Journal* (May 1978):303, 319–35.

glect. Some of these questions concern the insurers' ability or willingness to innovate; others deal with the state of competition in the commercial health insurance industry. In general, commercial insurers have remained wedded to the pure indemnity insurance approach, paying any claim that could not be rejected retroactively for some objective reason, and have eschewed shifting risks to insureds or providers as a way of curbing the effects of moral hazard. Although they have faced a difficult challenge requiring creative departures from traditional insurance practices, the commercial carriers individually and collectively have produced a singularly unimpressive list of cost-containment measures. For years the industry could talk—always collectively, it seemed[5]—only about such conventional and essentially marginal strategies as second opinions, $100 deductibles, 20 percent copayments, coordination of benefits, prevention and wellness programs, and broadened coverage of ambulatory surgery and such out-of-hospital services as preadmission testing and home care. An outsider looking for signs of entrepreneurial initiative was bound to be disappointed by the contrast between what seemed possible and what the industry and its individual members were doing or even talking about. Whether the industry's failure to innovate resulted from exogenous factors, from some market failure, from poor management, or from cartel behavior is considered below, but surely some explanation is needed.

Further evidence suggesting poor industry performance can be found in the contrast between insurers' pusillanimous efforts to control medical costs and what many of the same companies were doing to control moral hazard in other lines of insurance. Auto insurers were tough in dealing with body shops,[6] and dental insurers found predetermination of benefits to be effective long before the strategy was tried in financing hospital and medical care.[7] Direct contracting with providers was standard operating procedure in many prepayment plans for dental, pharmacy, optometric, auto repair, burial, and legal services, but was used only by Blue Cross and Blue Shield plans for hospital and

5. See text accompanying notes 40–45.

6. See *Quality Auto Body, Inc. v. Allstate Insurance Co.*, 1981–2 Trade Cases (CCH) ¶64,303 (7th Cir. 1981); *Chick's Auto Body v. State Farm Mutual Auto Insurance Company*, 168 N.J. Super. 68, 401 A.2d 722 (1979), *aff'd per curiam*, 176 N.J. Super. 320, 423 A.2d 311 (1980).

7. See Council on Wage and Price Stability, Executive Office of the President, *The Complex Puzzle of Rising Health Care Costs: Can the Private Sector Fit It Together?* (Washington, D.C.: Government Printing Office, 1977), pp. 115–18

medical insurance. In view of the large stakes, the (until very recently) total neglect of these strategies by commercial health insurers does not seem to be adequately explained simply by the added administrative difficulties of carrying them out in connection with medical services.

That competing insurers could have done more than they did to control health care costs is also suggested by historical evidence. The medical profession openly recognized at an early date the threat that the cost-containment impulses of lay-controlled insurers posed to physician interests, and early insurers bore out the doctors' fears by embarking on aggressive cost-containment programs. Evidence from antitrust cases shows how those early efforts were stifled, suggesting one possible explanation for later insurer passivity.[8] Nevertheless, one can ask whether the commercial carriers did not accept too readily the passive role into which the medical profession attempted to force them. For whatever reason, the insurance industry finally came to embrace the medical profession's view (some insurers stated it as a philosophy) that their job was not to influence medical practice but only to pay claims. The doctors' argument that the patient's "free choice" of physician should not be violated was accepted by insurers even to the extent of not using incentives to steer patients to lower-cost providers. In general, costs were seen as being beyond the insurers' control and as the responsibility of either individual physicians guided by ethical norms or the organized, self-regulating medical profession. Questionable claims were usually referred to professional organizations for "peer review," and insurers were pleased to adopt profession-sponsored fee schedules.[9] More recently the commercial carriers, recognizing that profession-sponsored cost controls were inadequate to silence the public's complaints, have vigorously embraced various proposals for government cost-containment regulation.

Publicly, the position of the commercial health insurance industry has always been that it supports private cost containment in theory and is doing all that is within its power to implement it. Nevertheless, the industry has always seemed to want someone else to do the cost-containment job, as long as the insurers could continue to handle the money. The most cynical interpretation of the industry's record is that

8. See text accompanying notes 45–48.
9. See text accompanying notes 52–55.

insurers have supported professional and government cost-containment measures with the full knowledge that those measures would be less successful at reducing industry revenues than the efforts of individual insurers aggressively competing in cost containment.

EXPLAINING THE INDUSTRY'S RECORD

What may seem to be poor performance by the health insurance industry of its cost-containment responsibilities may not have been the fault of the health insurers at all. Perhaps the problem lay with the industry's obtuse customers, who may have had strong preferences for things other than cost containment. Or it may be that government subsidized perverse behavior, impaired insurers' freedom of action, or fostered conventional ways of thinking about the problem to an extent that made innovation impossible. Perhaps health insurers were constrained by other forces impeding normal competitive behavior. Indeed, it may have been a complex combination of these factors that undermined insurers' ability and willingness to fight the cost battle. The following discussion offers some hypotheses that might explain commercial health insurers' seemingly poor performance as consumer agents in the search for effective cost containment that impairs neither the consumer's essential financial protection nor his or her access to good-quality medical care.[10]

Is Health Care Insurable at All?

One possibility is that insurance is the wrong vehicle for financing medical care. More precisely, it is possible that the moral hazard problem is so great and the tools needed to counter its effects so cumbersome that the insurance model is doomed. If so, what we have seen is simply the increasing manifestation of the obsolescence of the products of an industry that is destined to wither away as more efficient mechanisms, better at integrating the financing and delivery of care, displace it.

In some sense, the obsolescence of the traditional system of insured

---

10. Earlier attempts to explain insurers' failure to do more to control moral hazard include Mark Pauly, *The Role of the Private Sector in National Health Insurance* (Chicago: Health Insurance Association of America, 1979), pp. 30–41; Jon Gabel and Alan Monheit, "Will Competition Plans Change Insurer-Provider Relationships?" *Milbank Memorial Fund Quarterly* 61, no. 4 (1983):614, 623–35.

fee-for-service medicine is an underlying premise of this discussion. Indeed, the precise issue being explored is why traditional insurance mechanisms have not evolved more rapidly into a more suitable form. Some of the most promising techniques for solving the problem of moral hazard involve fundamental departures from the traditional insurance model and the integration of financing and delivery through contracts between payers and providers. Other approaches that are somewhat truer to the insurance model (in focusing on better benefit design and administration of claims) may nevertheless turn out to be much easier to implement if the insurer has explicit arrangements with individual doctors or hospitals. Perhaps the most logical approach for insurers to follow is to combine pure insurance, featuring unlimited choice of provider, with incentives for insureds to patronize a more organized health plan—a so-called preferred-provider organization (PPO)—comprising providers who have contracted with the insurer or otherwise demonstrated that they are trustworthy and efficient. The analysis thus begins by recognizing that pure casualty insurance is an obsolete vehicle,[11] then proceeds to ask why insurers have been so slow either to scrap it or to revamp it to meet the apparent requirements of the modern consumer.

For most of the 1970s, the only recognized alternative to traditional health insurance was the HMO, an integrated health plan offering extensive financial protection while also featuring delivery and provider compensation arrangements that were highly conducive to efficiency. Unfortunately, government intervention in support of HMOs, as well as other factors, including the characterization of HMOs as "alternative delivery systems," perpetuated a belief that the traditional system was itself immutable and could not be reformed from within. As a result, such innovative impulses as existed, including those of a number of leading commercial insurers, were channeled into the difficult and costly task of HMO development. The overemphasis on HMOs left largely unexplored the wide spectrum of possibilities for private reform that lay between HMOs at one extreme and traditional financing and delivery arrangements at the other. It is hard to say whether it was government's role in defining the reform agenda, the

---

11. See Alain Enthoven, *Health Plan: The Only Practical Solution to the Soaring Cost of Medical Care* (Menlo Park, Calif.: Addison-Wesley, 1980), pp. 1-12; Gabel and Monheit, "Insurer-Provider Relationships," pp. 624–25.

perceptions of the insurance industry's customers, insurers' or providers' collective resistance to change, or some other factor that accounted for the force of conventional wisdom and the lack of attention to reforming private health insurance.

Whether private health insurers will survive in a form even remotely resembling the traditional model of the passive reimburser of patients' incurred charges remains an open question. Consumers are beginning to have not only HMOs but a variety of hybrid forms, especially PPOs, as meaningful alternatives to traditional health insurance. Employers and employment groups are beginning to see the benefits of exploring these alternatives. If traditional insurance is indeed unfit for its customary role, the marketplace is gradually developing the capacity to render that verdict.

Is There a Demand for Cost Containment?

Insurers have repeatedly claimed that they have always been ready and willing to assume a larger cost-containment role but that their customers, primarily large employers, did not demand it. The insurers' excuse was that, although employers talked about high costs, they were reluctant to cut back on employee benefits, to limit employee options, or to have the insurer do anything aggressive that might be construed as a denial of an employee's entitlement. A skeptic listening to insurers' excuses throughout the 1970s might have said that they were simply making self-fulfilling prophecies about what employers and employees would stand for instead of pursuing the usual competitive approach of producing innovations and persuading customers of their merits. But while it sometimes looked as though insurers were waiting for their customers to design the industry's products, there is some evidence that until quite recently purchasers of health insurance were unwilling to consider insurance packages that appeared, in theory, to be well designed to meet the consumer's need for basic financial and health protection at a reasonable price.[12] Even today, many employers wring their hands about the cost problem without being willing to embrace any radical change in the insurance they purchase.

---

12. See Harvey Sapolsky et al., "Corporate Attitudes toward Health Care Costs," *Milbank Memorial Fund Quarterly* 59, no. 4 (1981):561.

The Tax Subsidy.   The leading explanation for the apparently weak demand for insurer cost containment lies in the substantial tax subsidy for private health insurance. This subsidy takes the form of an exclusion from employees' taxable income (under federal and state income taxes and the federal Social Security tax) of employer contributions to private health insurance. This subsidy is estimated to exceed $36 billion dollars in 1987 in the form of revenue forgone,[13] and it has the practical effect of giving the average employee a discount of roughly 40 percent—the sum of the average combined marginal federal and state income tax rate and the aggregate FICA tax rate—on any health bill that is paid out of employer-funded insurance rather than out of pocket. The impressive size of this discount means that people have a powerful incentive to pay as much of their health care bill as possible through employer-purchased insurance. As a result, coinsurance and deductibles are unattractive, and employees seek coverage for routine services that could readily be budgeted and paid for out of pocket. Under the prevailing tax system, most health insurance is valued not only as a means of obtaining essential financial protection but also as a way of obtaining government help in paying for care.

In addition to discouraging cost-sharing and encouraging overly comprehensive coverage, the tax subsidy also encourages liberality on the part of insurers in paying claims and discourages dollar limitations on indemnity payments. In general, it reduces interest in all cost-containment efforts by third parties, since the savings from such efforts would be taxable income if passed on in wages; a penny saved through health care cost containment is not a penny earned. Moreover, because employees have not been asked to bear much of the premium cost of insurance out of their after-tax incomes, they have been rendered unconscious of plan costs and lulled into an entitlement mentality that makes cost-saving initiatives that much more difficult to implement.

The health insurance industry has been in the awkward political position of excusing its members' neglect of cost containment on the grounds that their customers are not interested in it while failing to

---

13. See Congressional Budget Office, *Reducing the Deficit: Spending and Revenue Options,* Report to the Senate and House Committees on the Budget (Washington, D.C.: Government Printing Office, 1985):285–87.

identify what is certainly the main reason for this attitude. The industry has aggressively opposed any change in the tax subsidy, and opposition has come from employers and employee groups as well.[14] When forced to defend their political position on policy grounds, these interests usually claim that the nature and extent of insurance coverage would not change even if the tax law did not encourage overinsurance. To show that consumers are wedded to comprehensiveness, they cite the purchasing propensities of federal employees under the Federal Employees Health Benefits Program and of Medicare beneficiaries in buying supplemental "Medigap" coverage. On the basis of this evidence, the industry and other beneficiaries of the tax subsidy argue that eliminating it would not lead to increased cost-containment efforts.

These arguments are unpersuasive. The evidence cited is equivocal because it involves atypical, risk-averse populations that have not been offered a full range of insurance options; nor have they been educated as to where their true interest lies. Because it is impossible to believe that *no* change would occur at the margin if the tax subsidy were capped, the only issue is one of magnitude. Even assuming that consumers would cling to inefficient forms of coverage, it is not clear why these middle- and high-income persons should have their peculiar preferences subsidized (more heavily for higher-bracket taxpayers) by a federal government badly in need of revenues to reduce a worrisome budgetary deficit.

The only possible policy justification for a subsidy of this kind is that it encourages people to do something that is in the larger public interest. Although some analysts have turned the issue around and asked whether limiting the subsidy can be proved to have beneficial effects,[15] the burden of proof should be on the defenders of an unlimited subsidy to show that it is affirmatively beneficial; it is insufficient to argue, as they do, that the distortions caused by the unlimited subsidy are small because consumers would buy the same insurance even in its absence. Viewed in this light, there is no reason

14. See Julie Kosterlitz, "Broad Coalition Prepares to Do Battle on Taxing Employee Fringe Benefits," *National Journal* 17, no. 18 (1985):956.

15. See Health Insurance Association of America, *The Case against the Taxation of Employee Health Benefits* (Chicago: HIAA, 1985), pp. 12–14; Gabel and Monheit, "Insurer-Provider Relationships."

why the nation should grant regressive tax subsidies for overinsurance that contributes more than anything else to wasting societal resources on unjustified and inefficiently produced health care. Of all the sources of new tax revenue currently available to government, this one alone promises to have incentive effects that would improve efficiency and increase aggregate national wealth. Thus, as a policy matter, there would seem to be no argument whatsoever against capping or altering the tax subsidy for private health insurance in a way that would discourage both underinsurance and overinsurance.[16] The politics of the question are, of course, something else again.[17]

Employer and Employee Attitudes. It is far from clear that the tax subsidy accounts entirely for the insurance industry's poor performance of its cost-containment responsibilities. Although the tax subsidy substantially shifts the margin at which cost containment becomes desirable, one may still doubt whether insurers have undertaken as much cost control as subsidized consumers would find optimal. Conditions on the demand side of the market suggest some other reasons for suspecting inadequate cost containment. These additional problems lie in the complex politics of employee health benefits within a given firm.

Group health insurance has customarily been designed to meet the expectations of the majority of workers in the group. In circumstances where no choice is offered,[18] even a sizable minority willing to give up some protection for more take-home pay is likely to have its preference ignored. Thus, a high level of employee sophistication is needed

16. The most equitable form of subsidy, and the one most effective in inducing coverage of lower-income employees, would be a limited tax credit.

17. See notes 14–15. Failure of the 1986 Tax Reform Act to limit the tax subsidy was a major setback. The case illustrates economist Mancur Olson's thesis that abuses of the political process by well-organized interest groups not only can result in the transfer of others' wealth to themselves but can reduce the aggregate wealth of the whole society. See Mancur Olson, *The Rise and Decline of Nations: Economic Growth, Stagflation, and Social Rigidities* (New Haven, Conn.: Yale University Press, 1982).

18. In 1982, only 18 percent of workers with job-related health coverage could choose from among alternative plans. Pamela Farley and Gail Wilensky, "Options, Incentives and Employment-Related Health Insurance Coverage," *Advances in Health Economics and Health Services Research* 4 (1983):57. The second option was almost always an HMO, not a cost-controlled insurance plan.

before economizing reforms can become attractive.[19] Moreover, many employers rely upon their health benefits plans as a principal symbol of their beneficence toward their employees, and they have consequently been reluctant to appear to be retracting benefits previously conferred, to cultivate rational perceptions on the part of their workers, or to offer employees choices. In unionized firms, the problem is even greater. Union leaders, often abetted by employers anxious for their cooperation, uniformly point to the health plan as proof of the good things that they have been able to accomplish for the rank and file. Union members are naturally led to perceive the health plan as a hard-won benefit, an entitlement not to be given up without a fight. Although these attitudes and practices have changed significantly in recent years,[20] for a long time cost containment was not the main objective of purchasers of employment-based health insurance.[21]

Dispassionate review of an existing employer-purchased health benefits program is made exceedingly difficult by the symbolism of health care, by an intrafirm political context conducive to exaggerated paternalism, by the dominance of an entitlement mentality, and by the health plan's value both to union leaders seeking to justify their positions and to employers seeking to live with or stave off unionization. Even when employers and workers have felt intense economic pressures—as in the 1981-82 recession—it has usually remained unthinkable that employees might be better off with fewer health benefits, more cost containment, less freedom in selecting a provider, and more take-home pay.[22] A strong argument for eliminating the tax

19. On the issue of whether individual purchasers of health insurance are willing to accept cost-containment measures or behave rationally when purchasing insurance, see Gabel and Monheit, "Insurer-Provider Relationships," pp. 617–21, 631–32; and John Hershey et al., "Health Insurance under Competition: Would People Choose What Is Expected?" *Inquiry* 21, no. 4 (1984):349.

20. See Lewin and Associates et al., *Synthesis of Private Sector Health Care Initiatives,* Report for the Department of Health and Human Services, March 1984; and John Iglehart, "American Health Care and Business," *New England Journal of Medicine* 306, no. 2 (1982): 120.

21. See Sapolsky et al., "Corporate Attitudes."

22. On the desirability of restricted freedom of choice, see Avedis Donabedian, "Perspectives on the Free Choice of the Source of Personal Health Care," *Milbank Memorial Fund Quarterly* 59, no. 4 (1981):586; Mancur Olson, "Introduction," in Mancur Olson, ed., *A New Approach to the Econommics of Health Care* (Washington, D.C.: American Enterprise Institute, 1981), p. 1; and Gabel and Monheit, "Insurer-Provider Relationships," pp. 631–32.

subsidy for employer-purchased health insurance is that it would finally force reexamination of these matters. By the same token, it can be observed that taxpayers are currently bearing much of the additional cost that employers and union leaders incur in using their health plans for purposes that are essentially political. Ironically, many employers and union leaders, unable or unwilling to retract workers' health benefits openly, work actively for state or federal regulation that would significantly reduce the value of the ostensibly sacrosanct benefits package.

There is no question that employees have come to accept comprehensive health insurance as an entitlement and have been generally encouraged in this respect by those to whom they look for decisions on the nature and extent of coverage. In these circumstances, new forms of health coverage, such as HMOs, have been offerable only when it has been possible to preserve the old form as an available option. Although many employees have begun to learn the value of economizing in such multiple-choice settings, a major educational job remains to be done, and it remains unclear whether employers and unions are entirely reliable intermediaries, able to act in consumers' true economic interest. Thus, a powerful case can be made for reducing tax subsidies and strengthening competitive conditions as a way of starting the process of reeducation that is needed if more rational kinds of insurance are to become attractive. Severe problems do indeed appear to exist on the demand side of the market for private health insurance and to explain, at least in part, why insurers have not introduced the kinds of innovations that outside observers have thought both desirable and feasible. These problems could be solved, however, by clearly thought-out measures, political courage, and a little bit of luck.

Are Insurers Too Small?

Commercial health insurers have regularly argued that they are poorly situated to negotiate cost controls and lower prices with providers.[23] Because these insurers write numerous contracts covering scattered

---

23. See Gabel and Monheit, "Insurer-Provider Relationships," pp. 629–31. The authors misinterpret the situation somewhat in order to support the thesis that the insurance market will not change appreciably under competition. For example, the authors present the conventional view that Blue Cross discounts reflect only buying power rather than the actions of a

employees of national firms, they may insure only small numbers of patients in many markets. Thus, they claim that they lack the clout necessary to get providers' attention. On the basis of these claims, the insurers have periodically sought an antitrust exemption that would allow them to confront local doctors and hospitals collectively. They observe that Blue Cross plans frequently possess market shares that enable them to negotiate discounts, while commercial insurers, committed to reimburse their insureds on the basis of hospital charges incurred, are poorly positioned to resist the "cost-shifting" that may occur when hospitals find payers unwilling to cover the full cost of treating their own beneficiaries.

It is not clear that the commercial insurers' problem arises solely from low market shares. Certainly there are many markets in which the single insurer of one or more large employment groups could exert substantial bargaining power if it chose to do so. Moreover, although there are undoubtedly economies of scale in localized cost containment, solutions to the problem should not be difficult. There should be no antitrust or other impediment, for example, to collective action by a few insurers seeking to organize on a scale sufficient to permit effective negotiation with the providers in a community.[24] Finally, it does not appear that a substantial market share is necessary to enable effective bargaining with providers. Hospitals are very sensitive to occupancy rates, and any insurer with the ability to move even a small percentage of patients to another facility would have no trouble getting the attention of a hospital administrator. Unfortunately, commercial health insurers have been unwilling to influence their insureds' choice of hospital either by excluding services at a given institution from coverage or by attaching a higher copayment obligation if the patient should choose a higher-cost hospital. As long as they exercise no influence over where their patients go, commercial insurers should not be surprised when hospitals ignore their pleas for cost restraint.

Despite the insurers' claims of helplessness, it can be seen that their

---

hospital cartel. (See text accompanying notes 57–67.) They also appear to miss the close connection between freedom of choice and insurers' ability to negotiate.

24. The Department of Justice has lately been at pains to encourage procompetitive joint ventures. See "Antitrust Division Chief's November 2 Speech on Joint Ventures," *Antitrust & Trade Regulation Report* (BNA), 8 November 1984, p. 872.

problem lies not in their lack of market share but in the inefficient insurance policies they are writing. Fortunately, PPO developments—which, interestingly enough, have originated more often with providers and employers than with the insurers themselves—are beginning to give even small employment groups the ability to obtain significant concessions from hospitals and physicians. There is certainly no need for antitrust relief for insurers.

One factor that has made it hard for insurers to change their traditional philosophy and approach has been their lack of an effective presence in local markets for medical care. The HMO movement has demonstrated that health services can be efficiently organized and integrated with financing only at the local community level, where providers can be dealt with individually. Commercial insurers, whatever the size of their insured population in a given market, have seldom been equipped to function at the local level. As a result, much of the insurance industry's slowness in facing the challenge of cost containment probably reflects the fact that shifting from the pure insurance model to a hybrid or HMO arrangement requires a major effort to develop a presence and new capabilities in the myriad localities in which the insureds reside. Several leading insurers have not shrunk from this challenge, although they have had to concentrate their HMO development efforts in a few places. Perhaps those who criticize insurers for their apparent inaction have underestimated the magnitude of the task of developing the personnel and relationships needed to be effective at the local level.

Are Insurers Unable to Capture the Benefits of Their Cost-Containment Innovations?

Some economists have offered a technical explanation for insurers' hesitancy to innovate in cost containment.[25] Cost containment, they argue, has characteristics of a public good, meaning that its benefits may be shared by others who contribute nothing to the cost of achieving the savings. Thus, an insurer in a position to cause providers to operate more efficiently might refrain from making the needed effort

---

25. See Mark Pauly, "Paying the Piper and Calling the Tune: The Relationship between Public Financing and Public Regulation of Health Care," in Mancur Olson, ed., *New Approach,* pp. 67–86; idem, *Role of the Private Sector,* pp. 9–10, 37–38; Gabel and Monheit, "Insurer-Provider Relationships," pp. 626–29.

because it would gain no advantage over other insurers underwriting care by those same providers. The problem would exist only if the measures to be taken would cause providers to alter their style of practice with respect to all their patients, not just those insured by the innovating insurer. Thus, certain cost-containment measures, such as publicizing more efficient treatment modalities, would not be rewarding to a particular insurer. Similarly, if physicians could not or did not distinguish between patients on the basis of their insurers, an innovating insurer would find it hard to capture the benefits of its innovation. The problem arises in part because insurers deal with providers who also treat patients covered by competing insurers. In contrast, an HMO of the prepaid group practice variety can easily confine the benefit of its innovations to its own subscribers.

A related problem concerns the ease of imitation. If an insurer should alter its benefit package in some strategic way and persuade its customers to accept its innovation, it might simply be smoothing the way for competitors to introduce comparable innovations. Because competitors would not face the same costs of innovation and promotion, they could "ride free" on the innovator's successful efforts. Given the nature of the product, there is no way for an innovating insurer to preserve an intellectual property interest in new concepts.

To the extent that free-rider and public-good problems preclude innovators from recouping the costs of desirable innovations, such problems can explain the hesitancy of insurers to undertake major innovations. The fact that many PPOs have been developed by providers rather than by individual insurers indicates that insurers may indeed be inhibited from moving ahead with promising ideas. Although the magnitude of the problem is difficult to assess, it seems great enough to suggest an important role for employer coalitions[26] as well as for providers or insurers acting collectively[27] to develop beneficial cost-containment strategies that might not be rewarding to competing insurers. On the other hand, because there are many strategies that an insurer could adopt with only minimal spillover benefits

26. See Lewin and Associates, "Private Sector Health Care Initiatives," chap.5.

27. See note 24. Although antitrust law is not clear, competitor collaboration may sometimes be defensible on the grounds that market failure exists and that collaboration yields results closer to those that would result if the market functioned smoothly. Phillip Areeda, *The "Rule of Reason" in Antitrust Analysis: General Issues* (Washington, D.C.: Federal Judicial Center, 1981).

for its competitors, this explanation for industry inaction seems not to cover the full range of insurer inactivity.

Are Insurers Constrained by Law and Regulation?

Some departures from the traditional insurance model may violate insurance laws or regulatory restrictions under which the industry operates. In particular, insurers have frequently claimed that state regulation prevents them from limiting or influencing their insureds' choice of provider. They have also cited antitrust risks as another reason for their hesitancy to exclude or discriminate against particular providers who may wish to serve an insured group.

In each case, the insurers have overstated the breadth of the prohibitions under which they operate. Only a few states flatly prohibit insurers from influencing an insured's choice of provider.[28] Although many states do require that certain nonphysician providers be eligible to provide insured services,[29] those statutes do not appear to prohibit selectivity except along occupational lines; for example, although an insurer could not refuse to cover podiatrists' services altogether (assuming that it pays physicians for similar care), it would not be statutorily bound to pay for the services of any podiatrist (or physician) whom the patient might select.[30] Insurers who pleaded state law as their excuse for not interfering with absolute freedom of choice also cited federal antitrust law as an obstacle to discrimination among providers of insured services even on the basis of price. Although the law was unclear and did pose certain risks,[31] sound legal reasoning

28. See Elizabeth Rolph et al., *State Laws and Regulations Governing Preferred Provider Organizations*, Report for the Department of Health and Human Services and the Federal Trade Commission, August 1986; "Selected State Statutory Provisions Relating to the Insured's Choice of Provider and to Reimbursement Practices," *State Health Legislation Report* 11, no. 1 (1983):7; New Mexico Attorney General Opinion No. 77-13 (1977). California and Utah previously had such laws but have amended them.

29. See "Selected State Statutory Provisions."

30. See *Insurance Commissioner v. Mutual Medical Insurance, Inc.*, 241 N.E. 2d 56 (Ind. S. Ct. 1968).

31. The real legal problems surrounding the legality of discriminating against providers on the basis of price and the claim that monopsony power was being exerted were overcome in such cases as *Group Life & Health Insurance Co. v. Royal Drug Co.*, 440 U.S. 205 (1979); *Kartell v. Blue Shield*, 749 F.2d 922 (1st Cir. 1984); *Pennsylvania Dental Association v. Medical Service Association of Pennsylvania*, 745 F.2d 248 (3d Cir. 1984); *Sausalito Pharmacy v. Blue Shield*, 1981–1 Trade Cases (CCH) ¶63,885 (N.D. Cal. 1981), *aff'd per curiam*, 675 F.2d 502 (2d Cir. 1982); *Medical Arts Pharmacy v. Blue Cross and Blue Shield*, 518 F. Supp. 1100 (D. Conn. 1981), *aff'd per curiam*, 675 F.2d 502 (2d Cir. 1982).

would have inspired confidence that these problems could be over-come. Subsequent events have now firmly established that under the antitrust laws even very large insurance plans are free to drive hard bargains with providers and to reflect in their coverage provisions the willingness of particular providers to cooperate in cost containment.[32]

The interesting question here is not the legal obstacles to innovation themselves but the possibility that regulation was used by the insurers as an excuse for not doing what they did not wish to do. One inter-pretation might be that the industry hit upon a unique cartel strategy, coordinating their business practice by agreeing informally on restric-tive interpretations of legal rules. Perhaps, however, the insurance industry, famous for its caution in the face of uncertainty, was sincere in its legal fears. If the insurers' uniform behavior reflected only each insurer's individual interests and its independent reading of the legal situation rather than a concern for the industry's collective welfare, no conspiracy charge would stick.[33]

Although one may wonder at the unanimity with which commercial insurers avoided actions that might embroil them in lawsuits—even lawsuits that they stood a good chance of winning—innocent expla-nations for their individual unwillingness to challenge regulatory re-strictions may be found in the public-good and free-rider problems mentioned earlier. Probably because their larger market shares allow them to capture more of the benefits of successful litigation, Blue Cross and Blue Shield plans have been quicker to test the limits of restrictive laws than have commercial insurers. The Blues have borne the brunt of antitrust challenges to procompetitive restrictions on con-sumer free choice, ultimately triumphing in every case.[34] With respect to antidiscrimination requirements in state insurance laws, commer-cial carriers have sometimes worked to change these limitations, but they have usually been moved to act only because the law did not bind self-insured employers and thus created an added incentive for

32. See note 31.

33. See *Theatre Enterprises v. Paramount Film Distribution Corp.*, 346 U.S. 537, 541–42 (1954); *Interstate Circuit v. United States*, 306 U.S. 208, 226–27 (1939); *Bogosian v. Gulf Oil Corp.*, 561 F.2d 434, 445–47 (3d Cir. 1977), *cert. denied*, 434 U.S. 1086 (1978); George Hay, "Oligopoly, Shared Monopoly, and Antitrust Law," *Cornell Law Review* 67, no. 3 (1982):439; Richard Posner, "Oligopoly and the Antitrust Laws: A Suggested Ap-proach," *Stanford Law Review* 21, no. 6 (1969):1562, 1576–78; Donald Turner, "The Def-inition of Agreement under the Sherman Act: Conscious Parallelism and Refusals to Deal," *Harvard Law Review* 75, no. 4 (1962):655.

34. All of the health care cases cited in note 31 involved Blue Cross or Blue Shield plans.

large employers to drop their traditional coverage.[35] Similarly, the commercial carriers seldom sought repeal of "freedom of choice" statutes. Only in California, where a well-advanced HMO movement presented a serious competitive challenge to the commercials, did the industry actively seek legislation that legalized PPOs and selective contracting.[36] On the record, it appears that, for whatever reason, the insurance companies have been content to live with legal constraints on their own competitive behavior except where those constraints did not bind their competitors as well.

Another possible obstacle to some insurer cost-containment measures is the doctrine of insurance law under which insurance policies are regarded as contracts of adhesion, allowing courts to invalidate exclusions and limitations that have the effect of disappointing the insured's "reasonable expectations"; insurers may also be liable for punitive damages if they are deemed in retrospect to have acted in bad faith in not paying a claim.[37] Although these legal doctrines prevent insurers (appropriately) from laying traps for the unwary in fine print and from insisting too rigorously on their contractual rights, they are unlikely to be invoked if the insurer acts reasonably and makes reasonable disclosure—perhaps through provision for predetermination of benefits. A limited-benefit plan would also stand a good chance of being administered according to its terms if it were offered by the employer as one option in a multiple-choice situation. If a traditional plan offering comprehensive benefits was also available (at extra cost), the insured should be precluded from arguing that he did not freely assume the risk that he later regrets having to bear.[38] It appears once again that commercial insurers acquiesced in legal restrictions that they might have aggressively sought to overcome or circumvent.

Was There Collusion, Explicit or Tacit?

The commercial health insurance industry's longstanding failure to depart from traditional insurance practices in pursuit of cost contain-

---

35. For a description of such an effort by commercial insurers, see *Metropolitan Life Insurance Co. v. Massachusetts,* 471 U.S. 724 (1985).

36. Cal. Ins. Code §10133 (West Supp. 1985).

37. See Kenneth Abraham, "Judge-made Law and Judge-made Insurance: Honoring the Reasonable Expectations of the Insured," *Virginia Law Review* 67, no. 5 (1981):1151.

38. See Clark Havighurst, "Decentralizing Decision Making: Private Contract versus Professional Norms," in Jack Meyer, ed., *Market Reforms in Health Care: Current Issues, New Directions, Strategic Decisions* (Washington, D.C.: American Enterprise Institute, 1983), pp. 22, 39–41.

ment has reflected a high degree of what antitrust lawyers call "conscious parallelism."[39] The question thus arises whether industry adherence to common business policies, under circumstances that appeared to invite more competitive behavior, was the result of an express agreement not to compete. An alternative explanation for the insurers' parallel conduct, however, is that no individual firm could see any net benefit to itself from innovation because of the likelihood that its competitors would quickly imitate the competitive move, thus making the entire industry worse off while not significantly benefiting the initiator of the innovation. The phenomenon of oligopolistic inter-dependence, though imperfectly understood, can produce parallelism without agreement in concentrated industries, because individual firms recognize their collective stake in maintaining the status quo and therefore forbear from making competitive moves.[40] In some circumstances, it may be legally permissible to find unlawful collusion even without an express agreement, on the ground that the individual firms relied upon each other to act similarly and, instead of aggressively pursuing their individual self-interest, tailored their actions to serve the interests of the industry as a whole.[41] In other circumstances, however, the firms' refusals to compete may not be culpable, because they result from a recognition that innovation would not pay, even in the short run.[42] As noted earlier, a health insurer might hesitate to incur the costs and risks of innovation if its competitors could readily imitate its successes while leaving it to bear the consequences of its failures.

In addition to engaging in conscious parallelism, the health insurance industry, through the Health Insurance Association of America (HIAA), engages in a great deal of mutual consultation on competitive strategies. Cost-containment measures—coverage of second opinions, for example—are regularly examined in HIAA forums, with individual insurers apparently disclosing rather than withholding the results of their experience. Moreover, insurers frequently tell the world and each other what the industry—as opposed to its individual members—is doing about the cost problem. Some years ago, when Dr. Paul M. Ellwood, Jr., proposed the concept of "Health Alliances"—

39. See note 33.
40. See Turner, "Definition of Agreement."
41. See Posner, "Oligopoly and the Antitrust Laws."
42. See *E. I. Du Pont Nemours & Co. v. Federal Trade Commission*, 729 F.2d 128 (2d Cir. 1984).

mechanisms comparable to PPOs[43]—the HIAA convened a committee to examine the proposal. I subsequently asked members of that committee if I could see the results of their discussions, but was told that, on advice of antitrust counsel, the report was not available. It is reasonable to wonder about the state of competition in an industry where the desirability of particular competitive initiatives was examined by industrywide committees. Just as the industry seemed to strive for consensus on what was legally too risky to undertake, there also appeared to be an attempt to reach general agreement on what was feasible in cost containment.

Attributing the poor performance of the commercial health insurance industry to collusion, tacit or explicit, is, in the final analysis, difficult. Since the top five carriers hold only about one-third of the commercial group health insurance business, the industry is not concentrated to a degree that makes collusion feasible or likely. Moreover, the total number of competitors in the industry is substantially larger than is normally thought compatible with the maintenance of an effective conspiracy; in an industry populated by so many firms, the individual competitors would seem to lack the degree of interdependence necessary to stifle independent initiative. In addition, although the number of competitors in any given local market is smaller than the total number of firms in the industry as a whole, entry into specific local markets is relatively easy, requiring no investment in fixed assets and a scale of operation only large enough to realize the limited economies of scale. Finally, the commercial carriers have long faced substantial competition from Blue Cross and Blue Shield plans and from HMOs, indicating that collusion would not be a successful policy in any event.

Despite the numerous factors casting doubt on the existence of collusion actionable under the Sherman Act, one is still left with the impression that the health insurance industry's sense of its collective welfare is strong and may well have discouraged innovation beneficial to consumers. Perhaps the explanation for the questionable state of competition in the industry lies in the regulatory climate in which insurers operate.[44] Regulation has frequently contributed to cartel-like

---

43. See, e.g., James Reynolds, "A New Scheme to Force You to Compete for Patients," *Medical Economics,* 21 March 1977, p. 23.

44. See Gabel and Monheit, "Insurer-Provider Relationships," pp. 632–34.

performance in other regulated industries, and the special antitrust exemption for "the business of insurance" contained in the McCarran-Ferguson Act has fostered a high and probably unhealthy degree of consultation and collaboration among insurers. Whether or not anything approaching a conspiracy ever existed in fact, the weak entrepreneurial instincts and paradoxical aversion to risk-taking evinced by health insurers are similar to the attributes of other industries that have been closely regulated and relieved of accountability under the antitrust laws. It is ironic that the industry holds out the hope that it will perform better if its antitrust exemption is broadened.

Was Innovation Restrained by the Medical Profession?

It seems undeniable that, at least historically, the medical profession's strong preferences concerning the nature of private health insurance substantially governed industry performance. At an early date, the medical profession expressed strong feelings about the nature of lay-controlled insurance plans and threatened to boycott insurers that stepped out of the passive role that the physicians prescribed.[45] Insurers were peculiarly susceptible to physician boycotts—even poorly organized or incomplete ones—because their subscribers, most of whom were enrolled as members of employment groups rather than through individual choice, expected a wide range of choice among available practitioners. Thus, an employer would find his employees discontented if a significant number of physicians in a community refused to treat patients insured by the group's carrier or to accommodate those patients by submitting their claims directly to the insurer instead of billing the patient, who would then have to apply for reimbursement. There are signs that, during the period when the medical profession felt most free to agitate against unwanted cost-containment measures, those health plans that depended most on relations with local fee-for-service hospitals and physicians were inhibited in their actions. By the same token, the HMOs most successful in controlling costs were those that, like the Kaiser Foundation Health Plan, Inc.,

---

45. "The American Medical Association: Power, Purpose and Politics in Organized Medicine," *Yale Law Journal* 63 (1954): 937, 976–96. Early attitudes were revealed in the AMA's position with respect to the 1932 work of the Committee on the Costs of Medical Care. See *In re AMA*, 94 F.T.C. 701, 1011–16 (1979), *modified and enforced*, 638 F.2d 443 (2d Cir. 1980), *aff'd by an equally divided Court*, 455 U.S. 676 (1982).

and the Group Health Cooperative of Puget Sound, were largely self-contained, possessing their own hospitals and full-time specialists. Because these plans were less dependent on community resources, they were less susceptible to physicians' retaliatory action.

The evidence of professional restraints on early insurer behavior is fairly substantial. Lawrence Goldberg and Warren Greenberg reviewed the record in an early antitrust case against the Oregon State Medical Society[46] and found that substantial cost-containment efforts by private health plans were eventually discontinued as a result of professional opposition.[47] Perhaps the most egregious boycott was that by the Michigan State Medical Society, which resulted in a cease and desist order by the FTC in 1983.[48] Disturbed by certain cost-containment measures undertaken by the local Blue Shield plan, the society solicited its members' powers of attorney authorizing it to withdraw them as participating physicians from the Blue Shield program. Armed with these proxies, the society negotiated a more acceptable method of administering insurance coverage, only to be found guilty of an unlawful group boycott. Another case brought by the FTC dealt with collusion among a group of Indiana dentists who agreed not to grant insurers access to X-rays needed to determine the appropriateness of the treatment being rendered at insurer expense.[49] Although professional power has only rarely been used as blatantly as it was on these occasions, there would appear to be enough historical evidence of professional restraints to explain a great deal of the health insurance industry's failure to pursue cost containment aggressively.[50]

Although the medical profession took the initiative in restraining competition among health insurers, it can be asked whether commercial insurers did not acquiesce too quickly in the role that the profession prescribed for them. The impression that emerges from a study of the behavior of physicians and insurers during the long era

46. See *United States v. Oregon State Medical Society*, 343 U.S. 326 (1952).

47. See Lawrence Goldberg and Warren Greenberg, "The Effect of Physician-Controlled Health Insurance: *U.S. v. Oregon State Medical Society*," *Journal of Health Politics, Policy & Law* 2, no. 1 (1977):48.

48. *In re Michigan State Medical Society*, [1979–1983 Transfer Binder] Trade Reg. Rep. (CCH) ¶21,991 (FTC DKT 9129, February 17, 1983).

49. *See Federal Trade Commission v. Indiana Federation of Dentists*, 106 S. Ct. 2009 (1986).

50. See Havighurst, "Professional Restraints."

of professional exemption from meaningful antitrust enforcement is that two relatively loose cartels found mutually advantageous ways to accommodate each other's interests. The medical profession, on its side, welcomed the expansion of health insurance as long as such expansion served to increase the demand for medical care and did not substitute a sophisticated and powerful buying agent for the relatively uninformed consumer. The insurance industry, for its part, elected not to challenge the medical profession's monopoly, choosing instead to submit to its discipline. In this way, insurers avoided the unsettling competition that would otherwise have ensued among carriers seeking to minimize the effects of moral hazard. Interestingly, both parties had a great deal to gain if competition in the other's market were minimized. Together they were able to maintain for a long time the quiet life that monopolists are said to prefer.

One manifestation of insurer submission to physician dictation has been the widespread adoption by insurers of the medical profession's own cost-containment machinery. Unable to deny the need for some mechanism to prevent physician overcharging and unnecessary care, local medical societies set up peer review committees to which insurers were invited to refer disputes. Although these committees appeared to simplify insurers' problems in challenging questionable claims, they were unlikely—because they were organized by and accountable to physicians—to make a major dent in the overall cost problem.[51] Nevertheless, insurers generally accepted such peer review, not only because they knew that physicians would resent and possibly resist insurers' own efforts to impose stricter limits, but also perhaps because they found it convenient not to have to compete among themselves in the difficult business of cost containment.

Another example of insurer acquiescence in the cost-control programs of organized medicine appeared in *Arizona v. Maricopa County Medical Society*.[52] In that case, two physician organizations called "foundations for medical care" established schedules of fees that participating physicians agreed to accept as maximum limits on their

51. See Clark Havighurst and James Blumstein, "Coping with Quality/Cost Trade-offs in Medical Care: The Role of PSROs," *Northwestern University Law Review* 70, no. 1 (1975):6–68. For a case revealing insurer use of such a peer review mechanism, see *Union Labor Life Insurance Co. v. Pireno,* 458 U.S. 119 (1982).

52. See *Arizona v. Maricopa County Medical Society,* 457 U.S. 332 (1982).

charges for treating beneficiaries of foundation-approved insurance plans. A significant number of insurers sought foundation approval in order to benefit from the physicians' pricing self-restraint. The Supreme Court, finding the maximum fee schedules unlawful under the Sherman Act, stated, "Even if a fee schedule is . . . desirable, it is not necessary that the doctors do the price fixing."[53] It then proceeded to suggest that those who pay for services, including the insurers, should assume the responsibility for negotiating prices—that is, that they should compete in cost containment.[54]

There is now ample legal authority for prosecuting health care professionals who act collectively to coerce insurer behavior.[55] As a result, the insurance industry can no longer claim fear of professional retaliation as an excuse for refraining from aggressive cost containment. Moreover, insurers can no longer count on medical professionals to restrain competition among themselves. It is probably not coincidental that innovation in health insurance has significantly increased since the antitrust enforcement effort began in earnest in the late 1970s. Indeed, with the removal of provider-imposed constraints on insurer behavior, it is far less clear today than previously that the insurance industry is not performing in a reasonably competitive fashion. Certainly the industry is responding more creatively to demand-side signals and consumer preferences than ever before. There is a great deal of circumstantial evidence that antitrust enforcement is the predominant reason why competition has become a meaningful force in the health care industry and why health insurers no longer insulate health care providers so effectively from cost pressures.

Are the Blues the Ultimate Source of the Problem?

The failures of commercial insurers to control health care costs were for a long time insignificant in comparison with the cost-escalating practices followed by the prepayment plans belonging to the Blue Cross and Blue Shield system. Blue Cross plans, which generally cover only hospital services, originated under hospital sponsorship in

---

53. Ibid., p. 352.
54. Ibid. Significantly, the Court relied on the practice of using insurer-provider agreements, as revealed in *Group Life & Health Insurance Co. v. Royal Drug Co., Inc.,* 440 U.S. 205 (1979), involving pharmacies.
55. See notes 48–49.

the 1930s and were long controlled by hospitals; their policy of paying hospitals their retrospectively determined costs had the effect of insulating patients from having to consider cost differences when selecting a hospital, and thus enhanced hospitals' pricing and spending freedom. Similarly, Blue Shield plans, which cover medical services, were developed by and closely allied with state medical societies; their methods of paying physicians—most commonly by paying "usual, customary, and reasonable" fees—made it easier for a physician to set high prices without driving patients away. Given the Blues' origins, it should be no surprise that their payment policies were tailored primarily to serve provider rather than consumer interests. Because the Blues occupied a predominant market position in many states, they tended to set the overall tone in the health insurance market. In serving as models of insurer behavior, they may have been a more fundamental cause of the industry's cost problems than were the commercial carriers.

Although any proprovider bias reflected in the Blues' payment policies would seem to create market opportunities for commercial insurers, a number of factors, some of them explained earlier, inhibited commercial insurers from departing significantly from provider-approved practices. A major problem for the commercials was their inability to enter into direct contracts with providers, as the Blues routinely did. This inability resulted in part from ethical restrictions on physician contracting with lay-controlled insurers and in part from legal questions about such contracts. Even without legal barriers, however, an insurer seeking to contract directly with hospitals or doctors was likely to confront a concerted refusal to deal, explicit or tacit. A boycott of insurers who pursued policies objectionable to providers was an important factor in the stifling of early cost containment in Oregon, as shown by Goldberg and Greenberg.[56] As noted earlier, even an imperfect boycott could frustrate an insurer's initiative.

Another factor possibly enabling the Blues to set the standards for insurer conduct was their enjoyment of certain cost advantages over their commercial rivals. These advantages gave the Blues a price-cutting capacity that could be used to repel any move by a competing insurer that was threatening to the controlling provider interests. One significant cost advantage that could be put to such use was the ex-

---

56. Cal. Ins. Code §10133 (West Supp. 1985).

emption from premium taxes (typically around 2 percent) that the Blues enjoyed in many states. In addition, the Blues may have had generally lower loading (sales) costs and the benefit of scale economies. Although some have argued that, as nonprofit corporations not accountable to investors, the Blues squandered their cost advantages by tolerating administrative slack,[57] another type of cost advantage enjoyed by the Blues by virtue of their close relationship with providers gave them a unique power to discipline their competitors.

As long as the Blues were under provider control, it was easy for them to reduce their payments to participating providers whenever the controlling interests found it expedient to mount a response to some competitive initiative. By agreeing in effect to take less than 100 cents on a dollar for their claims, physicians or hospitals could equitably tax themselves in order to subsidize the Blue plan's counterattack. The potential effectiveness of this strategy can be sensed in the early experience of Oregon, where a new Blue Shield plan, Oregon Physicians Service (OPS), which was created to compete with payers whose cost controls were objectionable to physicians, quickly gained a two-thirds share of the health insurance market. Although the evidence is only suggestive, it has been speculated that, "during the period in which OPS was competing for subscribers and seeking to become the model of insurer conduct, the doctors underwrote the plan's losses by taking less than their full fees allowable under OPS schedules. The [competing insurers], unable to compete against the temporarily low price, submitted to the doctors' rule, thereafter regaining some of the market share they had lost."[58] As long as the Blues were under provider control, they were useful to providers as a "fighting ship" with which to engage in disciplinary price-cutting against any private payer that adopted unacceptable cost-containment practices.[59]

Although provider control was undoubtedly the crucial factor in establishing the Blues as market leaders, their influence continued even after direct provider influence over the plans began to decline

57. See H. E. Frech III and Paul B. Ginsburg, "Competition among Health Insurers," in *Competition in the Health Care Sector: Past, Present, and Future* (Germantown, Md.: Aspen Systems Corp./Federal Trade Commission, 1978), p. 210.

58. See Havighurst, "Professional Restraints," p. 315.

59. See Clark Havighurst and Glenn Hackbarth, "Enforcing the Rules of Free Enterprise in an Imperfect Market: The Case of Individual Practice Associations," in Mancur Olson, ed., *New Approach*, pp. 377, 391–92.

in the 1960s as increasing numbers of public representatives were added to the boards of many plans. Despite the attenuation of their influence, hospitals continued to grant Blue Cross plans substantial discounts, causing commercial insurers to complain about "cost-shifting." According to the commercial carriers, the discounts granted Blue Cross forced other payers to bear a disproportionate share of hospital costs and thus to face a serious competitive disadvantage. Those discounts continue to this day and no longer seem attributable in any measure to provider control. Although numerous cost justifications have been offered for the discounts, they have never been adequately explained on this or any other basis.

In a 1973 antitrust case, a commercial carrier challenged the discounts enjoyed by Blue Cross of Western Pennsylvania.[60] The court found, however, that, "in its negotiating with hospitals, Blue Cross has done no more than conduct its business as every rational enterprise does, i.e., [to] get the best deal possible."[61] The court also found that "the economic inducements which made the Blue Cross contract acceptable to hospitals did not amount to 'coercion.'"[62] Possibly confirming the passivity attributed to commercial insurers in this chapter, the court found that the "evidence suggests not that Travelers [the plaintiff] was unable to obtain any price reductions from hospitals, but rather that Travelers assumed its inability to do so and, therefore, did not press the matter."[63] Questions remain as to why the hospitals in the *Travelers* case gave Blue Cross a price break, and why Travelers thought that the same hospitals would not do the same for it. The commercials' claim was that Blue Cross, which possessed a 62 percent market share, had superior bargaining power.[64] In fact, however, the hospitals were not forced to grant the discounts by competition for Blue Cross's business. Instead, the discount was "negotiated jointly"[65] by an association representing all the hospitals. A more complex explanation for the discounts must therefore be sought.

60. See *Travelers Insurance Co. v. Blue Cross of Western Pennsylvania*, 481 F.2d 80 (3d Cir. 1973).

61. Ibid., p. 84.

62. Ibid.

63. Ibid., p. 85.

64. For an antitrust case rejecting a challenge to a similar plan's alleged use of its bargaining power, see *Kartell v. Blue Shield*, 749 F.2d 922 (1st Cir. 1984).

65. *Travelers Insurance Co. v. Blue Cross of Western Pennsylvania*, 481 F.2d at 84.

Why would a hospital cartel grant a large discount to one favored buyer? One possible explanation is that Blue Cross, though no longer under hospital control, retained its willingness to advance hospitals' interests and thus served as their cat's-paw in warding off payers who threatened to become aggressive purchasers able to force hospitals into intense price competition yielding even larger discounts. Although this explanation probably contains important elements of truth, another possibility is that the hospitals perceived that, by granting the biggest purchaser a standard discount, they could reduce the competitive pressure on themselves as individual sellers to grant that buyer even bigger discounts. In other words, the hospitals may have seen an advantage in collectively agreeing on the amount of discount that the largest insurer would be allowed. The benefit to the hospitals— and to Blue Cross itself, it will be noted—would lie in the preservation of their gentlemen's agreement to contract directly with no other payers and to grant no other discounts. Fortunately, agreements of this type are now breaking down, but the hypothesis offered to explain the discounts granted exclusively to Blue Cross in the past seems highly plausible.

Early antitrust experience with volume discounts under the Robinson-Patman Act confirms that a cartel policy of recognizing the entitlement of large buyers to special discounts may be rational and has manifested itself in other market settings. In the leading Robinson-Patman case, *Morton Salt Co. v. Federal Trade Commission,*[66] a major seller of salt maintained a schedule of volume discounts benefiting those who purchased large amounts over the course of a year. Given the homogeneous nature of the product and the oligopolistic nature of the industry, other sellers must have maintained identical pricing schedules. These schedules served the oligopolists as what antitrust analysts today would call "facilitating devices"—mechanisms that make it easier for the oligopolists to coordinate their practices, reduce each seller's temptation to break ranks, and otherwise foster adherence to the existing schedule.[67] By acknowledging and institutionalizing buying power, the volume discount schedule reduced the potential gains

---

66. *Morton Salt Co. v. Federal Trade Commission,* 334 U.S. 37 (1948).

67. See Hay, "Oligopoly, Shared Monopoly," pp. 453–57, describing "facilitating practices." As far as I know, a volume discount schedule has never been categorized as a facilitating device, but as analyzed here it has all the earmarks of one.

to large buyers from attempting to obtain an even better price, an effort that might open competition to an extent that would allow their smaller competitors actually to narrow or even eliminate the prevailing price differential. At the same time, each seller, having agreed to discounts for its most valued customers, was less likely to be tempted to shade prices further to gain their business, thus destroying the oligopolistic pricing structure. The result was a foreclosure of active price competition among sellers and an artificial cost disadvantage for smaller purchasers.

The remedy proposed by commercial insurers for discriminatory hospital discounts to their competitors has been state legislation that would prohibit hospitals from making price concessions to any nongovernment third-party payer unless the price differential could be justified by demonstrating a specific benefit of commensurate value conferred on the hospital by the payer.[68] The campaign for such legislation featured the claim that it would enhance competition. It should be clear, however, that preserving inefficient competitors, such as insurers wedded to old ways of paying hospitals, and preventing payers from benefiting from hard bargaining with hospitals would be neither procompetitive nor in the public interest. In supporting such legislation, the HIAA has once again revealed its members' disturbing preference for avoiding competition among themselves in procuring hospital services for their insureds on advantageous terms. Fortunately, fast-moving events are opening up new possibilities for insurer competition in cost containment.

One development ameliorating many of the problems identified here has been the application of the antitrust laws to challenge the control of the Blues and other prepayment plans by powerful provider organizations.[69] Another essential remedy, however, which has so far been pursued in only one case,[70] is antitrust enforcement against hospital collective bargaining with Blue Cross. Without collective action

---

68. Bills to this effect were introduced in several legislatures (e.g., Ohio and Alabama) in 1981 and 1982.

69. See Federal Trade Commission, Bureau of Competition, Staff Report on Medical Participation in Control of Blue Shield and Certain Other Open-Panel Medical Prepayment Plans, April 1979. (Unpublished.)

70. *Ohio v. Greater Cleveland Hospital Association,* 1983–2 Trade Cases (CCH) ¶65,685 (N.D. Ohio 1983) (consent decree). The case was subsequently settled, and no other like it has been brought.

by the hospitals, each would have to decide for itself what discounts to grant. Under these conditions, commercial insurers, once they developed the capacity to bargain at the local level and to steer patients to lower-cost institutions, should have no trouble competing with Blue Cross on reasonably equal terms; forced to act independently, hospitals would be eager for any insurer's business because of their need to retain or attract even small numbers of patients in order to maintain occupancy levels and to generate revenues helpful in covering their fixed costs. In addition to these antitrust initiatives, other remedies for the problems identified here include legislative action to eliminate the different treatment of Blue Cross and commercial insurers under state premium taxes and other competitive disadvantages under which the latter may operate because of different legislative treatment. Competitive conditions could also be improved by removing artificial incentives for employers to self-insure their employee health benefits, a policy move that would require amending the federal Employee Retirement Income Security Act (ERISA), which currently prevents states from regulating employer plans to the same extent that they regulate insurers.[71]

CONCLUSION: THE POLICY IMPLICATIONS

This chapter has advanced a series of untested but plausible hypotheses to explain why commercial carriers appeared for a long time to be nearly useless in combating the influence of moral hazard on the cost of insured health services. The most interesting aspect of the explanations offered here, aside from their inherent insidiousness and complexity, is that very few of them are mutually exclusive. Instead, they are cumulative in their impact and leave one with the impression that, even if some of the theories suggested are incorrect or practically unimportant, the total picture painted of the industry's poor performance cannot be seriously inaccurate. Another important point is that many of the theories offered absolve commercial insurers from blame for neglecting cost containment. There are, however, several points at which industry members might have opted to compete but chose instead to adhere to traditional patterns. Despite the plausibility of

71. See *Metropolitan Life Insurance Co. v. Massachusetts*, 471 U.S. 724 (1985).

some of the industry's excuses for behaving as it did, its overall performance can be fairly criticized.

The relevance of this discussion for the current policy debate would seem to lie in several areas. In general, it appears that the most serious problems identified are remediable by policy moves that are well within the realm of political feasibility. Capping the tax subsidy for private insurance is essential if private insurers are to pursue cost containment to an optimal degree, and the public will assuredly pay a significant cost if it persists in thinking that the subsidy relieves rather than contributes to its overall cost burden. Antitrust enforcement has already freed innovating insurers from retaliatory threats by organized providers, and the law has been clarified so that it now supports insurers' prudent purchasing and such innovations as PPO development. Additional measures to relieve commercial carriers of cost and regulatory burdens, including those not borne equally by their competitors, are very much in order and are being taken in many state legislatures. Earlier discussion identifies other points at which government might make helpful policy adjustments.

One point that emerges with great clarity is the potential for harm to the public interest in the HIAA's legislative agenda. Again and again, health insurers have advocated policies aimed at reducing the competitive pressures on themselves to change their antiquated practices. Perceiving themselves to be disabled from competing effectively in cost containment, they have invested more resources in seeking legislation to suppress or obviate such competition than in overcoming their disadvantages. In general, the insurers' strategy has been to minimize the adverse competitive consequences of their own deficiencies as payers for health services by depriving those who do business differently from enjoying any competitive advantage as a result. The industry's advocacy of tax subsidies that impair their customers' cost consciousness, of both state and federal regulation of hospital rates, of prohibitions against discounts to aggressive buyers, and of an expanded antitrust exemption for themselves indicates that they are hoping to avoid the necessity of fundamentally changing the way they write and administer coverage.

Fortunately, recent events have not gone the insurers' way. Employers' increased awareness of cost burdens, the increasing sophistication of insurance purchasers (developed in part by employer coalitions), and antitrust enforcement's new challenge to professional restraints on innovation in health care financing have unleashed new market forces, culminating in faster HMO growth, direct contracting by insurers with providers, and insurer- and provider-sponsored PPOs. These and other developments are finally making purchasers face the need to adapt themselves to economic realities. Now that government, both at the federal level and in all but a few states, has lost interest in regulating private health care costs, private purchasers of health care benefits are acutely aware that they cannot rely on government to solve their problems. Commercial insurers, if they are to have any future at all, must respond to the new demands for cost control; a few are doing so in ways that are all the more impressive when they are contrasted with insurer inaction in the recent past. But whether the commercial carriers survive in anything like their traditional form should be a matter of supreme indifference to the general public, which should do all that it can to expose those who persist in marketing obsolete insurance products to the full competitive consequences of that persistence.

SELECTED BIBLIOGRAPHY

Abraham, Kenneth S. "Judge-made Law and Judge-made Insurance: Honoring the Reasonable Expectations of the Insured." *Virginia Law Review* 67, no. 5 (1981):1151.

Council on Wage and Price Stability, Executive Office of the President. *The Complex Puzzle of Rising Health Care Costs: Can the Private Sector Fit It Together?* Washington, D.C.: Government Printing Office, 1977.

Donabedian, Avedis. "Perspectives on the Free Choice of the Source of Personal Health Care." *Milbank Memorial Fund Quarterly* 59, no. 4 (1981): 586.

Farley, Pamela, and Gail Wilensky. "Options, Incentives and Employment-Related Health Insurance Coverage." *Advances in Health Economics and Health Services Research* 4 (1983):57.

Federal Trade Commission, Bureau of Competition. Staff Report on Medical Participation in Control of Blue Shield and Certain Other Open-Panel Medical Prepayment Plans, April 1979. (Unpublished.)

Feldstein, Martin. "The Welfare Loss of Excess Health Insurance." *Journal of Political Economy* 81, no. 2 (1973):251.

Frech, H. E. III, and Paul Ginsburg, "Competition among Health Insurers." In Warren Greenberg, ed., *Competition in the Health Care Sector: Past, Present and Future,* pp. 210–37. Germantown, Md.: Aspen Systems Corp./ Federal Trade Commission, 1978.

Gabel, Jon R., and Alan C. Monheit, "Will Competition Plans Change Insurer-Provider Relationships?" *Milbank Memorial Fund Quarterly* 61, no. 4 (1983):614.

257

Goldberg, Lawrence, and Warren Greenberg. "The Effect of Physician-Controlled Health Insurance: *U.S. v. Oregon State Medical Society.*" *Journal of Health Politics, Policy & Law* 2, no. 1 (1977):48.

Havighurst, Clark C. "The Role of Competition in Cost Containment." In Warren Greenberg, ed., *Competition in the Health Care Sector: Past, Present and Future.* Germantown, Md.: Aspen Systems Corp./Federal Trade Commission, 1978.

——. "Professional Restraints on Innovation in Health Care Financing." *Duke Law Journal* (May 1978):303.

Havighurst, Clark C., and Glenn M. Hackbarth. "Private Cost Containment." *New England Journal of Medicine* 300, no. 23 (1979):1298.

Health Insurance Association of America. *The Case against the Taxation of Employee Health Benefits.* Chicago: HIAA, March 1985.

Hershey, John C., Howard Kunreuther, J. Sanford Schwartz, and Sankey V. Williams. "Health Insurance under Competition: Would People Choose What Is Expected?" *Inquiry* 21, no. 2 (1984):349.

Lewin and Associates, et al. *Synthesis of Private Sector Health Care Initiatives.* Report prepared for the Department of Health and Human Services, March 1984.

Newhouse, Joseph, and Vincent Taylor. "How Shall We Pay for Hospital Care?" *Public Interest* 23 (Spring 1971):78.

Pauly, Mark V. *The Role of the Private Sector in National Health Insurance.* Chicago: Health Insurance Association of America, 1979.

Rolph, Elizabeth, J. Peter Rich, Paul Ginsburg, Susan Hosek, Karen Keenan, and Gary Gertler. *State Laws and Regulations Governing Preferred Provider Organizations.* Report prepared for the Department of Health and Human Services and the Federal Trade Commission, August 1986.

Sapolsky, Harvey, Drew Alman, Richard Greene, and Judith Moore. "Corporate Attitudes toward Health Care Costs." *Milbank Memorial Fund Quarterly* 59, no. 4 (1981):561.

7

THE DECLINING PRICE OF HEALTH INSURANCE

Jody L. Sindelar

INTRODUCTION

The escalating costs of medical care and health insurance premiums have been analyzed, scrutinized, deplored, lamented, and cursed. Employers, academics, government analysts, and politicians are all searching for policies to reduce the mounting cost of health insurance premiums, medical prices, and expenditures on medical care. In surprising contrast to rising prices for most medical goods and services, the price of health insurance has experienced a downward trend over the last several decades. Like most reductions in prices, this phenomenon may provide benefits to society. In the case of health insurance, however, a lower price can result in higher prices for medical care because individuals may buy more health insurance in response to the lower price. The greater coverage would result in increased demand and fuel spiraling medical prices.

This chapter documents the previously undetected declining price, introducing and empirically analyzing potential causes of the decline. Analysis is useful because the declining price of health insurance (1) has not previously been demonstrated and analyzed, (2) is contrary to all other price trends in the medical care field, (3) may be a part of the cause of increasing medical prices and health insurance premiums, and (4) has important welfare effects.

259

The "price" of insurance is measured here as the ratio of premiums to benefits; in other words, the amount that must be spent in premiums, on average, to get one dollar back in benefits. State data from 1959 to the 1980s show that the overall decrease in the price of health insurance can be attributed to changes in the price of commercial insurance; the price of Blue Cross/Blue Shield insurance remained stable from 1959 to the 1980s.

The rest of the chapter is organized as follows. Pertinent institutional factors and characteristics of the market are presented in the following section. Then we discuss measurement of the price of insurance and document the secular and cross-sectional variations in the price for the nonprofit and for-profit sectors. The fourth section discusses factors that may account for the overall declining price of insurance and endeavors to explain why the price of nonprofit insurance has remained stable while the price of commercial insurance has declined. The fifth section defines the variables and states the empirical methods used to investigate potential explanations of the price trends. The sixth section presents the results, and the chapter is summarized in the final section.

INSTITUTIONAL ASPECTS OF THE INSURANCE MARKET

Several institutional aspects of the health insurance market are relevant to understanding the price of health insurance. The market is believed to be basically competitive, although some noncompetitive elements exist because of the presence of the nonprofit sector and because of the tax and regulatory policies of the various states. The market comprises many buyers and sellers: More than a thousand firms sell health insurance.[1] These range from large nationwide companies that sell a diversified line of insurance to smaller firms that sell in a limited geographic location. Although all firms may not sell insurance in the same location, they are sufficiently numerous in any one location to constitute a competitive market. Furthermore, firms that sell

---

1. The *National Health Insurance Resource Book*, Subcommittee on Health, House of Representatives (Washington, D.C.: Government Printing Office, 1976), pp. 218–49, estimates that 916 firms were selling health insurance in 1970. According to the *Life Insurance Fact Book* (Washington, D.C.: American Council of Life Insurance, 1984), there were 1,895 firms selling life insurance in 1979. Many of those sold health insurance.

health insurance are poised to enter new geographic markets if the opportunity arises, and firms selling other lines of insurance are poised to enter the health insurance market.

Both nonprofit and for-profit firms sell health insurance.[2] Blue Cross/ Blue Shield plans comprise the nonprofit sector. The Blues were started by medical care providers and still retain some of their original relationships and control despite public inquiry into the nature of the relationship.[3]

The Blues differ from the commercial sector in the coverage they offer, what they maximize, who the residual claimants are, how they operate, and how they are taxed and regulated. The Blues have claimed, and others have concurred, that the Blues offer coverage that is competitive with—but differentiated from—that of the private commercial sector. For example, the Blues offer more complete and comprehensive coverage (e.g., with lower deductibles); they generate discounts on hospital bills; and they typically pay providers directly.[4] The direct payment of providers has developed the idea that Blues pay for "services" rather than financial benefits. This view has been used to justify lower reserve requirements for the Blues than for the commercial sector. The Blue Cross/Blue Shield plans are also different in that they rarely compete against each other. They have generally segmented the market so that their markets do not overlap, either geographically or by product line.

Insurance as a line of business has been exempted from federal taxation and regulation; it is taxed and regulated only by the states.[5] State taxation and regulation policies produce some barriers to entry. All states impose a tax on suppliers of insurance. Since the tax is

---

2. The for-profit, or commercial, sector is composed of mutual companies and stock companies. These two types cannot be distinguished from each other in the data and, since we have no a priori reason to predict different behavior, there is no need to make a distinction between them.

3. See David Kass and Paul Pautler, *Physician Control of Blue Shield Plans* (Washington, D.C.: Federal Trade Commission, November 1979).

4. See Sylvia Law, *Blue Cross: What Went Wrong?* (New Haven, Conn.: Yale University Press, 1976); and H. E. Frech III, "Blue Cross, Blue Shield, and Health Care Costs: A Review of Economic Evidence," in Mark Pauly, ed., *National Health Insurance: What Now, What Later, What Never?* (Washington, D.C.: American Enterprise Institute, 1980), pp. 250–64.

5. For further information on regulation and taxation of the supply of health insurance, see *National Health Insurance Resource Book*, 1976; and R. Eilers, *Regulation of Blue Cross and Blue Shield Plans* (Homewood, Ill.: Irwin for S. S. Heubner Foundation, 1963).

typically a fixed percentage of sales (rather than of profits, as in state corporate income tax), even a small tax on premiums is equivalent to a relatively large tax on profits. Because each state has the power to set tax and regulatory policies, there is considerable variation across states in the tax rates for each type of insurer. Most states exempt Blue Cross/Blue Shield from taxes (as nonprofit corporations); tax domestic companies (domiciled within the state) at a rate of about 1 to 2 percent; and tax foreign insurers (domiciled outside the state) at a higher rate, say 2 to 3 percent.

In addition to the competitive advantage given the Blues through premium taxes, the Blues also have other tax advantages. Commercial insurers must pay property tax and federal and state corporate income tax, while the Blues are typically exempt from these taxes. Even with these tax advantages, the Blues have not taken over the market. Two views have been advanced to explain why this has not occurred. One view is that, as nonprofit firms, the Blues suffer from managerial slack, which increases their administrative costs. Another is that they use their tax advantage to achieve other goals, such as increasing coverage, rather than to maximize profits.[6]

State taxation of insurers provides general revenues as well as financing the states' development and enforcement of insurance regulation. Private insurers are often required to file their policy forms with the state. The state commission reviews the language of the policy forms, e.g., the language guaranteeing renewability. Typically,

---

6. For an explanation of, and evidence on, these views, see H. E. Frech III, "The Property Rights Theory of the Firm: Empirical Results from a National Experiment," *Journal of Political Economy* 84, no. 1 (1976):143–52; and D. Eisenstadt and T. Kennedy, "Control and Behavior of Nonprofit Firms: The Case of Blue Shield," *Southern Economic Journal* 48, no. 1 (July 1981):26–36. Frech finds that nonprofit firms have higher administrative expenses per dollar paid in claims, all else being equal, than do for-profit firms in administering Medicare claims. This finding is consistent with the idea of administrative slack in the nonprofit sector. Although at first glance it is seemingly inconsistent with the findings of this chapter that the Blues have lower prices, our conclusion is not necessarily inconsistent with Frech's: The Blues' prices may be lower because they encourage purchase of more insurance coverage and more complete coverage instead of profit maximization. Thus, they can be inefficient from society's perspective, but may be maximizing different goals. Furthermore, not only do Blues pay lower premium taxes, they are also exempt from many state and local taxes, such as those on property and sales. These advantages can be used to maximize special goals, not to maximize profits.

states do not regulate premium rates, coverage, or benefits paid.[7] Although premium rates are not regulated for the commercial firms, in some states the rates of the Blues' policies for individuals must be approved prior to implementation.

The demand for all types of health insurance is increased by the favorable federal tax treatment of expenditures on health insurance. Health insurance that is provided as a fringe benefit of employment is tax deductible to the employer. This explains, in part, why most health insurance policies are now sold through employer groups. In addition, a portion of individuals' expenses on health insurance premiums is deductible from personal federal income tax under some conditions.

TRENDS IN PRICES

Examining changes in the price of health insurance, especially as compared to other prices, can help identify developments in the market (Table 7–1). We will examine changes in the overall price of health insurance and then delineate the market into the for-profit and nonprofit insurers on the grounds that the two constitute segmented markets.

How Price Is Measured

In this chapter price is defined as a standardized per unit measure that corresponds to underlying economic principles. Price is measured as the ratio of premiums to benefits per annum. This ratio tells us how much must be paid in premiums to receive, on average, one dollar paid in claims. A price of $1.35, for example, indicates that for one dollar expected to be paid out in claims, an individual would pay, on average, $1.35 in premiums. The 35 cents is called the loading

---

7. Loss ratio of the insurance company is sometimes analyzed by state commissions as an indicator of exceedingly high charges relative to claims paid. Previously, a ratio of less than 50 percent indicated the possibility of excessive charges by an insurance company. See *National Health Insurance Resource Book*, 1976. A loss ratio of less than 50 percent would be more of an outlier today than in 1959, when the average loss ratio for all commercial firms was 64 percent (the inverse of the price, in Table 7–2). By 1979 it had increased to 70 percent.

Table 7–1.   Prices of All Medical Care and Health Care Items, 1959–1981.

	All Items[a]	Medical Care[a]	Medical Care Services[a]	Medical Care Com- modities[a]	Price of Health Insur- ance[b]
1959	87.3	76.4	72.0	104.4	1.35
1960	88.7	79.1	74.9	104.5	1.38
1961	89.6	81.4	77.7	103.3	1.34
1962	90.6	83.5	80.2	101.7	1.35
1963	91.7	85.6	82.6	100.8	1.34
1964	92.9	87.3	84.6	100.5	1.32
1965	94.5	89.5	87.3	100.2	1.30
1966	97.2	93.4	92.0	100.5	1.30
1967	100.0	100.0	100.0	100.0	1.26
1968	104.2	106.1	107.3	100.2	1.26
1969	109.8	113.4	116.0	101.3	1.24
1970	116.3	120.6	124.2	103.6	1.19
1971	121.3	128.4	133.3	105.4	1.24
1972	125.3	132.5	138.2	105.6	1.26
1973	133.1	137.7	144.3	105.9	1.29
1974	147.7	150.5	159.1	109.5	1.25
1975	161.2	168.6	179.1	118.8	1.24
1976	170.5	184.7	197.0	126.0	1.16
1977	181.5	202.4	216.7	134.1	1.23
1978	195.4	219.4	235.4	143.5	1.21
1979	217.4	239.7	258.3	153.8	1.17
1980	246.8	265.9	287.4	168.1	1.11
1981	272.4	294.5	318.2	186.5	1.12
Ratio of 1981 to 1959	3.1	3.8	4.4	1.8	.83
Continuously compounded annual growth rate (%)	0.05	0.06	0.07	0.03	−0.01

SOURCES: Blue Cross–Blue Shield Association, *Blue Cross–Blue Shield Fact Book* (Chicago: BCBSA, various years); CPI Data Tape, U.S. Department of Labor, Bureau of Labor Statistics, Washington, D.C.; *Source Book of Health Insurance Data* (Washington, D.C.: Health Insurance Association of America, yearly).

[a]CPI for all urban consumers (city average).

[b]Calculated as the ratio of health insurance premiums to health insurance benefits, 1959–1982.

fee.[8] Premiums (*PREM*) are set to cover the expected benefits to be paid out [*E(BEN)*] as well as marketing and administrative expenses (*ADMIN*), taxes (*TAX*), and a normal return of capital and residual risk-taking (*PROFITS*), as well as, in a noncompetitive market, excess profits.

Dividing premiums by price shows that price is equal to one plus the loading factor, which covers all expenses and incorporates forecast errors.

$$PREM = E(BEN) + ADMIN + TAX + PROFITS$$

$$\text{Price} = \frac{PREM}{BEN} = 1 + \frac{e + ADMIN + TAX + PROFITS}{BEN}$$

where: $E(BEN) = BEN + e$,

where e is the forecast error.

This method of measuring price is chosen to correspond to underlying economic concepts, e.g., as price declines, quantity demanded increases. It is also preferred here because it is a per unit, or standardized, measure. Contrast this measure of price to premiums. Premiums measure total expenditure, i.e., price times quantity. Premiums do not constitute a per unit measure, and demand is not a function of price. In contrast to price, premiums have increased in real and nominal terms, as seen in Table 7–2. Nominal premiums grew over the time period 1959 to 1982 by a factor of 12.8, or at an annual continuously compounded rate of 11 percent. Real premiums more than tripled over this period, which, with a declining price, indicates that quantity of coverage increased.

Comparison to Other Price Trends

Table 7–1 displays the often-discussed increasing medical care prices of the last few decades and demonstrates the little-known declining price of health insurance. The first column shows that, for all items, the Consumer Price Index (CPI) increased by a factor of approximately three from 1959 to 1981—an increase corresponding to an average continuously compounded growth rate of 5 percent. The med-

8. The loading fee could have been used as the measure of price without any substantive changes in the results or conclusions, as it is only a variant of the same measure.

Table 7–2. Price of Health Insurance and Health Insurance Premiums, 1959–1982.

	Price		Premiums Per Capita	
	Blue Cross/ Blue Shield	Commercial	Nominal	Real (1972 $)
1959	1.10	1.55	34	51
1960	1.11	1.59	38	55
1961	1.10	1.53	41	59
1962	1.08	1.55	45	63
1963	1.08	1.54	48	68
1964	1.07	1.51	53	73
1965	1.09	1.48	58	77
1966	1.10	1.45	60	79
1967	1.06	1.43	64	80
1968	1.09	1.39	70	84
1969	1.07	1.36	81	93
1970	1.06	1.31	93	101
1971	1.09	1.40	104	108
1972	1.09	1.42	117	117
1973	1.11	1.47	133	126
1974	1.05	1.43	147	128
1975	1.03	1.47	171	136
1976	1.07	1.26	185	140
1977	1.11	1.37	210	150
1978	1.12	1.31	235	156
1979	1.09	1.26	255	157
1980	1.04	1.18[b]	328	162
1981	1.04	1.18[b]	369	176
1982	1.05	1.19[b]	435	186
Ratio 1979/1959[a]	.99	.81	7.5	3.1
Growth rate	−.0004	−.009	.10	.05
Ratio 1982/1959	.95	.77	12.79	3.6
Growth rate	−.0021	−.011	.11	.05

SOURCES: Blue Cross–Blue Shield Association, *Blue Cross–Blue Shield Fact Book* (Chicago: BCBSA, various years); CPI Data Tape, U.S. Department of Labor, Bureau of Labor Statistics, Washington, D.C.; *Source Book of Health Insurance Data* (Washington, D.C.: Health Insurance Association of America, yearly).

[a]A slightly different method of calculating premiums may account for a downward bias for the years 1980–1982.

ical care component of the CPI, seen in the second column, increased by 3.8 times (a 6 percent growth rate). The medical care services component has increased 4.4 times over the same period (third column C:—a 7 percent growth rate). In contrast, the price of health insurance in 1981 was only 83 percent of that in 1959 (fifth column). This corresponds to a continuously compounded growth rate of -1 percent. Thus, while all other prices in the health insurance field have been increasing rapidly, health insurance prices have been decreasing.

Blue Cross/Blue Shield versus Commercial Firms

Table 7–2 shows the change in prices for both Blue Cross/Blue Shield and commercial insurance from 1959 to 1982. The price of the Blues' insurance has historically been lower than that of commercial insurance. For example, in 1959 the price of the Blues was $1.10, while the price of commercials was $1.55, a 41 percent difference. However, from 1959 to 1979, the price of the commercial firms declined substantially, by a significant 23 percent.[9] Over the same period, the price of Blues has remained basically stable at the national level. Despite the significant decline in the price of commercial insurance, the Blues' price of $1.09 in 1979 is still lower than the price of $1.26 for commercial insurers in the same year. The differences in the level and change in price across the segments is consistent with differentiated markets across the nonprofit and for-profit sectors, although the convergence of their prices indicates that the sectors may be becoming more similar.

Table 7–3 demonstrates that the price decline for commercial insurance has been robust across different methods of measurement. Columns one, three, and five measure the price of all commercial, and Blues' insurance, respectively, at the national level with each state equally weighted. Columns seven through nine display price levels weighted by the magnitude of premiums in each state. In columns three and eight it can be seen that the price of commercial insurance has exhibited similar declines for both measures. The overall price level has also declined similarly across the two measurement methods (columns one and seven). The Blues' price, measured either way (columns five and nine), exhibited almost no significant change over this period.

9. Data are not available by state for Blues and commercial insurers after 1979. Another source of data must be used to extend the national estimates to 1982. There was an apparently larger decline in price from 1959 to 1982, as seen at the bottom of Table 7–2. However, this may be an overestimate of the decline, as the figures for 1980 to 1982 are calculated by a slightly different method (they could not readily be made comparable). Also note that states are equally weighted in these calculations.

Table 7–3.   Prices of Commercial and Blue Cross/Blue Shield Health Insurance: Comparative Measures.

	States Equally Weighted						States Weighted by Premiums		
	All		Commer-cial		Blues		All	Com-mer-cial	Blues
	μ	SD	μ	SD	μ	SD	μ	μ	μ
1959	1.35	0.10	1.55	0.12	1.10	0.05	1.30	1.48	1.08
1960	1.38	0.10	1.60	0.11	1.11	0.07	1.32	1.52	1.07
1961	1.34	0.11	1.53	0.11	1.10	0.08	1.29	1.48	1.08
1962	1.35	0.11	1.55	0.12	1.09	0.05	1.30	1.49	1.09
1963	1.34	0.10	1.54	0.11	1.08	0.06	1.29	1.48	1.07
1964	1.32	0.10	1.51	0.11	1.07	0.05	1.27	1.45	1.07
1965	1.30	0.09	1.48	0.11	1.09	0.05	1.26	1.42	1.07
1966	1.30	0.09	1.45	0.12	1.10	0.10	1.25	1.40	1.07
1967	1.26	0.09	1.43	0.11	1.06	0.09	1.22	1.38	1.03
1968	1.26	0.08	1.39	0.10	1.09	0.05	1.22	1.35	1.07
1969	1.24	0.10	1.38	0.10	1.09	0.10	1.21	1.35	1.06
1970	1.19	0.10	1.31	0.10	1.08	0.18	1.16	1.27	1.04
1971	1.24	0.13	1.40	0.14	1.11	0.19	1.21	1.35	1.08
1972	1.26	0.08	1.42	0.13	1.10	0.06	1.22	1.35	1.10
1973	1.29	0.07	1.47	0.10	1.11	0.05	1.25	1.40	1.10
1974	1.25	0.10	1.42	0.13	1.06	0.16	1.21	1.35	1.06
1975	1.24	0.09	1.47	0.16	1.03	0.04	1.20	1.40	1.02
1976	1.16	0.06	1.26	0.11	1.07	0.03	1.14	1.22	1.06
1977	1.23	0.06	1.37	0.12	1.11	0.03	1.21	1.34	1.11
1978	1.21	0.07	1.31	0.10	1.12	0.07	1.21	1.27	1.16
1979	1.17	0.05	1.26	0.08	1.09	0.04	1.16	1.23	1.09

Ratio of μ 1979/1959:

	.87		.81		.99		.89	.83	1.01

Continuously compounded annual growth rate:

	−.007		−.01		−.0005		−.006	−.009	.004

SOURCES: Blue Cross–Blue Shield Association, *Blue Cross–Blue Shield Fact Book* (Chicago: BCBSA, various years); CPI Data Tape, U.S. Department of Labor, Bureau of Labor Statistics, Washington, D.C.; *Source Book of Health Insurance Data* (Washington, D.C.: Health Insurance Association of America, yearly).

The price of Blues can be further disaggregated into separate prices for Blue Cross and Blue Shield. These data are available only for 1969 to 1979 and are measured in a somewhat different manner from the previous figures. They produce slightly lower prices for Blues overall, as seen in Table 7–4. Also, the data show a small but insig-

Table 7–4. Price of Blue Cross and Blue Shield Insurance (Calculated Separately).

| | *States Weighted Equally* | | | | *States Weighted by Premiums* | |
| | *Blue Cross* | | *Blue Shield* | | *Blue Cross* | *Blue Shield* |
	μ	SD	μ	SD	μ	μ
1969	1.05	0.05	1.13	0.08	1.02	1.09
1970	1.04	0.04	1.32	1.51	1.01	1.16
1971	1.06	0.05	1.11	0.08	1.06	1.11
1972	1.10	0.06	1.15	0.09	1.09	1.15
1973	1.10	0.05	1.14	0.06	1.10	1.12
1974	1.07	0.05	1.10	0.05	1.05	1.08
1975	1.02	0.05	1.05	0.06	1.01	1.03
1976	1.06	0.04	1.32	1.44	1.05	1.22
1977	1.10	0.04	1.14	0.05	1.10	1.13
1978	1.12	0.05	1.15	0.05	1.10	1.13
1979	1.08	0.04	1.15	0.38	1.07	1.14

SOURCES: Blue Cross–Blue Shield Association, *Blue Cross–Blue Shield Fact Book* (Chicago: BCBSA, various years); CPI Data Tape, U.S. Department of Labor, Bureau of Labor Statistics, Washington, D.C.; *Source Book of Health Insurance Data* (Washington, D.C.: Health Insurance Association of America, yearly).

nificant increase in the prices of both Blue Cross and Blue Shield over time. Table 7–4 also shows that the price for Blue Cross is somewhat lower than that for Blue Shield. Loading fees are typically lower for hospital (as opposed to physician) coverage, presumably because hospital coverage involves larger, less frequent claims. If the costs of handling a claim are invariant to the size of the claim, then the loading fee (price) for hospital insurance would tend to be smaller than that for physician insurance, as the average claim is higher for hospital care.

Table 7–5 displays the prices and price changes of insurance for each state by several measures. The previously discussed relationships hold for each state as well as for the national averages. In Table 7–5, prices are displayed in sets of: the overall price, the commercial price, the Blues price, the Blue Cross price, and the Blue Shield price. The first column of each set gives the price in 1959; the second column gives the price for 1979; and the third gives the ratio of 1979 to 1959 prices. The same is true for the columns showing Blue Cross/Blue Shield prices, except that the first year of available data is 1969 instead of 1959.

Table 7–5.   Prices of All, Commercial, Blues, and Blue Cross and Blue Shield Insurance for Each State.

	All			Commercial			Blues			Blue Cross			Blue Shield		
	1959	1979	1979/ 1959	1959	1979	1979/ 1959	1959	1979	1979/ 1959	1969	1979	1979/ 1969	1969	1979	1979/ 1969
Ala.	1.34	1.17	0.87	1.51	1.26	0.83	1.12	1.08	0.97	1.04	1.10	1.05	1.04	1.10	1.05
Alaska	1.31	1.21	0.93	1.36	1.22	0.90	1.15	1.17	1.02	—	—	—	—	—	—
Ariz.	1.31	1.17	0.89	1.42	1.20	0.85	1.09	1.10	1.01	1.09	1.16	1.07	1.13	1.16	1.03
Ark.	1.40	1.14	0.81	1.52	1.24	0.81	1.14	1.04	0.92	1.06	1.04	0.98	1.06	1.04	0.98
Calif.	1.27	1.10	0.86	1.34	1.14	0.85	1.13	1.06	0.94	1.05	1.12	1.07	1.15	1.17	1.02
Colo.	1.25	1.23	0.98	1.52	1.33	0.87	1.07	1.11	1.04	1.07	1.13	1.06	1.20	1.13	0.94
Conn.	1.24	1.08	0.87	1.36	1.13	0.83	1.11	1.03	0.93	0.95	1.03	1.08	1.10	1.03	0.93
Del.	1.26	1.13	0.90	1.93	1.13	0.58	1.02	1.12	1.10	1.01	1.13	1.12	1.10	1.13	1.03
D.C.	1.24	1.16	0.94	1.74	1.31	0.75	1.08	1.12	1.04	1.06	1.05	1.00	1.06	1.13	1.06
Fla.	1.54	1.21	0.79	1.73	1.22	0.71	1.08	1.16	1.08	1.04	1.12	1.08	1.21	1.22	1.01
Ga.	1.57	1.20	0.76	1.67	1.24	0.74	1.11	1.10	0.99	1.08	1.08	1.00	1.16	1.11	0.96
Hawaii	1.33	1.11	0.84	1.65	1.12	0.68	1.13	1.11	0.98	—	—	—	1.09	1.04	0.95
Idaho	1.49	1.25	0.84	1.60	1.43	0.89	1.13	1.11	0.99	1.10	1.13	1.03	1.15	1.10	0.96
Ill.	1.31	1.20	0.91	1.47	1.26	0.86	1.02	1.09	1.07	1.00	1.10	1.09	1.10	1.10	1.00
Ind.	1.36	1.18	0.86	1.52	1.27	0.84	1.12	1.08	0.97	1.03	1.04	1.02	1.08	1.07	0.99
Iowa	1.42	1.20	0.84	1.62	1.35	0.83	1.13	1.08	0.96	1.06	1.06	1.00	1.21	1.07	0.89
Kan.	1.38	1.09	0.79	1.65	1.18	0.72	1.07	1.03	0.96	1.08	0.98	0.91	1.12	1.07	0.96
Ky.	1.39	1.16	0.84	1.64	1.32	0.80	1.11	1.06	0.95	1.02	1.07	1.05	1.17	1.07	0.91
La.	1.35	1.13	0.84	1.42	1.17	0.83	1.13	1.05	0.93	1.06	1.06	1.00	—	—	—
Maine	1.32	1.16	0.88	1.54	1.27	0.83	1.06	1.08	1.02	1.07	1.08	1.01	1.23	1.08	0.88
Md.	1.30	1.12	0.87	1.59	1.14	0.72	1.01	1.10	1.09	1.05	1.06	1.01	1.12	1.16	1.04
Mass.	1.25	1.13	0.91	1.44	1.18	0.82	1.11	1.11	1.00	1.02	1.07	1.05	1.04	1.12	1.08
Mich.	1.20	1.12	0.93	1.35	1.24	0.92	1.09	1.06	0.97	1.05	1.06	1.01	0.93	1.06	1.14
Minn.	1.30	1.27	0.97	1.51	1.38	0.92	1.07	1.10	1.03	1.04	1.10	1.07	1.01	1.10	1.09
Miss.	1.42	1.21	0.85	1.56	1.26	0.80	1.16	1.09	0.94	1.08	1.09	1.01	1.09	1.09	1.00
Mo.	1.36	1.16	0.85	1.51	1.20	0.79	1.14	1.12	0.98	0.96	1.08	1.13	1.16	1.19	1.03
Mon.	1.45	1.24	0.85	1.51	1.27	0.84	1.28	1.20	0.93	1.12	1.17	1.04	1.11	1.23	1.11
Neb.	1.50	1.25	0.83	1.64	1.44	0.88	1.14	1.05	0.92	1.03	1.07	1.04	1.13	1.07	0.95
Nev.	1.39	1.18	0.85	1.39	1.20	0.86	—	1.09	—	—	—	—	—	1.07	—
N.H.	1.32	1.12	0.85	1.66	1.23	0.74	1.09	1.04	0.96	1.07	1.04	0.97	1.26	1.04	0.82
N.J.	1.25	1.16	0.93	1.48	1.28	0.86	1.04	1.07	1.03	0.88	1.03	1.18	1.12	1.13	1.01
N.M.	1.48	1.20	0.81	1.55	1.24	0.80	1.12	1.11	0.99	1.09	1.10	1.02	1.09	1.10	1.01
N.Y.	1.22	1.18	0.97	1.42	1.23	0.87	1.05	1.16	1.11	0.98	1.07	1.09	1.11	1.09	0.98
N.C.	1.52	1.23	0.81	1.68	1.38	0.82	1.12	1.07	0.95	1.09	1.08	0.99	1.09	1.08	0.99
N.D.	1.40	1.19	0.85	1.66	1.25	0.75	1.14	1.16	1.03	1.00	1.11	1.10	1.02	1.16	1.14
Ohio	1.24	1.13	0.91	1.46	1.17	0.81	1.05	1.10	1.05	1.01	1.07	1.06	1.18	1.14	0.97
Okla.	1.44	1.18	0.82	1.66	1.23	0.74	1.08	1.09	1.00	0.99	1.09	1.10	1.12	1.09	0.97
Ore.	1.33	1.16	0.87	1.63	1.27	0.78	1.08	1.09	1.01	1.11	1.09	0.98	1.14	1.15	1.01
Penn.	1.25	1.13	0.90	1.53	1.26	0.82	1.05	1.08	1.02	1.04	1.04	1.00	1.16	1.12	0.97
P.R.	1.08	1.13	1.05	1.53	1.29	0.84	0.98	1.10	1.12	0.99	1.11	1.12	1.00	1.02	1.02
R.I.	1.61	1.24	0.77	1.70	1.36	0.80	1.17	1.10	0.94	1.03	1.10	1.07	1.15	1.10	0.95
S.C.	1.44	1.35	0.94	1.50	1.39	0.93	1.13	1.22	1.08	—	—	—	1.33	1.17	0.88
S.D.	1.40	1.14	0.82	1.56	1.22	0.78	1.15	1.05	0.92	1.10	1.06	0.97	1.10	1.06	0.97
Tenn.	1.38	1.16	0.84	1.45	1.19	0.82	1.15	1.11	0.97	1.08	1.08	1.00	1.29	1.17	0.91
Texas	1.30	1.20	0.92	1.47	1.28	0.87	1.09	1.10	1.01	1.06	1.07	1.01	1.18	1.15	0.98
Utah	1.30	1.15	0.88	1.54	1.35	0.88	1.09	1.03	0.95	—	—	—	—	—	—
Vt.	1.42	1.16	0.81	1.68	1.27	0.75	1.03	1.07	1.04	1.07	1.03	0.96	1.25	1.08	0.86
Va.	1.33	1.18	0.89	1.55	1.29	0.83	1.13	1.13	1.00	1.12	1.10	0.98	1.11	3.69	3.33
Wash.	1.34	1.10	0.82	1.64	1.25	0.76	1.06	1.02	0.96	1.07	1.01	0.94	1.20	1.05	0.87
W.Va.	1.29	1.26	0.97	1.46	1.44	0.99	1.07	1.13	1.06	1.06	1.09	1.03	1.12	1.12	1.00
Wis.	1.38	1.19	0.86	1.55	1.30	0.84	1.15	1.05	0.92	1.12	1.15	1.02	1.26	0.75	0.60
Wyo.	1.38	1.19	0.86	1.55	1.30	0.84	1.15	1.05	0.92	1.12	1.15	1.02	1.26	0.75	0.60

SOURCES: Blue Cross–Blue Shield Association, *Blue Cross–Blue Shield Fact Book* (Chicago: BCBSA, various years); CPI Data Tape, U.S. Department of Labor, Bureau of Labor Statistics, Washington, D.C.; *Source Book of Health Insurance Data* (Washington, D.C.: Health Insurance Association of America, yearly).

UNDERSTANDING THE DECLINING PRICE

In the previous section we showed that the price of insurance has been declining over time. The puzzling aspect of this decline is that it can be attributed to a decline in the prices of commercial firms alone; the prices of the Blues have been stable. It is easy to imagine that reduced costs of communication and travel and increasingly sophisticated technology would reduce the costs of providing insurance for all firms. But what could explain the declining price of commercial firms' insurance in light of the relatively stable price of the Blues?

In order to find the answer, we will look toward supply and demand characteristics, as these determine the price. Demand has increased over this period, which would, other factors held constant, result in an increased price. We must therefore consider other factors to explain the declining price. Consequently, we will focus on competition in the market and on the factors that would reduce the costs of supplying insurance. Because the markets are believed to be somewhat segmented, changes in the competitiveness of the commercial sector or in the costs of supplying commercial insurance might explain the differentially changing price. We will advance several possible explanations and bring indirect evidence to bear, when possible. The potential explanations will be tested in regression analysis when data permit.

Increased Competition

Increased competition in the health insurance market could reduce the price of health insurance. The efficient firms would begin to dominate the market; inefficient firms would drop out. Firms would increasingly be looking for ways to cut administrative costs, and extra-normal profits would be reduced.

Since the Blues and the commercial insurers may sell a differentiated product, it is possible that the increased competition could have occurred primarily in the commercial sector. Although this idea is appealing on conceptual grounds, some indicative data on for-profits over this period are inconsistent with a systematic increase in competition. Table 7–6, column two, shows that profits of commercial insurance companies as a percentage of premiums did not systematically decline over this period. In addition, even though the Blues

Table 7–6.   Corporate Profits, Profit Rate, Percentage
Compensation, and Rate of Return, 1959–1981.

	Corporate Profits After Tax (000,000)	Profits/ Premiums	Compensation/ Premiums	Rate of[a] Return
1959	460	—	—	0.0143
1960	422	0.0564	0.5945	0.0116
1961	376	0.0454	0.5625	0.0144
1962	284	0.0309	0.5380	0.0149
1963	−226	−0.0225	0.5280	0.0144
1964	−485	−0.0437	0.5157	0.0232
1965	−601	−0.0496	0.5032	0.0197
1966	47	0.0037	0.5125	0.0136
1967	−180	−0.0133	0.5268	0.0113
1968	−673	−0.0447	0.5156	0.0046
1969	−1093	−0.0632	0.4810	0.0045
1970	−271	−0.0136	0.4606	0.0098
1971	410	0.0180	0.4283	0.0099
1972	592	0.0226	0.4088	0.0041
1973	28	0.0010	0.4073	−0.0175
1974	−1766	−0.0544	0.4003	−0.0378
1975	−2352	−0.0636	0.3835	−0.0114
1976	−226	−0.0052	0.3547	0.0026
1977	2773	0.0550	0.3396	−0.0156
1978	3172	0.0542	0.3316	−0.0171
1979	2176	0.0333	0.3309	−0.0262
1980	3540	0.0474	0.3221	−0.0105
1981	1629	0.0192	0.3119	0.0533

SOURCES: Blue Cross–Blue Shield Association, *Blue Cross–Blue Shield Fact Book* (Chicago: BCBSA, various years); CPI Data Tape, U.S. Department of Labor, Bureau of Labor Statistics, Washington, D.C.; *Source Book of Health Insurance Data* (Washington, D.C.: Health Insurance Association of America, yearly); R. Ibbotson and R. Sinquefield, *Stocks, Bonds, Bills and Inflation* (Charlottesville, Va: Financial Analysis Research Foundation, 1984); U.S. Chamber of Commerce, *Survey of Current Business* 59, no. 8 (Washington D.C.: Bureau of Economic Analysis):30–31 and 60, no. 4 (Washington D.C.: Bureau of Economic Analysis):25.

[a]U.S. Treasury bill inflation-adjusted total returns.

hold some monopoly power, it seems unlikely that over a twenty-year period the competitive effects would be felt only in the commercial sector, without spillover to the Blues.

Errors in Forecasting Claims

The price of insurance could decline if insurers consistently underestimated the magnitude of the claims they would have to pay. This error could occur because of repeated, unexpected increases in covered individuals' use of, or the price of, medical care, resulting in unexpectedly large claims. The negative profits that commercial insurers have suffered during some years is consistent with the existence of some forecast errors, but not of systematic or repeated errors. It seems unlikely that systematic errors would occur for only the commercial sector and not the Blues.

Decreasing Taxes

Taxes imposed on health insurers raise the costs of supplying insurance and consequently raise the price of insurance, all else being equal. A decrease in the statutory (or effective) tax rate over this time period could account for a decline in the price of insurance. Furthermore, since the Blues are generally exempt from taxes, a decrease in taxes would have a greater effect on commercial insurers and could explain the differential decline in the price of the commercials.

The effective federal corporate income tax rate declined from 41.4 percent to 25.4 percent over the time period in question; the statutory rate declined only slightly, from 52 to 46 percent.[10] Statutory state corporate income taxes, which are of smaller magnitude than the federal tax, increased. In 1960, the rate was 3.59 percent on average (equally weighted by state). By 1979 the rate had risen to 6.15 percent. The corresponding effective tax rates for state taxes are not readily available to determine whether or not effective taxes have increased at the same rate, or at all.

Premium taxes on both Blues and the commercial sector were stable over the period. The average premium tax on Blues was generally 0.52 percent in 1959 and 0.62 percent in 1979. For the commercial sector the rates were 1.44 percent and 1.40 percent, respectively, for in-state firms, and 2.32 percent and 2.36 percent for out-of-state firms.

Administrative Costs

If administrative costs were to decline, the price of commercial insurance would be expected to decline in the competitive market. There are several types of administrative costs to consider.

---

10. See Joseph Pechman, *Federal Tax Policy* (Washington, D.C.: Brookings Institution, 1983), p. 144.

Change in Technology.   Advances in computer technology and communications could reduce administrative costs and consequently reduce the price of insurance. These advances could even reduce the cost of adverse selection and moral hazard by reducing the informational costs of detecting high risks, monitoring coordination of benefits clauses, and monitoring unnecessary or exorbitant claims.

Although we have little direct data on this, data on the percentages of premiums paid as salaries may be an indicator of administrative costs; the lower percentage flowing to labor could indicate a higher productivity of non-labor inputs, e.g., of capital. The decline in the percentage of premiums allocated for compensation of commercial insurers' employees is consistent with the greater productivity of capital (see Table 7–6, column three). However, the increased productivity of capital would be available to both for-profit and nonprofit insurers. Even if the Blues were relatively slow to adapt because of administrative slack attributed to their nonprofit status, they would be expected to respond over two decades.

Growth of Group Insurance.   Insuring through a group reduces the per capita costs of supplying insurance by reducing the per capita administrative and marketing costs as well as reducing the costs of adverse selection. The percentage of insurance sold through groups has increased over the last several decades and could explain the declining price of commercial insurance—if group coverage grew faster in the commercial sector.[11] Unfortunately, there is little direct empirical evidence on the differential percentage of group sales by profit status over time.

Expansion of the Market and Economies of Scale.   At face value, if economies of scale occur in the production of insurance as the size of the market increases, more firms might be able to benefit by reaching their optimal lower-cost size as the market increases in size. Prices would consequently decline. Although the market has grown over time, the logic of this hypothesis does not hold up under scrutiny. We would expect both Blues and commercial firms to reap benefits from econ-

---

11. The percentage of group enrollment appears to be high and similar for both sectors; for example, in 1977 the percentages were 83 for commercial, 82 for Blue Cross, and 80 for Blue Shield.

omies of scale available in the larger market, so this does not appear to explain the differential change in prices. More important, however, is that, except for the artificial constraints on Blues, firms would be expected to move toward their optimal size even without growth in the sector. Furthermore, larger market does not ensure larger size of firms; additional firms may appear, each competing to achieve a larger size.[12]

Increased Claim Size.   Increased claim size could result in declining prices if the costs of administering claims did not rise by as much as the average claim. The real costs of health care have increased substantially over time. For example, in 1972 dollars, the average cost per stay in the hospital increased from $340 in 1959 to $912 in 1979. There is some evidence that the costs of administering a claim have not increased as much as has claim size. The fact that the price index for health care has grown faster than the CPI is consistent with this possibility (as the CPI may indicate costs of administering claims) and would result in declining prices. However, the effect would be expected to be similar for both sectors. If anything, Blues' average claim size might be expected to increase relatively faster, as they are increasingly more likely to offer deductibles than they did in the past, which would eliminate the small claims.

Costs of Regulations and Reserves.   The costs of supplying insurance may be affected by state regulations. There is the generalized red tape of filing policies and loss ratios and the licensing of sales staff. In addition, regulations on the size and type of reserves may impose significant opportunity costs to the firm.[13] The size of reserves required by the states may be in excess of the profit-maximizing size. States also restrain the type of investment, mandating only "prudent"

12. Because the Blues have geographic monopolies, increased market size may increase their firm size, while in the commercial sector there may be more firms but not necessarily larger firms. One way in which the commercial firms, but not the Blues, might benefit through economies of scale could be through an expansion of the entire insurance market, i.e., commercial firms can sell more than one type of insurance, while Blues sell only health insurance.

13. The greater the reserves, the greater the chance that consumers will get their claims paid, even in the case of extraordinary total claims. However, the chance that investors will be paid their return is reduced, increasing the default risk to investors or lowering the option value of the firm. Firms might prefer to have no reserves and reduce the default risk to investors.

investments. These regulations impose both direct and opportunity costs on the firm and may make supplying insurance more costly. Changes in regulations and requirements could affect the costs of supplying insurance, and consequently the price. Changes in the rate of return on investments could also change the opportunity costs of the reserve requirements.

Input Prices.   Declining prices of capital and labor could account for the decline in the price of commercial health insurance. However, these should affect the for-profit and nonprofit sectors approximately equally.

DATA AND METHODS OF EMPIRICAL ANALYSIS

Data

A data set has been developed appropriate to empirical analysis of the price of health insurance and its changes over time. The data set includes information on premiums and benefits for each of the Blues and for commercial firms, sales tax rates on each sector as well as corporate income taxes, and socioeconomic and demographic variables. The state is used as the unit of observation because it is appropriate to these markets (which are segmented to some extent by, for example, state taxation and regulation) and because relevant data are available over time at the state level. In the few states in which there is more than one Blue Cross or Blue Shield plan, a single observation is made for the state by aggregating the plans. (Note that the Blue Cross/Blue Shield business of New Hampshire and Vermont is administered by one plan but treated as two observations in the empirical analysis.) Using this data, some of the above-mentioned hypotheses can be examined.

Estimation Methods

Reduced-form equations of the price of insurance are estimated for the nonprofit and for-profit sectors, respectively. The regressions are estimated separately for the nonprofit and for-profit sectors because these are believed to be segmented markets and because each sector may respond differently to the independent variables. We want to allow the coefficients to take on different values, and are especially interested in estimates of the commercial sector, as this is the sector with the declining price.

The reduced-form equations are initially estimated separately for each year. The cross-sectional and time-series estimates will be pooled if the coefficients are stable over time and if there is no significant loss in making the coefficients the same for each year. Pooling enhances the degrees of freedom and may reduce the standard errors of the estimates. Another advantage of pooling is that the estimated coefficients will give a summary statistic of the effects we are seeking to measure. Because there are too few years of data, we cannot effectively perform time-series analysis.

The general form of the reduced-form pooled equation is as follows:

$$P_{it} = a + B_k X_{kit} + v_k Y_{kt} + e_{it} \quad \text{for}$$
$$i = 1 \ldots n, t = 1 \ldots T, k = 1 \ldots K$$

Where: i is for each state

t is for each year

a is the intercept term

P_{it} is the price in state i for time period t

X_{kit} is the value of independent variable k for it.

B_k is the coefficient of X_k

Y_{kt} is the value of the independent variable k that is available only at the national level

v_k is the coefficient of y_k

e_{it} is the error term that is assumed to have zero mean and constant variance

From this general formulation we will examine alternative specifications to find the most appropriate formulation.[14] We will compare this general specification to error component models and fixed effects (allowing each year and each state or region to have a separate effect). Dummy variables on regions have the advantage over those on states in that they allow more degrees of freedom. As seen in Table 7–5, states in the same region have similar price declines and may thus be grouped together.

---

14. For a discussion of the pooling of cross-sectional and time-series data, see George G. Judge et al., *The Theory and Practice of Econometrics*, 2d ed. (New York: Wiley, 1980), chap. 8.

Dependent Variable: Price of Health Insurance

The price of commercial insurance is calculated as the ratio of yearly premiums to yearly benefits.[15]

Independent Variables

Independent variables are entered into the reduced-form estimates to correspond to some of the hypotheses and to control for other supply and demand. The symbols, means, and standard deviations of the independent variables are displayed in Table 7–7.

State and Federal Corporate Income Tax Rate. As the effective federal corporate tax rate declines, so could the price of commercial health insurance. Although the effective rate may vary by state, data are not available; the effective rate is reported at the national level.[16] This variable is entered into the equation for each sector. The tax rate would directly raise the costs of supplying commercial insurance while affecting the Blues' price indirectly by increasing the demand for Blues. Thus the tax rate is expected to produce a positive coefficient for Blues' as well as for commercial firms.

Premium Taxes on Commercial Insurance. The price of insurance could vary with the state sales tax imposed on premiums. Each state's tax rates on out-of-state and in-state commercial insurance as well as on Blues are entered as explanatory variables. A positive coefficient is predicted for all coefficients in both sectors. The argument for including all taxes in regressions for both sectors is parallel to that discussed for corporate tax.

---

15. Premiums are recorded on an earned basis; benefits are recorded as they are paid out in claims. Therefore, premiums are recorded contemporaneously and benefits are recorded with a comparative lag. The partially lagged benefits could be a good predictor of expected benefits, but empirically the lag does not have much of an effect on the regression results.

Excluded from the measure of premiums and benefits is insurance provided directly by the government (e.g., Medicaid, Medicare, Veterans Administration benefits) and self-insurance conducted by corporations. Administrative services only (ASO) contracts sold through insurers are included in the premiums and produce a downward bias in price because premiums do not cover risk-taking. However, any bias introduced by the growth of ASO contracts is expected to be small, as they were a small part of the insurance market in the years studied.

16. Pechman, *Federal Tax Policy*, p. 144.

Table 7–7. Dependent and Independent Variables: Symbol, Definition Means, and Standard Deviation.

Symbol	Definition	Mean	S. D.
Dependent			
COMPRI	The price of commercial insurance	1.43	.15
BLUPRI	Price of Blues insurance	1.08	.11
Independent			
OUTSTTAX	Tax rate on out-of-state commercial insurers	2.33	.49
INSTTAX	Tax rate on in-state commercial insurers (%)	1.43	.93
BLUETAX	Tax rate on the Blues (%)	.45	.76
CORPTAX	State corporate profits tax rate (%)	4.67	2.90
FEDTAX	Federal corporate tax rate (national)[a]	33.21	4.52
INCRPL	Real per capita income, logged	5.95	.24
EMPLOY	Proportion of the population employed	.32	.05
AVCOSTR	Real average cost per stay to the hospital	1.69	.48
POPL	The log of the population of the state	5.53	1.01
AGE65	Percentage of population 65 years or over	.10	.02
REGU	Prior approval of state necessary for Blues to change individual rates (=1)	.71	.45
INFMORT	Infant deaths per 100,000 births	.20	.06
USTBILL	U.S. Treasury bill rate	.004	.018
LK	Percentage of premiums paid toward employee compensation[b]	.44	.09

Sources: Blue Cross–Blue Shield Association, *Blue Cross–Blue Shield Fact Book* (Chicago: BCBSA, various years); CPI Data Tape, U.S. Department of Labor, Bureau of Labor Statistics, Washington, D.C.; *Source Book of Health Insurance Data* (Washington, D.C.: Health Insurance Association of America, yearly); R. Ibbotson and R. Sinquefield, *Stocks, Bonds, Bills and Inflation* (Charlottesville, Va.: Financial Analysis Research Foundation, 1984); National Association of Life Underwriters, *Survey of Extent of Regulation and Taxation of Blue Cross–Blue Shield Plans* (Washington, D.C.: NALU, various years).

Note: The means and standard deviations apply to all 21 years. Real dollars are calculated in 1972 dollars. Alaska and Nevada are dropped from these calculations and the regressions, as they are both outliers. Neither had in-state Blue Cross in the early years.

[a]These data are found in Table 7–6, column four.
[b]These data are found in Table 7–6, column three.

Average Cost Per Stay in the Hospital.   If the cost of administering claims is relatively invariant to claim size, as the average size of the claim increases, the price should decline. The average cost per stay in the hospital is used as a proxy for the size of the claims. Hospital costs may be a good proxy for overall costs because they are a higher percentage of all costs and may be correlated with other medical care prices. Average cost per stay would be predicted to reduce costs of supplying insurance and thus to have a negative coefficient. However, average cost per stay could also affect the demand for insurance possibly offsetting the negative effect.

Size of Market: State Population.   The population of the state is entered as a proxy variable for the potential size of the insurance market. If there are significant economies of scale, the proxy could have a negative coefficient.

Percentage of Population Employed.   The percentage of the population that is employed (from census data) is included as a proxy for group purchase of insurance. Direct observations of the percentage of group sales are not available by state. Selling insurance through a group reduces administrative costs and would be expected to have a negative coefficient. The percentage employed could also increase demand as more insurance is provided to take advantage of tax subsidies, resulting in a positive effect on price that would at least partially offset the effects of group insurance.

Regulations.   Whether prior approval of the state is needed for Blues to increase their rates on individual policies is used as a proxy for the costs imposed by regulations. This variable takes on the value of one if approval is needed and zero otherwise. As a proxy for the red tape of regulations, this variable is predicted to raise the costs of supplying insurance for each sector. However, in the short run at least, it may constrain increases in Blues' prices.

Forecast Error.   Price is also affected by the accuracy of insurers' forecast of claims. A proxy for forecast accuracy (error) was developed. It is the ratio of the average growth rate in claims over five years to the growth rate in the last year. As this ratio gets smaller (i.e., faster recent growth and hence underestimation of claims), price can be expected to decline.

Cost of Capital/Rate of Return on Reserves.   The price of commercial insurance could be affected by the cost of capital/rate of return in several different ways. An increase in the cost of capital, as it is an input price, could increase the price of insurance. Alternatively, an increase in the cost of capital, which is also the rate of return, could decrease the price of commercial insurance as the return on investments rises. Because the reserve requirement is higher for commercial insurers, it may have a larger effect on commercial firms. A proxy for the cost of capital/rate of return on reserves, which must be of prudently low risk, is the rate of return on U.S. Treasury bills, a low-risk asset. Because this financial market is primarily national, only a national rate of return is used in estimation.

Percentage Employee Compensation. The percentage of the premium that goes toward employee compensation (see Table 7–6, column three) is used as a proxy for the change in technology. As capital-intensive technology such as computers increases productivity, one would expect that the percentage of total expense (using premiums as an approximation of the total expense) flowing to employee compensation would decrease. Thus, we predict a positive relationship between employee compensation's share of the premium and price of health insurance.

Other Demand Variables. Other variables are entered to control for demand. Income per capita is used as a control both because demand increases with income (due to the pure income effect) and also because of the increased value of the tax subsidy in purchasing insurance. This variable is so highly correlated with wages that it may also act as a control on labor input prices. It is also highly correlated at the state level with Medicaid coverage and may control for the extent of Medicaid coverage. Percentage of the population over the age of sixty-five is entered, as it is highly correlated at the state level with Medicare coverage. It may also serve as a proxy (along with the infant mortality rate) for health status, as health status can affect (or be affected by) the demand for insurance.

RESULTS

Tests showed that the cross-sectional and time-series data could be pooled without significant loss of explanatory power for both the commercial firms and the Blues. The estimated coefficients of the separate cross-sectional estimates were insignificantly different over time. The magnitude of the coefficients of the pooled results typically fell within the range of the estimates of the separate cross-sectional coefficients, but were estimated with smaller standard errors.

Pooled cross-sectional and time-series regressions are estimated for the price of Blue Cross/Blue Shield, on the one hand, and commercial insurance on the other. The results are displayed in Table 7–8. Since we are especially interested in the results for the commercial sector, we will compare the results for commercial insurance to that of the Blues to see if the price of the Blues would remain stable under similar circumstances, i.e., to see if they have different coefficients.

Table 7–8.   Regression Results: Pooled Cross-Section and Time Series.

Variable	COMPRI		BLUPRI	
	Coefficient	T	Coefficient	T
INTERCEPT	3.38	9.50	1.04	3.26
OUTSTTAX	0.02	2.12	−0.02	2.38
INSTTAX	0.00	0.24	0.01	2.35
BLUETAX	−0.02	3.42	0.01	2.02
CORPTAX	0.00	1.96	−0.00	0.49
FEDTAX	−0.01	0.34	0.01	2.63
INCRPL	0.01	0.11	−0.03	0.61
EMPLOY	0.11	0.70	−0.33	2.31
AVCOSTR	−0.14	5.14	0.00	0.03
POPL	−0.06	10.89	−0.02	4.40
AGE65	0.45	2.26	0.45	2.54
REGU	−0.00	0.15	0.01	0.78
INFMORT	−0.05	0.34	0.09	0.72
USTBILL	−0.63	10.30	0.10	0.31
TIME	−0.03	5.62	0.01	1.22
TIME2	−0.00	5.03	0.00	1.41
LK	−0.02	7.50	0.00	0.06
Mid Atlantic	0.06	3.21	0.06	3.58
East North Central	0.00	0.05	0.06	3.15
West North Central	−0.01	0.62	0.03	2.33
South Atlantic	0.05	3.09	0.03	2.02
East South Atlantic	0.01	0.64	−0.00	0.18
West South Atlantic	−0.08	3.30	0.03	1.42
Mountain	−0.11	6.78	0.01	0.68
Pacific	−0.04	1.88	0.07	3.56
R^2	.60		.10	

SOURCES: Blue Cross–Blue Shield Association, *Blue Cross–Blue Shield Fact Book* (Chicago: BCBSA, various years); CPI Data Tape, U.S. Department of Labor, Bureau of Labor Statistics, Washington, D.C.; *Source Book of Health Insurance Data* (Washington, D.C.: Health Insurance Association of America, yearly); R. Ibbotson and R. Sinquefield, *Stocks, Bonds, Bills and Inflation* (Charlottesville, Va.: Financial Analysis Research Foundation, 1984); National Association of Life Underwriters, *Survey of Extent of Regulation and Taxation of Blue Cross–Blue Shield Plans* (Washington, D.C.: NALU, various years).

We compared fixed effects and error component models and found the fixed effects models to have better explanatory power. The specification of the pooled model that we present in Table 7–8 has effects for each of ten geographical regions (New England is the omitted region). Using the fixed effects for regions appeared to give more reasonable results than using the complete set of state effects. State effects overcontrolled for the variation across states, and the coefficients on the other explanatory variables became insignificant. A variable for time and time squared is the preferred specification to control for variations over the years. Separate dummies for each year were too highly correlated with the national-only data.

A potential advantage to pooling is that we can use independent variables that are available only at the national level. However, in this case, the national-only variables all tended to exhibit similar trends. Thus, the national level variables (*USTBILLS, LK,* and *FEDTAX*) are highly correlated with each other and with the time and time-squared variables, which means that the coefficients of these variables may be unstable and may pick up some of the effects that should be attributed to the other national-only variables.

The proxy variable for forecast error is omitted from the displayed results because the coefficient was insignificant in the regressions and using it necessarily eliminated the first four years of data that were required to estimate it. Thus, it seemed preferable to retain the extra four years of observations and omit the variable forecast error.

Table 7–8 shows that a reasonable amount of the variation in the price of commercial insurance (an R^2 of .60) can be explained by the set of independent variables. In contrast, the same variables are able to explain relatively little of the variation in the Blues' price (R^2 of .09).[17] The greater explanatory power in the commercial sector may occur because that sector is more sensitive to market forces (e.g., no tax advantage and less monopoly power) and/or because we have a better understanding of the behavior of the for-profit than of the non-profit sector.

The regression results show that several of the hypothesized factors are significant in explaining the variation in price. However, only a

17. The R^2 for the separate regressions for each year for Blues were higher than the pooled R^2, ranging from 0.11 to 0.45. The R^2 for the Blues were reduced by pooling. However, the tests for the restrictions of pooling did not reject pooling. In contrast, the R^2 for the commercial sector was somewhat increased by pooling.

few of them can simultaneously explain the decline in the price of commercial insurance and the stable price of the Blues.

The tax variables are typically significant in explaining both commercial and Blues' price. However, with the exception of the effective federal tax rate (*FEDTAX*), the taxes did not change much over the period of observation and consequently cannot account for the declining price of commercial insurance. The coefficients of taxes were all expected to be positive. However, the coefficient of tax on the Blues in the estimate of commercial insurance and the tax on out-of-state premiums in the Blues' regression were both negative.

The results support several hypotheses under the general rubric of economies of scale, including economies of scale that occur with growth in size of claims as well as growth in the size of the market. The average cost per hospital stay (in 1972 dollars) has a negative and significant effect in estimates of commercial insurance, as predicted. Over this time period, the real average cost per stay increased 2.75 times. Using this change, the estimated coefficient of −0.14, and a linearity assumption, we can account for the entire decline in the price of commercial insurance over this period. In addition, the coefficient of *AVCOSTR* is insignificant in the regression of Blues' price. Thus, the increasing average cost of real claims could account for the declining price of commercial insurance in the face of an unchanging price of Blues if for some reason Blues are truly unaffected by the increased size of claims.

The state's total population also has a negative and significant effect on price, as would be predicted if population is a proxy for the potential size of the market and markets are segmented by state taxes and regulations. As population grows, so does the size of the market, hence the possibility of economies of scale. Population has increased over this period, so the growth in population could account for the declining price. Although the coefficient of population was negative for the estimates of both prices, Blues' coefficient was about a third of the absolute size of that of the commercial sector. The coefficients of population were surprisingly significant, so much so that one wonders whether they might be controlling for other, unobserved factors correlated with population. In the case of large interstate commercial firms, the size of a single state would not be expected to matter except for the regulation and tax barriers to entry.

Contrary to expectations, the coefficient of employment (as a proxy for group sales) did not have a significant effect on the price of commercial insurance.[18] It did have a significant and negative effect on the Blues' price. As employment increased over this period from 27 to 40 percent, one would have expected the price of the Blues to decline, *ceteris paribus*.

The coefficient of regulation is insignificant in both the regressions. Alternative measures of the degree of regulation did not increase the significance of the coefficient. Unfortunately, more comprehensive measures of the costs of regulation are not readily available.

Of the three independent variables that are measured at the national level—*LK*, *USTBILL*, and *FEDTAX*—the first two are found to affect the price of commercial insurance negatively and significantly. The negative coefficient of *USTBILL* is consistent with its effect as a proxy for the rate of return on investments. As was expected, *USTBILL* is more important in commercial insurance than it is in the Blues. The negative coefficient of *LK* runs contrary to the positive effect that it was predicted to have. As mentioned above, the national variables are all highly correlated with each other and with the time trend; as a result each coefficient may be unstable.

CONCLUSIONS

We have shown that the overall price of insurance has decreased over the last two decades. We have also shown that the decline is due entirely to the change in the price of commercial insurance; the price of Blue Cross/Blue Shield insurance has remained stable over the same period. The downward trend in the price of commercial insurance and the stable price of Blues insurance are in sharp contrast to the rising prices of health care in general. As the price of commercial insurance has declined, the prices of commercial and Blues insurance have approached each other. The increased similarity in price may reflect the fact that the two sectors are becoming more alike over time.

We have offered explanations of the differential decline in the price of insurance in the nonprofit and the commercial sector. Several hypotheses would explain the decline in the overall price of insurance.

---

18. The insignificance may be attributed to the relatively high correlation of income and employment, or because employment has offsetting effects on price.

Only a few of these are, at face value, consistent with both the decline in the price of commercial insurance and the stable price of the Blues. Other factors may explain the differential price changes, as they could apply systematically to only the commercial sector. The for-profit and nonprofit sectors may differ in their goals, their methods, and the services they offer. They are believed to offer differentiated services and to constitute related but segmented markets, as they are taxed and regulated differently by the states.

Although we have not been able to resolve the puzzle, we have provided some insight and evidence. One empirical finding is that the same variables that explain the variation in the price of commercial insurance do not explain much of the variation in the Blues' price. This finding is consistent with a segmented market in which prices change differentially by sector over time. Furthermore, the same variables affect prices in the sectors differently.

We have provided some evidence that the declining price of commercial insurance is due to an increase in claim size, and that this significantly affects only the price of the commercial sector. Proxies for other types of economies of scale were found to affect the prices of both sectors significantly, but to affect the commercial sector with a greater magnitude.

Other hypotheses were advanced, but could not be systematically and directly evaluated empirically. These include increased competition in the commercial sector, increased enrollment of groups in the commercial sector, reductions in effective state corporate taxes imposed on commercial insurance, and slow adaptation of technology by the Blues because of administrative slack.

The newly observed declining price of health insurance is an important discovery, as it has a potentially significant effect on the welfare of society. From society's perspective, the declining price of health insurance, like most declining prices, is largely beneficial. Cost-saving changes in technology, increased competition, gains from economies of scale, or reduced costs of distorting regulations (e.g., restrictions on the size and type of reserves) would all be beneficial to society.

However, in the case of declining health insurance prices, society may suffer accompanying and perhaps partially offsetting losses. As the price of health insurance declines, more people purchase it, and they purchase more complete coverage. The additional coverage reduces the out-of-pocket price of medical care to consumers, but not the real cost to society. Thus, people use medical care in such a way that the value to them is less than the real cost to society. This produces welfare losses.

The extent of losses due to this moral hazard depends on the price elasticity of demand for health insurance as well as on the price elasticity of demand for medical care. The Rand Health Insurance Study[19] showed that the demand for medical care is increased by more complete insurance coverage. A recent study shows that the demand for commercial insurance is price elastic, while it is price inelastic for the Blues.[20] Thus, the declining price of commercial insurance may cause an increase in insurance coverage, increased utilization of medical care, increased medical care prices, and subsequent further declines in the price of insurance, with welfare losses accruing. Whether there will be net gains or losses to the declining price, and their magnitude, depends upon the importance of the offsetting effects.

19. Joseph P. Newhouse et al., "Some Interim Results from a Controlled Trial of Cost Sharing in Health Insurance," *New England Journal of Medicine* 305, no. 25 (1981): 1501–7.
20. J. L. Sindelar, "The Supply and Demand for Health Insurance: Empirical Estimates," working paper series, Yale Institution for Social and Policy Studies in Medical Economics, 1986.

SELECTED BIBLIOGRAPHY

American Council of Life Insurance. *Life Insurance Fact Book,* pp. 88–89. Washington, D.C.: ACLI, 1984.

Anderson, O. *Blue Cross Since 1929: Accountability and Public Trust.* Cambridge, Mass.: Ballinger, 1975.

Blair, R. D.; P. Ginsburg; and R. J. Vogel. "Blue Cross–Blue Shield Administrative Costs: A Study of Non-Profit Health Insurers." *Economic Inquiry* 13 (June 1975):237–51.

Blair, R. D.; J. R. Jackson; and R. J. Vogel. "Economies of Scale in the Administration of Health Insurance." *Review of Economics and Statistics* 57 (1975):185–89.

Blue Cross Association. *Enrollment and Utilization Data of Blue Cross Plans,* 4th Quarter, Appendix A, pp. 23–25. Chicago: Blue Cross–Blue Shield Association, 1978.

Eilers, R. *Regulation of Blue Cross and Blue Shield Plans.* Homewood, Ill.: Irwin for S. S. Heubner Foundation, 1963.

Eisenstadt, D., and T. Kennedy. "Control and Behavior of Nonprofit Firms: The Case of Blue Shield." *Southern Economic Journal* Vol. 48, no. 1 (July 1981):26–36.

Frech, H. E. III. "The Property Rights Theory of the Firm: Empirical Results from a National Experiment." *Journal of Political Economy* 84, no. 1 (1976):143–52.

———. "The Demand for Health Insurance: Comment." In R. Rossett, ed., *The Role of Health Insurance in the Health Services Sector,* pp. 156–60.

289

New York: Columbia University Press for the National Bureau of Economic Research, 1976.

————. "Market Power in Health Insurance: Effects on Insurance and Medical Markets." *Journal of Industrial Economics* 27, no. 1 (1978):55–72.

————. "Blue Cross, Blue Shield, and Health Care Costs: A Review of the Economic Evidence." In Mark V. Pauly, ed., *National Health Insurance: What Now, What Later, What Never?*, pp. 250–63. Washington, D.C.: American Enterprise Institute, 1980.

Frech, H. E. III, and Paul Ginsburg. "Competition among Health Insurers." In Warren Greenberg, ed., *Competition in the Health Care Sector: Past, Present, and Future*, pp. 210–37. Germantown, Md.: Aspen Systems Corp./Federal Trade Commission, 1978.

Greenspan, N. R., and R. J. Vogel. "Taxation and Its Effect upon Public and Private Health Insurance and Medical Demand." *Health Care Financing Review* 1, no. 4 (1980):39–45.

Health Insurance Association of America. *A Current Profile of Group Medical Expense Insurance in Force in the United States, December 1970.* Chicago: HIAA, 1982.

Judge, G.; W. Griffiths; R. C. Hill; H. Lutkepohl; and T. C. Lee. *The Theory and Practice of Econometrics*, 2d ed., sections 13.1–13.4. New York: Wiley, 1980.

Kass, D., and P. A. Pautler. "The Administrative Costs of Non-Profit Health Insurers." *Economic Inquiry* 19 (1981):515–21.

————. *Physician Control of Blue Shield Plans.* Washington, D.C.: Federal Trade Commission, November 1979.

Law, S. *Blue Cross: What Went Wrong?* New Haven, Conn.: Yale University Press, 1976.

Newhouse, J. P. "New Estimates of Price and Income Elasticities of Medical Care Services." In R. Rossett, ed., *The Role of Health Insurance in the Health Services Sector*, pp. 261–333. New York: Neale Watson Academic Publications, 1977.

Newhouse, J. P., and Charles E. Phelps. "Price and Income Elasticities for Medical Care Services." In M. Perlman, ed., *The Economics of Health and Medical Care*. London: Macmillan, 1974.

Newhouse, J. P.; Willard Manning, et al. "Some Interim Results from a Controlled Trial of Cost Sharing in Health Insurance." *New England Journal of Medicine* 305, no. 25 (1981):1501–7.

Pechman, J. A. *Federal Tax Policy.* Washington, D.C.: Brookings Institution, 1983.

Phelps, C. E. "Demand for Reimbursement Insurance." In R. Rossett, ed., *The Role of Health Insurance in the Health Services Sector*, pp. 115–156. New York: Neale Watson Academic Publications, 1976.

Sindelar, J. L. "The Disincentive Effects of Taxing Health Insurers," Medical Economics Group Working Paper Series, No. 5. New Haven, Conn.: Yale Institution for Social and Policy Studies in Medical Economics, July 1986.

————. "The Supply and Demand for Health Insurance: Empirical Estimates," Medical Economics Group Working Paper Series. New Haven, Conn.: Yale Institution for Social and Policy Studies in Medical Economics, 1986b.

U.S. House of Representatives, Subcommittee on Health. *National Health Insurance Resource Book*. Washington, D.C.: Government Printing Office, 1976.

Vogel, R. J. "The Effects of Taxation on the Differential Efficiency of Non-Profit Health Insurance." *Economic Inquiry* 15 (October 1977):605–9.

8

MONOPOLY IN HEALTH INSURANCE: THE ECONOMICS OF *KARTELL v. BLUE SHIELD OF MASSACHUSETTS*

H. E. Frech III

INTRODUCTION

In the spring of 1985, the U.S. Supreme Court denied certiorari in the case of *Kartell v. Blue Shield of Massachusetts,* thus preserving the previous ruling of the U.S. Court of Appeals for the First Circuit in favor of Blue Shield. This decision marked the end of a long, costly battle that the plaintiffs had first won in the federal district court. One never knows whether the denial of certiorari means that the Court agreed with the court of appeals. On any interpretation, the decision gives Blue Cross and Blue Shield health insurers more freedom from antitrust enforcement.

The plaintiffs in *Kartell* were individual physicians, supported by the Massachusetts Medical Society. The doctors sought to stop Blue Shield from regulating their fees through its reimbursement system. They did not question Blue Shield's right to set its own reimbursement schedule for physician services; they sought the right to charge the patient for the difference, if any, between the physician's fee and the insurance payment. Blue Shield prohibited this charge through a rule known as the ban on balance billing. The plaintiffs claimed that Massachusetts Blue Shield used its market power to drive physicians' fees well below market level, thus reducing competition among physicians, damaging them financially and professionally, and harming consumers.

Blue Shield responded by claiming that there was little competition for physician services and that driving prices charged to Blue Shield customers below market prices was beneficial because it reduced costs. Blue Shield also argued that as a purchaser of medical care it was within its rights to purchase that care as cheaply as possible.

The Lower Court and Appellate Opinions

Judge Andrew A. Caffrey largely agreed with the plaintiffs. He found that the Blue Shield system, with its ban on balance billing, had harmed both price and nonprice competition. As to price competition, he found that the system has the effect of fixing physician prices and "substantially reduces the level of price competition in the market for physician's services in Massachusetts."[1] He found no offsetting procompetitive effects. In the arena of nonprice competition, he found that the system discourages innovation and reduces quality. Judge Caffrey ruled, therefore, that "the ban on balance billing unreasonably restrains trade in the market for physician's services in Massachusetts in violation of Section 1 of the Sherman Act and that its further implementation should be enjoined."[2] Perhaps because he thought it unnecessary, Judge Caffrey rejected the plaintiffs' claim that the Blue Shield system reduced competition in the health insurance market.

The appellate opinion was written by Stephen Breyer, a well-known legal scholar specializing in economic regulation. Surprisingly, the decision to reverse was primarily based on narrow legal grounds. Judge Breyer viewed Blue Shield as the purchaser of medical care. He then argued that "the lawfulness of the term in question [balance billing] stems from the fact that it is an essential part of the price bargain between buyer and seller. Whether or not that price bargain is, in fact, reasonable, is, legally speaking, beside the point, even in the case of a monopolist."[3] The opinion ignored the district court's find-

1. *Kartell v. Blue Shield of Massachusetts*, 582 F. Supp 734, 755 (D.C. Mass. 1984).
2. Ibid.
3. *Kartell v. Blue Shield of Massachusetts*, U.S. Court of Appeals, 749 F.2d 922, 928 (1st Cir. 1984). For an excellent legal analysis of the opinions, see Thayer Freemont-Smith, "Recent Developments in Massachusetts" (Paper presented at the American Bar Association Conference on Antitrust, Washington, D.C., July 1985).

ings that Blue Shield did in fact impair competition. Judge Breyer rejected the plaintiff's argument that market power over physicians increased market power in the insurance market.

THE FACTS OF THE CASE

As is the case in most health insurance markets, Blue Shield of Massachusetts provides physician services insurance in cooperation with Blue Cross, which provides hospital insurance. Both were originally founded by their respective providers, the Massachusetts Medical Society in the case of Blue Shield, and the Massachusetts Hospital Association in the case of Blue Cross. Blue Shield has since become completely independent of the medical society. The Blues, as they are often called, are very successful in Massachusetts. They insure about 74 percent of those with private health insurance and about 60 percent of the state's population.[4] Blue Shield alone insures 56 percent of the population. Massachusetts' is one of the highest Blue Shield market shares in the country. In the typical state, Blue Shield has about 40 percent of the privately insured population, or about 32 percent of the total population. In the private health insurance market, the Blues compete directly with other insurers, including traditional insurers like Aetna and innovative ones like the Harvard Health Maintenance Organization.

Blue Shield pays physicians directly for services provided to about 90 percent of its customers. Participating physicians must agree to accept the Blue Shield allowance as their full payment. Doctors may not bill patients for any amount above the allowance. This constitutes the ban on balance billing. Physicians who have not agreed to this limitation are not allowed participating status. Nonparticipating physicians and their patients receive no payment whatsoever from Blue Shield unless the services were provided in an emergency or outside the commonwealth of Massachusetts. This system is unique to Massachusetts. Elsewhere, except for one of the Blue plans in Washington state, doctors can always bill for the balance and be paid, either directly or indirectly, by the local Blue Shield plan, whether or not they have participating status.

Given the high market share of the Massachusetts Blue Shield plan,

---

4. This section is primarily based on the opinion of Judge Andrew A. Caffrey, *Kartell v. Blue Shield of Massachusetts, supra,* 582 F. Supp at 737.

the refusal to remunerate nonparticipating physicians might violate antitrust law, but Judge Caffrey has ruled that it is mandated by Massachusetts law and hence is immune from antitrust attack. In their relationship with the physicians and hospitals, the Blues influence a second market, the market for health care. Judge Breyer viewed the Blues as a purchaser in this market. I prefer to consider the consumers as the purchasers. It seems more useful to think of the Blues and other insurers as financing and facilitating the transaction rather than purchasing the services and reselling them to the consumers. In that sense they are analogous to credit card companies, such as American Express.

History of Massachusetts Blue Shield

Blue Shield was created by the Massachusetts Medical Society under a special Massachusetts enabling act in 1942. Initially, it created two classes of subscribers. Lower-income subscribers received "unlimited" coverage, under which the doctor was not allowed to balance-bill. Higher-income consumers received "limited" coverage, under which balance billing was allowed. The allowance was set by a formal indemnity benefit schedule. In 1951, Blue Shield subdivided the "unlimited" class, charging higher premiums to the higher-income members of the original class and raising their allowances for physician payment. Initially, more than 90 percent of the subscribers were "unlimited" and thus could not be balance-billed. However, over the years inflation eroded the fixed-dollar income levels that divided the classes, so that by 1967 more than half of the customers were in the highest "limited" class and thus could be balance-billed. Inflation also eroded the level of the fixed allowances (unchanged since 1952) relative to actual market prices. By 1967, Blue Shield allowances were about 30 percent below market fees (charges). Physicians were dissatisfied with the level of reimbursement of their own Blue Shield insurance plan. Nonetheless, a 1966 survey showed that about 90 percent of physicians did not balance-bill any Blue Shield patients, regardless of the physicians' income.

Physician pressure led Blue Shield to eliminate the income distinctions and to base Blue Shield allowances on market fees. The result was the "usual, customary, and reasonable" system that was becoming increasingly popular with Blue Shield plans and that was adopted by Medicare. Under this scheme, a physician was paid the lowest of (a) the submitted charge, (b) the doctor's "usual" charge (the median of recent fees for the procedure), or (c) the "customary" charge in the area (the 90th percentile of the usual charges of all physicians for that procedure). In addition 5 percent was deducted for administrative costs. The ban on balance billing applied to all consumers insured under the system. Blue Shield promised to update the allowed fees at least once a year to reflect changes in market levels. Currently this plan applies to about 90 percent of Blue Shield's subscribers.

Massachusetts Blue Shield's policies require even less consumer out-of-pocket payment than do most other Blue Shield plans. The Massachusetts plans, for the most part, have neither deductibles nor coinsurance. Naturally, the combination of an automatic upward adjustment in insurance payments and 100 percent coverage for a large proportion of the population caused rapid increases in health care costs.

Blue Shield continued its annual updates from 1968 through 1975. By 1976, however, Blue Shield found itself simultaneously losing market share and losing money, thus reducing its reserves. As a remedy, Blue Shield simply skipped its 1976 update, which reduced its payments to physicians by several percentage points. In 1977, Blue Shield filed a new amended schedule of benefits with the insurance commissioner, giving it complete control over updates, with one exception: the annual increase would have to be less than the percentage increase of the Boston Consumer Price Index (excluding medical care). Since then, Blue Shield has depressed its allowance well below market fees. By 1981, the Blue Shield discount reached about 30.7 percent and has remained near that level. Not surprisingly, Blue Shield's market share, profits, and reserves have risen since 1977.

Most physicians find that they must accept these large price discounts from Blue Shield to survive financially in Massachusetts. While only about 13 to 14 percent of physician income comes from fees on which the ban on balance billing is directly applicable, physicians who do not agree to participate in Blue Shield are likely to sacrifice much more. Most directly, they lose the opportunity to receive other Blue Shield payments not subject to the ban. They also lose most older patients who originally were Blue Shield patients but have converted to Medicare. Also, many physicians will be leery of recommending another physician who cannot effectively treat most privately insured consumers. As a result, about 98 percent of Massachusetts physicians participate in Blue Shield.

BACKGROUND: THE NATURE OF COMPETITION IN HEALTH CARE

Competition among hospitals and physicians is imperfect, even in the largest cities with large numbers of competitors. There are two major reasons for the imperfection. First, consumers are poorly informed about alternative, lower-priced sources of medical care. Second, common types of health insurance provide many consumers with little or no incentive to shift to a lower-priced physician or hospital in response to a known price difference.

Traditional health insurance also exacerbates the information problem because there is little incentive to shop around. The effects are the worst with the most anticompetitive type of insurance—complete coverage. For consumers whose medical bills are paid 100 percent by the insurer, there is no incentive to respond to lower medical prices. If the consumer shifted to a lower-cost provider, only the insurer would benefit.

The Existence of Competition

First, all the empirical evidence points to the conclusion that health care demand over the whole market is relatively insensitive to price, with a price elasticity of demand of about -0.15. This finding is inconsistent with monopoly. *If health care were provided by a monopoly facing such a demand curve, that monopoly could raise revenue and lower costs by raising price. Some competition, however flawed, must be restraining the system.*

Second, the existence of competition requires that some consumers be sensitive to price. Consumers with relatively incomplete insurance should be more price sensitive; thus they should choose lower-priced providers. Surveys show that commercial insurance customers whose insurance requires more out-of-pocket payments select lower-priced hospitals than do Blue Cross customers.[5] More statistically sophisticated research by Joseph Newhouse and Charles Phelps also shows that less complete insurance leads to lower prices paid by consumers.[6]

5. Ronald Andersen and Odin W. Anderson, *A Decade of Health Services* (Chicago: University of Chicago Press, 1970), pp. 103–4.
6. Joseph P. Newhouse and Charles E. Phelps, "Price and Income Elasticities for Medical Care Services," in Mark Perlman, ed., *The Economics of Health and Medical Care:*

Perhaps the most powerful evidence for the existence of competition currently comes from Medicare physician services (part B) coverage. Until some recent changes, this coverage was structured much like Blue Shield would be if the plaintiffs in *Kartell* had prevailed. That is, Medicare benefits are heavily discounted from market prices, but they allow balance billing. In this context, a physician who does not balance-bill thereby offers a competitive discount to Medicare customers. In Massachusetts, about 80 percent of physicians did not balance-bill Medicare consumers. As Blue Shield President John Larkin Thompson noted in testimony to Congress, the percentage of doctors who do not balance-bill varies across the state according to the intensity of local doctor competition. In particular, Thompson noted that a lower proportion of physicians balance-bill Medicare patients in Worcester than on Cape Cod because competition is more intense in Worcester.[7]

Increasing Competition

When competition is imperfect, increasing it becomes all the more important. When a building's supporting columns are weak, you do not remove them, you reinforce them. Competition is important in allowing us to have a decentralized private health care system that is responsive to consumer wishes, values, and needs. Without competition, albeit imperfect, consumers have little influence. And because consumers alone know their own values, attitudes toward risk, and life style, such knowledge must enter into good medical decisions.

For example, whether to perform a coronary bypass operation is a common and important medical decision. It cannot be made on purely technical grounds. For most patients, life expectancy is about the same either way. The key to the decision is the patient's own value system. Consumers who forgo the operation face intermittent chest pain, particularly when exercising. Those who choose the operation can expect to live a virtually pain-free life, but not a longer one.

Many of the informational problems that make the competitive market

---

Proceedings of a Conference Held by the International Economic Association at Tokyo (New York: Wiley, 1973), pp. 139–61.

7. John Larkin Thompson, "Report Prepared for Presentation to the Advisory Council on Social Security," (Boston: Blue Shield of Massachusetts, April 6, 1983).

imperfect also make regulation imperfect, including private regulation by Blue Shield. If consumers have trouble judging medical care when their own health is at stake, imagine how hard it must be for regulators to do so far from the scene. Also, competition and regulation are not mutually exclusive. In a regulated system, one may think of competition as reducing the pressure on the regulations, thus helping the regulations to achieve their goals.

Coinsurance and Indemnity Insurance

Price competition makes sense only for the uninsured and for consumers with incomplete insurance benefits. Unfortunately, most of the less complete insurance has some anticompetitive effect. The most common form of incomplete insurance covers 80 percent of costs, requiring the consumer to pay the remaining 20 percent. Consumers with such insurance have some incentive to shift to lower-priced physicians or hospitals in response to a known price differential, but the incentive is weakened by the insurance.

For example, suppose that a consumer were well informed about two physicians, one of whom charges $1,000 for a given service while the other charges $500. For various reasons, many unrelated to technical medical concerns, the consumers may prefer the more costly physician. If the consumer had complete insurance, he would simply go to the more costly physician. If he had the common 20 percent coinsurance, he would save $100—20 percent of the actual savings of $500—by selecting the lower-priced physician. The $100 savings may not be enough to induce the consumer to choose the less costly alternative, but the entire savings of $500 might be enough.

There is only one kind of health insurance that prevents these anticompetitive effects. That is the type commonly called indemnity insurance, wherein the benefit is a fixed dollar amount per service. If the consumer chooses a less expensive provider, he keeps the entire savings himself. As long as the indemnity benefit is set below the price of most providers, indemnity benefits give consumers undiluted incentives to search for and respond to known lower-priced providers. Indemnity insurance also leads directly to more elastic demand curves, hence lower prices.[8]

8. See H. E. Frech III and Paul B. Ginsburg, *Public Health Insurance in Private Medical Markets: Some Problems of National Health Insurance* (Washington, D.C.: American Enter-

Balance Billing and Indemnity Insurance

Allowing balance billing would, in effect, transform the existing Blue Shield 100 percent coverage into an indemnity system. The current allowed fee would play the role of the indemnity insurance benefit. Consumers would be forced to choose among physicians with varying fees. Their out-of-pocket costs would no longer be uniformly zero. The balance bill itself would be the consumer copayment, and it would vary directly with the doctors' fees. The consumer would receive the total benefit of any price reduction that came about as a result of his or her choices.

THE ECONOMICS OF THE BAN ON BALANCE BILLING

The ban on balance billing has many effects on health care in Massachusetts. Although it seems counterintuitive, strict fee controls combined with the ban have raised costs, not controlled them. Further, the Blue Shield ban discourages competition, reduces access for the poor, rewards poor quality and a mechanistic, procedure-oriented style of practice, and retards innovation. All this occurs because of the way that Blue Shield affects two markets at once, the health care market and the health insurance market.

Blue Shield in Two Markets: The Vicious Circle

The share of Blue Shield plans in the health insurance market provides the basis for its power to extract discounts from physicians. Physicians fear the loss of a large part of their market if they do not go along. The large physician discount provides a competitive cost advantage for the Blue Shield plans. This advantage, in turn, allows them to raise their share in the insurance market, beginning the vicious circle over again. Only competition from other insurers, such as it is, prevents the vicious circle from progressing to completion with a 100 percent Blue Shield market share and even larger physician discounts.

---

prise Institute, 1978); and Frech and Ginsburg, "Imposed Health Insurance in Monopolistic Markets; A Theoretical Analysis," *Economic Inquiry* 13, no. 1 (March 1975):55–70.

Market Share and Physician Discount across States. It can be seen from data that became public during the *Kartell* trial that there is a strong positive statistical relationship between a Blue Shield plan's market share and the size of the physician discount imposed by that plan. The data are set out in Table 8–1, and the relationship is shown in schematic form in Figure 8–1. The line shows the average statistical relationship between Blue Shield market share and the Blue Shield physician discount.[9] The regression equation that generated this line is as follows:

Estimated Equation: *Expenditures = 668.0615 + 39.25877 × Discount*

t statistics: (17.01687) (2.247504)

F statistic for equation: 5.505127

Number of observations: 17

The odds against finding such a relationship by chance alone would be about 28 to 1.[10]

A similar strong positive relationship between market share and discount has been found by Killard Adamache and Frank Sloan, and by Roger Feldman and Warren Greenberg, for Blue Cross hospital insurance and hospital discounts.[11] This connection between Blue Shield/Blue Cross market power in the insurance market and monopsony power over providers was foreseen and intended by the founders of the plans.

Rufus Rorem, one of the original designers of the Blue Cross system, recently gave the rationale for the attempt to prevent competition among local Blue Cross plans: "Hospitals faced with the possibility of doing business with one of several Plans attempted to negotiate an agreement with the plan which imposed the least financial burden on the hospital and the greatest financial burden on the Plan. . . . The operation of only one Plan per service area helped the Plan obtain the participation of hospitals on terms which were favorable to the Plan

---

9. The discounts of the two Ohio Blue Shield plans were averaged for this analysis.

10. The relationship is statistically significant at the 0.0351 level, based on a one-tail test.

11. See Killard W. Adamache and Frank A. Sloan, "Competition between Non-Profit and For-Profit Health Insurers," *Journal of Health Economics* 2 (1983):225–43; and Roger Feldman and Warren Greenberg, "The Relation between the Blue Cross Share and the Blue Cross 'Discount' on Hospital Charges," *Journal of Risk and Insurance* 48 (1981):235–46.

Table 8–1. Market Share, Expenditures, and Physician Discount for Selected Blue Shield Plans.

Blue Shield Plan	Market Share 1980 (%)	Per Capita Total Health Care Expenditures 1978 ($)	Discount from UCR* 1980 (%)
California	23	904	12.9
Illinois (Chicago)	23	791	9.9
Florida	25	766	25.8
Wisconsin (Milwaukee)	29	742	3.0
Tennessee (Chattanooga)	37	675	1.0
Alabama	38	633	2.9
Ohio (Worthington)	38	738	1.9
Kentucky	40	542	8.9
Virginia (Richmond)	40	627	10.1
New York (New York City)	44	858	11.3
Indiana	46	671	10.5
Maryland	48	744	17.8
Iowa	51	724	4.0
New Jersey	51	699	18.3
Ohio (Cleveland)	53	738	9.6
Michigan	60	802	27.5
Massachusetts	64	935	28.2
Pennsylvania	69	756	20.1

SOURCES: Blue Cross–Blue Shield Association; Katharine R. Levit, "Personal Health Care Expenditures by State, Selected Years 1966–1978," *Health Care Financing Review* 4, no. 2 (December 1982):37.

*Usual, customary, and reasonable.

and its subscribers, thereby enhancing the Plan's attractiveness in the marketplace."[12]

The Discount and Competing Insurers. Ordinarily, one would expect a dominant firm's market power to weaken over time as it be-

12. C. Rufus Rorem, *Affidavit of C. Rufus Rorem, Ph.D., C.P.A.,* presented to the U.S. District Court for the District of Maryland regarding *State of Maryland v. Blue Cross and Blue Shield Association,* et al., Civil Action No. HM 84-3839 (May 14, 1985), pp. 13–14.

Figure 8–1.   Blue Shield Market Share and Discount.

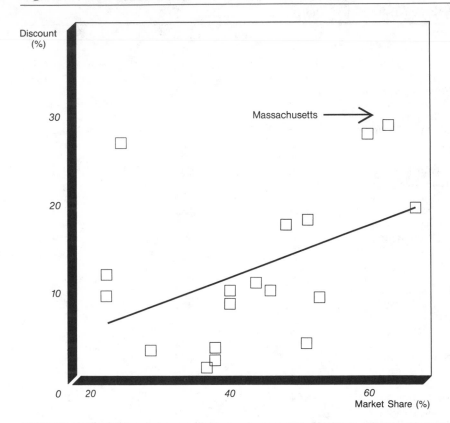

came undermined by the growth of competitors. However, this does not appear to have happened to the dominant Blue Cross/Blue Shield plans. There seems to be something special about the health care and health insurance markets that makes it hard for competitive insurers to grow, at least in markets with powerful Blue Cross/Blue Shield plans.

Blue Shield combines the demand of its members in the same way that a collusion or cartel of buyers would do, thereby creating the buying power necessary to induce physicians to accept its discount. Physicians, of course, would like to specialize in the better-paying, non-Blue Shield consumers. If enough of them did that, a profit opportunity for competing insurers would be created. But non-Blue Shield consumers are too few in number and cannot individually demand enough medical care to allow physicians to completely avoid Blue Shield subscribers.

Blue Shield itself prevents physicians from switching away from Blue Shield members. Physicians are forced to provide medical care to Blue Shield and competing patients on approximately the same terms (except for price) for a given medical problem.[13] Even without this Blue Shield policy, physicians would have problems in discriminating against Blue Shield customers. Referral relationships may require that physicians treat all customers more or less equally. Referring physicians are unlikely to send patients to physicians who might discriminate against their Blue Shield patients. Further, physicians are often not sure of the consumer's insurance status in advance. Because multiple insurance is so common, possession of a Blue Shield card is not conclusive.

Blue Shield's depression of the prices paid by its own subscribers does not benefit competing insurers. They do not share in the price reduction, which explains why competitive market forces are relatively weak in eroding Blue Shield's market power, even over time periods of several years.

The Blue Shield plan's depression of physician prices actually makes physicians as a group better off—up to a point. The price differential between what Blue Shield consumers must pay and the price paid by the uninsured and those with other, less complete insurance increases the market share of Blue Shield's very complete insurance, which raises the demand for medical care. The higher demand for medical care raises the incomes of physicians.[14] This higher demand has a very uneven impact on the medical profession, however. Physicians who have achieved the greatest market acceptance, for whatever reason (including high quality or important innovations) are hurt by the system, because they cannot charge the high fees that the market would

13. Enforcement is imperfect, so there is doubtless some small amount of better treatment for non–Blue Shield patients. But since it would be costly for Blue Shield to detect such favoritism, one would be surprised to find much direct evidence of it.

14. Blue Shield and Blue Cross plans were founded by physician and hospital organizations, respectively, and in most cases the plans were granted significant discounts from their inception. For an excellent analysis of how this contractual granting of a discount can raise physician income if it leads to the extension of insurance, see Keith Leffler, "*Arizona v. Maricopa County Medical Society:* Maximum Price Agreements in Markets with Insured Buyers," *Supreme Court Economic Review* 2 (1983):187–212.

allow. On the other hand, physicians with less market acceptance, those for whom high fees were never a possibility, could be made better off. That, no doubt, explains why the physician founders of Blue Shield built in a small discount from the beginning and did not object when the actual discount was in the neighborhood of 15 percent. Further, some discount is a common feature of Blue Shield plans, even where they are controlled by physicians.

Cost Containment in National Perspective

Massachusetts Blue Shield is unique. It alone can and does force physicians to accept a 25 to 30 percent discount and to abstain from balance billing. Defenders of the system argue that this power is necessary to control health care costs. Yet, Massachusetts health care costs are the highest in the nation. Table 8–2 reveals that in 1969 Massachusetts bypassed New York to become the state with the highest health care expenditures.

In the early 1970s, Massachusetts Blue Shield imposed drastic controls on its physician fee updates under the "usual and customary" system with its ban on balance billing. But that did not improve the state's dismal record of cost containment. In 1978, after years of stringent Blue Shield controls, Massachusetts health care costs were still the highest in the country, a full 25.5 percent above the average. It would seem to defy reason that Blue Shield's strict fee controls could have failed to contain costs.[15] Yet large Blue Shield discounts are associated with high health care costs, not low costs, across the nation.

---

15. In most industries, a successful monopsony reduces output. Therefore, examining the effect of a supposedly monopsonistic practice on output is typically a good indicator of whether competition has been hindered. In Massachusetts, however, Blue Shield's monopsony power allows it to suppress physician prices relative to those paid by consumers with competing insurance or without insurance. This cost advantage provides Blue Shield with the ability to use the potential monopoly (monopsony) profits to pursue its own goals.

In fact, Blue Shield uses its cost advantage to pursue two main goals: the promotion of very complete insurance and a large market share. Pursuing both goals raises the demand for health care. More complete Blue Shield insurance replaces commercial insurance that has deductibles, indemnity features, and coinsurance. That raises the volume of health care provided in the market and it can easily overwhelm the direct effect of the monopsony.

Overall, the impact of Blue Shield's policy is to raise medical output in the Massachusetts market. In most industries, that would be a good result, indicating that Blue Shield was operating in the public interest. However, in the health care industry, the main public policy problem is that of too much output, not too little. This is true both in terms of the quantity of health care and the resource intensiveness, or quality, of health care.

Table 8–2.   Personal Health Care Expenditures as a Percentage of the U.S. Average, 1966–1978.

	New England	*New York*	*Massachusetts*
Total Health Care			
1966	117.0	126.8	126.6
1969	117.7	128.8	129.3
1972	115.3	123.8	127.9
1976	113.3	122.8	125.6
1977	112.6	118.0	125.3
1978	112.4	115.2	125.4
Hospital Care			
1966	126.4	138.2	144.8
1969	127.3	144.2	149.6
1972	124.1	141.8	147.8
1976	120.8	135.7	144.0
1977	121.3	127.2	146.6
1978	119.7	123.4	144.1
Physician Care			
1966	104.2	129.8	104.5
1969	103.7	123.5	102.8
1972	98.1	113.5	98.6
1976	90.6	97.1	90.1
1977	87.8	95.9	87.5
1978	89.9	98.1	91.6

Source: Katharine R. Levit, "Personal Health Care Expenditures by State, Selected Years 1966–1978," *Health Care Financing Review* 4, no. 2 (December 1982):6, 38, 39.

Blue Shield Discounts and Total Expenditures across States.   The connections among the physician discount, high Blue Shield market share, and high expenditures hold across states as well as within Massachusetts. Figure 8–2 presents the data graphically. The dotted line shows the average statistical relationship (called the regression line) between the Blue Shield physician discount and total health care costs across states. The linear regression that produced the regression line is as follows:

Estimated Equation: *Discount = 0.151677 + 0.283658 × Share*

t statistics: (0.023)   (1.940)

F statistic for equation: 3.763

Number of observations: 18

Figure 8–2.   Discount and Expenditures Per Capita Across States.

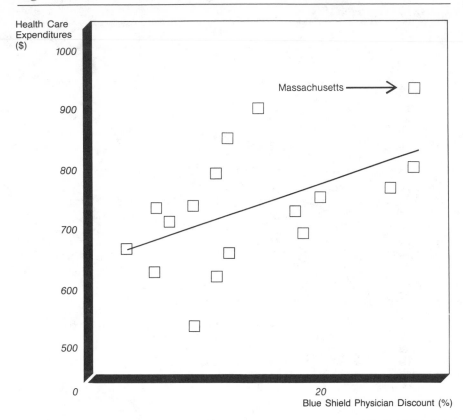

With these statistically strong results, the odds against the positive relationship we observed being a result of mere chance are about 80 to 1.[16]

As a general rule, large Blue Shield physician discounts appear to be counterproductive. This result is consistent with other research showing that large Blue Cross/Blue Shield market shares are strongly related to high health care costs.[17] We know that the Blue Shield discount is associated with high Blue Shield market shares. When we

16. This result is statistically significant at the 0.0125 percent level, based on a one-tail test.

17. On Blue Cross/Blue Shield market share and health care costs, see H. E. Frech III, "Market Power in Health Insurance: Effects on Insurance and Medical Markets," *Journal of Industrial Economics* 27, no. 1 (September 1978):55–72; Frech, "Blue Cross, Blue Shield

break down health care cost into its components, we can begin to see why Blue Shield physician discounts fail to control total expenditures.

Physician Expenditures.   Contrary to what one might expect, Massachusetts physician expenditures have never been particularly high. In 1966, they were only 4.5 percent above the national average. And, surprisingly, even under the unconstrained "usual and customary" system of the late 1960s and early 1970s, Massachusetts physician expenditures were declining relative to those of other states. By 1972, Massachusetts expenditures had fallen below the national average. The discounts mandated by Blue Shield in the 1970s accelerated the decline in expenditures, so that by 1978 Massachusetts physician services costs per capita were 8.4 percent below the national average.

The same picture of restraint in physician costs is reflected in physician incomes, shown in Figure 8–3 and Table 8–3. Despite the fact that Massachusetts boasts some world-famous teaching institutions and associated physicians, physician incomes in Massachusetts have always been low. Massachusetts physician income was about 14 percent below the national average in 1969. By 1982, New England physician income was about 17 percent below the national average. From 1969 to 1983 national physician income itself had declined about 1 percent in real terms. The uniquely restrictive policies of Blue Shield have harmed physicians, yet we see that they have not succeeded in containing costs. The data on hospital expenditures provide some insight into this phenomenon.

Hospital Expenditures.   Massachusetts hospital expenditures, as seen in Table 8–2, have always been, and still are, very high. The highest anywhere since 1969, by 1978 they were 44.1 percent above average.

---

and Health Care Costs: A Review of the Economic Evidence," in Mark V. Pauly, ed., *National Health Insurance: What Now, What Later, What Never?* (Washington, D.C.: American Enterprise Institute, 1980), pp. 250–63; H. E. Frech III and Paul B. Ginsburg, "Competition among Health Insurers," in Warren Greenberg, ed., *Competition in the Health Care Sector: Past, Present and Future* (Germantown Md.: Aspen Systems Corp./Federal Trade Commission, 1978), pp. 210–37; and Joel Hay and Michael J. Leahy, "Competition among Health Plans: Some Preliminary Evidence," *Southern Economic Journal* 50, no. 2 (January 1980): 831–46.

Figure 8–3.   Physician Real Income, 1983 Prices.

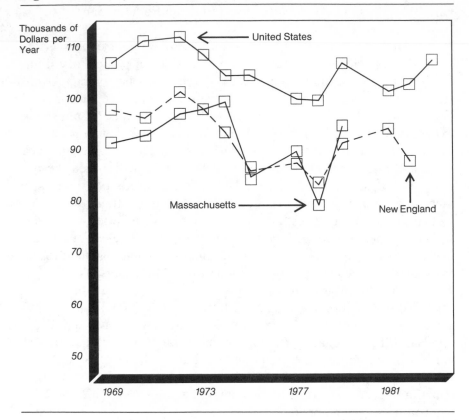

Because hospital care accounts for about twice the expenditures of physician services nationally, this figure accounts for Massachusetts' poor showing on overall costs. Blue Shield's fee controls have exacerbated the problem. Its exaction of large discounts from physicians is a dismal failure as a cost-containment policy.

Why the Blue Shield System Raises Costs.   Blue Shield's deep physician discounts, coupled with the ban on balance billing, provide a substantial competitive and marketing advantage for Blue Shield and Blue Cross. Blue Shield uses this advantage to increase its market share at the expense of the commercial insurers, health maintenance organizations, and so on. Blue Shield and Blue Cross strongly favor, on ideological or philosophical grounds, 100 percent, first-dollar health

Table 8–3. Physicians' Average Annual Real Income, 1969–1983 (1983 dollars).

	United States	New England	Massachusetts
1969	107,927	99,228	93,247
1970	111,905	97,532	93,938
1971	—	—	—
1972	112,443	103,391	99,341
1973	108,993	99,126	99,574
1974	105,091	93,571	99,836
1975	104,437	87,401	84,254
1976	—	—	—
1977	100,651	87,329	88,480
1978	100,060	83,867	79,895
1979	107,449	91,276	93,469
1980	—	—	—
1981	101,910	93,144	—
1982	102,735	84,872	—
1983	106,300	—	—

SOURCE: American Medical Association Periodic Survey of Physicians, Socioeconomic Monitoring System (Chicago: AMA, various dates).

insurance. This type of insurance leads to high demand for health care and discourages competition. Thus the high market share of its overly complete health insurance leads to the cost-containment failure of Massachusetts Blue Shield and Blue Cross.

In most of the nation, the Blue Shield/Blue Cross plans do not have the market power to force such perverse 100 percent insurance on so much of the market. Further, consumer copayment is becoming more and more popular as a cost-containment device, as is shown by a dramatic reversal in the historical trend of ever more complete health insurance that has occurred in the years since 1975. Figures 8–4, 8–5, and 8–6 and Table 8–4 document the changes.[18] Physician care insurance and especially hospital care insurance make increasing use of consumer out-of-pocket payments as a crucial cost-control mechanism. Further, a recent survey of large employers shows that the percentage of firms offering 100 percent reimbursement for hospital care fell from 89 percent in 1979 to 75 percent in 1983.[19]

18. The percentage of total health care costs paid out of pocket in Figure 8–6 and Table 8–6 shows little change because the coverage of newly insured services like dental care was increasing while the completeness of coverage of hospital and physician care was decreasing.

19. Bruce Keppel, "Recession, Costs Spur Changes in Health Benefits," *Los Angeles Times,* 21 February 1984, pp. 2,9.

Figure 8–4.   **Percentage Out-of-Pocket Physician Care.**

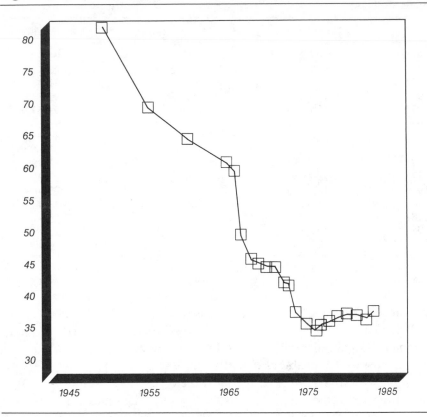

The Cost Savings from Allowing Balance Billing.   It is obvious that more complete physician services insurance would increase demand for ambulatory physician care. It is not so clear what would happen to the demand for hospital care. Since ambulatory care can, to some extent, substitute for hospitalization, it seems that more coverage for ambulatory care might actually reduce the demand for hospital care. However, the Rand Corporation health insurance experiment, directed by Joseph Newhouse, found that more complete ambulatory insurance causes increases in demand for both physician and hospital care. Comparison of two deductible plans, one for ambulatory care only and one for both, indicates that copayment reduces demand for hos-

Table 8–4. Percentage of U.S. Health Care Costs Paid Out of Pocket, 1929–1983.

	All Health Care	*Physician Care*	*Hospital Care*
1929	88.4	—	—
1935	82.4	—	—
1940	81.3	—	—
1950	65.5	83.2	29.9
1955	58.1	69.8	22.3
1960	54.9	65.4	19.8
1965	51.8	61.4	17.2
1966	49.2	59.9	15.6
1967	42.5	50.3	10.0
1968	40.9	47.0	10.0
1969	40.2	46.4	10.0
1970	39.9	45.1	10.0
1971	38.6	44.9	9.2
1972	38.6	42.4	10.9
1973	38.6	41.8	11.9
1974	36.1	37.9	10.4
1975	33.4	36.2	8.2
1976	32.6	35.1	8.3
1977	32.8	35.7	9.3
1978	32.5	36.6	8.6
1979	32.7	37.2	9.9
1980	32.9	38.0	10.9
1981	32.2	37.7	11.1
1982	31.5	37.3	12.1
1983	32.2	38.8	12.5

SOURCES: Robert M. Gibson, Daniel R. Waldo, and Katharine R. Levit, "National Health Expenditures," *Health Care Financing Review* 5, no. 1 (Fall 1983):8–10; and *Sourcebook of 1982–1983 Health Insurance Data: 1984 Update* (Washington, D.C.: Health Insurance Association of America, 1984), p. 16.

pital and ambulatory care by about the same percentage, whether it is concentrated on ambulatory care or not.[20]

By assuming that we can treat general coinsurance as if it applied only to outpatient care, we can actually calculate the cost savings that we would expect from eliminating the ban on balance billing. One of

20. Joseph P. Newhouse et al., "Some Interim Results from a Controlled Experiment in Health Insurance," *New England Journal of Medicine* 305, no. 25 (December 17, 1981): 1501–7. One of the benefit structures tested was a small deductible ($150 per person, $450 per family in 1974–78 dollars) for outpatient care only; inpatient care was free. Still, when compared to 100 percent coverage, the policy reduced the probability of hospitalization by 12 percent and reduced total health care expenditures by 23 percent. This overall savings was

Figure 8–5.   Percentage Out-of-Pocket Hospital Care.

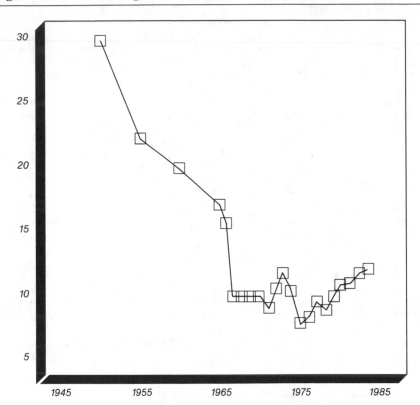

the insurance plans studied by the Rand Corporation provided co-insurance of 25 percent, which is comparable to the current Blue Shield discount. For those Massachusetts physicians who would balance-bill to the full extent of the discount, we can apply the experimental results to the effects of ending the ban on balance billing. The researchers found that coinsurance at this level reduced total health care expenditures by 19 percent, a 20 percent decline in ambulatory use and an 18 percent decline in hospital use.

---

composed of a 25 percent reduction in ambulatory spending and a 22 percent reduction in hospital expenditure. A similar but much larger deductible (about $1,000 per family) was applied to both ambulatory care and hospital care. It cut total expenditures by 31 percent; 39 percent for ambulatory care and 24 percent for hospital care.

Figure 8–6. Percentage Out-of-Pocket, All Health Care.

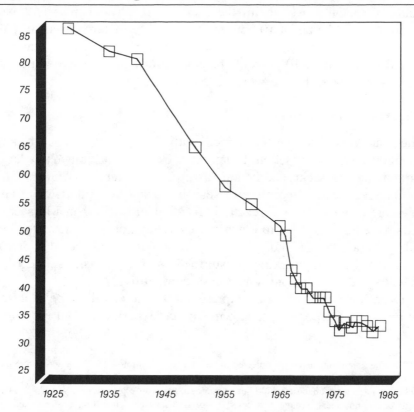

The consumer who faced this extent of balance billing would experience a 33 percent rise in physician care prices and a 20 percent decline in quantity,[21] which would cause about a 6 percent increase in costs for physician services. However, since hospital costs are about

21. The proportional change for physician services expenditures is calculated in the following way:

$$P(1) \times Q(1) = [1.33 \times P(o)] \times [0.80 \times Q(o)] = 1.064 \times [P(o) \times Q(o)]$$

where $P(1)$, $Q(1)$ are the price and quantity with balance billing, $P(o)$, $Q(o)$ are the price and quantity without balance billing. We know from the Rand experiment that 25 percent coinsurance (which corresponds to a 33 percent price rise from a 25 percent discount) leads to a 20 percent decline in quantity demanded.

twice as large as physician care costs, the 18 percent decline in hospital costs would overwhelm the increase in physician costs.[22] Net savings would be about 10 percent of total health care costs. In reality, both the higher prices of physician care and the overall savings would be less than 10 percent, because many physicians would not balance-bill even if there were no ban.

Effects on Competition

The Blue Shield system combined with the ban on balance billing enable Blue Shield to sell its 100 percent coverage insurance to a large part of the Massachusetts health insurance market. This kind of insurance reduces the incentive to search out and reward efficient and low-cost providers. As a result, individual physicians in Massachusetts have less incentive to lower prices. They know that lower prices will make absolutely no difference to consumers who have Blue Shield coverage. Thus, by making consumers less price sensitive, the Blue Shield system makes physicians less competitive.

The effects of this relationship are subtle and could not be captured by the Rand Corporation health insurance experiment. But they may

---

22. The defendants in *Kartell* objected to this analysis, claiming that if one were to reduce the consumer demand for hospital services, the same resources would still be employed by the hospital and therefore costs would not be reduced; the costs of empty beds would be passed on to other consumers through cost-based hospital insurance. Therefore, cost containment requires a regulatory reduction in the number of hospitals and/or hospital beds. Fortunately, this pessimistic argument is flawed.

Consider the expectations of the hospital. If it expects a bed to be occupied, it will plan for staff and other resources to care for the occupant. In this case, the costs of the unexpected empty bed would be a high proportion of the costs of an occupied one. However, systemwide cost containment would lower the expected occupancy. Thus, hospitals could and would reduce staffing and other input purchases. As a result, the costs of a bed emptied by demand reduction would be a small fraction of the costs of an occupied bed. Only very small further savings would accrue from reducing the number of beds by regulation or other means.

The idea that the cost of empty beds is high is based on incorrectly interpreted economic research. Most of the older econometric research on the cost of an empty bed related observed costs to observed occupancy rates. However, the cost associated with the observed occupancy rate applies to some mix of expected and unexpected empty beds. That explains why the typical finding was that an empty bed cost about half as much as an occupied bed. Recent research, including careful analysis of the hospital's expectations about occupancy, finds the costs of an expected empty bed to be very small, about 7 percent of the costs of an occupied bed. See Bernard Friedman and Mark V. Pauly, "Cost Functions for a Service Firm with Variable Quality and Stochastic Demand: The Case of Hospitals," *Review of Economics and Statistics* 63, no. 4 (November 1981):620–24.

be more important, in the long run, than what *could* be measured in the experiment. The ban on balance billing also prevents physicians from competing by providing a more costly and higher-quality service to consumers who are willing to pay an additional amount for such care. For example, a physician might prefer to spend a great deal of time with each patient and charge something extra for the service. The ban on balance billing directly reduces the choices that physicians and consumers can make. Less competition means that prices and the type of practice are too uniform, cutting off the choices that a minority of consumers and physicians might make for higher-quality and higher-priced care.

Other Effects of the Ban on Balance Billing

Innovation. Incentives for innovation are often dulled by the current Blue Shield system. Blue Shield is properly very conservative in deciding how much to pay for innovative procedures. But, given the ban on balance billing, when it sets its own allowance too low, it also sets the price too low. The low price retards the development and spread of new procedures, which is particularly unfortunate when an innovation both improves quality and saves costs, as in the development of orthoscopic procedures. A system of balance billing would encourage innovation, even if Blue Shield were to err and set the allowance too low, because physicians could charge patients the market fee. If the procedure were really an important advance, the procedure would succeed in spite of the Blue Shield error. Further, the success of the procedure in itself would provide information to Blue Shield that would be helpful in setting the allowance properly in the future.

A striking example of the Blue Shield system retarding innovation was presented at the *Kartell* trial in the testimony of the late Dr. Steven Hedberg, an expert in surgery and endoscopy at Massachusetts General Hospital and a clinical professor of surgery at the Harvard Medical School. He introduced an outpatient procedure, colonoscopy (with and without polypectomy), that replaced a far more expensive and dangerous inpatient surgical procedure. The new procedure allowed the physician to inspect the colon and remove polyps without performing a laparotomy, an abdominal wall incision requiring general anesthesia. Dr. Hedberg's charge for the procedure in the early 1970s, when it was introduced, was $500. Blue Shield paid $170 and prohibited balance billing, while other private insurers paid $425 and allowed balance billing. By the time of the trial, Blue Shield had corrected its error and was paying almost $700 of Dr. Hedberg's $800 charge. The financial cost of the medically inferior surgical alternative was then about $6,000. In his opinion, Judge Caffrey stated: "Blue Shield's reluctance to provide full remuneration for innovative procedures, coupled with its ban on balance billing, discourages physicians from undertaking the training and purchasing the equipment necessary to learn and offer the safer, innovative and relatively inexpensive procedure. As a result, doctors in Massachusetts have been reluctant to learn the new colonoscopy with polypectomy procedure."[23]

Blue Shield argued that insufficient data and incorrect filings by physicians were responsible for the very low fees initially set. In short, Blue Shield's intentions were good but their information was poor. According to Judge Caffrey's opinion, that argument misses the point: "The crucial point in plaintiff's argument is not that Blue Shield's fee determination was ultimately unreasonable (although it may have been), but that the low initial fee, in conjunction with the ban, in fact deterred physician adoption of the new procedure. Precisely, because a low fee determination by Blue Shield, even if made in good faith, can have these deleterious effects, it is especially important that during the early, formative development of a medical technique, the market, not Blue Shield, should determine the relative value of a procedure."[24]

Quality.　　The Blue Shield system is biased against high-quality medical care. Not only does the insurance reimbursement itself fail to recognize quality in any way, but the higher-quality providers are prevented from seeking additional payment from the consumers themselves. There is no incentive for physicians to take the time and effort to provide higher-quality services or to procure the necessary training and equipment to do so. By analogy, if the government were to give everyone $7,000 toward the purchase of an automobile but were to

23. *Kartell v. Blue Shield of Massachusetts*, 582 F. Supp. at 752.
24. *Kartell v. Blue Shield of Massachusetts, supra*, 582 F. Supp. at 753 n25.

forbid manufacturers to charge more than that, obviously only the lower-quality automobiles could succeed.

Massachusetts Blue Shield has traditionally frowned upon procedures performed in the office, a policy that aggravates not only the problem of quality but that of cost as well. Many insurers have taken steps to encourage the provision of services, tests, and surgery in the physician's office in order to reduce costly, unnecessary, and unpleasant hospitalizations. On the other hand, Blue Shield of Massachusetts has discouraged office-based services by, for example, refusing to pay for the costs of equipment and technician's labor in the office. However, while that has been the traditional Blue Shield view, new policies announced since the trial appear to recognize the savings of ambulatory and office-based procedures.

That is one example of the danger inherent in a nonprofit monopoly: It may persist for a long time in imposing a narrow ideology or philosophy on the market because its market power insulates it from the judgment of consumers and providers expressed in the market. A profit-seeking monopoly, on the other hand, has strong incentive to cater to consumer and provider demands and values so that it can earn more profits. Thus, even though managed by public-spirited citizens, a nonprofit monopoly can be more oppressive than a profit-seeking one.

An important aspect of quality is the time the physician takes with the patient, trying to become more clearly informed about the patient's problem. This is called cognitive medicine. Under the current Blue Shield "usual and customary" system, there is no reward for the physician taking more time, even if that would be better or cheaper for the patient. At the *Kartell* trial, Dr. Henry Brown, a distinguished hand surgeon and Harvard professor, told of leaving Blue Shield at personal financial cost because of his objection to this feature of its policy. Now outside the Blue Shield system, he is forced to commute to New Hampshire part of the time to support himself.[25]

The Ban and the Poor. The ban on balance billing makes Massachusetts less attractive to physicians than it would otherwise have been. Therefore, the physicians who do locate here will be more busy and

---

25. *Kartell v. Blue Shield of Massachusetts, supra,* 582 F. Supp. at 751.

less willing and able to devote themselves to charity and Medicaid care. Access to physician care is more difficult for the poor than it would be absent the ban.

From a superficial view, Blue Shield subscribers may appear to benefit from the ban, since they obtain physician care at a discount. But the subscribers are relatively well-to-do. Most Blue Shield insurance is an expensive part of an employment package. The poor, of course, do not have Blue Shield health insurance. At best, they have Medicaid insurance; at worst, none at all.

CONCLUSION

Massachusetts Blue Shield's ban on balance billing, in the context of its market power and other policies, leads to insurance with insufficient consumer copayment. Predictably, this causes a poor record for cost containment. The system also has more subtle harmful effects on quality and innovation and on the style of medical practice. Whether or not Judge Breyer is right in saying that Blue Shield should be viewed as a purchaser and that purchasers should be allowed to exploit their market power as they see fit, the ban is bad public policy. Although the immediate appeal of lower prices is clear enough, the ultimate effects are bad for Massachusetts consumers, the poor, physicians, and competing health insurers. The only real beneficiary is Massachusetts Blue Shield itself.

SELECTED BIBLIOGRAPHY

Adamache, Killard W., and Frank A. Sloan. "Competition between Non-Profit and For-Profit Health Insurers." *Journal of Health Economics* 2 (1983):225–43.

Andersen, Ronald, and Odin W. Anderson. *A Decade of Health Services.* Chicago: University of Chicago Press, 1970.

Feldman, Roger, and Warren Greenberg. "The Relation between the Blue Cross Share and the Blue Cross 'Discount' on Hospital Charges." *Journal of Risk and Insurance* 48 (1981):235–46.

Frech, H. E. III. "Market Power in Health Insurance: Effects on Insurance and Medical Markets." *Journal of Industrial Economics* 27, no. 1 (September 1978):55–72.

———. "Blue Cross, Blue Shield and Health Care Costs: A Review of the Economic Evidence." In Mark V. Pauly, ed., *National Health Insurance: What Now, What Later, What Never?* pp. 250–63. Washington, D.C.: American Enterprise Institute, 1980.

———. "Preferred Provider Organizations and Health Care Competition." This volume.

Frech, H. E. III, and Paul B. Ginsburg. "Imposed Health Insurance in Monopolistic Markets: A Theoretical Analysis." *Economic Inquiry* 13, no. 1 (March 1975):55–70.

———. *Public Health Insurance in Private Medical Markets: Some Problems of National Health Insurance.* Washington, D.C.: American Enterprise Institute, 1978.

———. "Competition among Health Insurers." In Warren Greenberg, ed., *Competition in the Health Care Sector: Past, Present, and Future,* pp. 210–37. Germantown, Md.: Aspen Systems Corp./Federal Trade Commission, 1978.

Freemont-Smith, Thayer. "Recent Developments in Massachusetts." Paper presented at the American Bar Association Conference on Antitrust, Washington, D.C., July 1985.

Friedman, Bernard, and Mark V. Pauly. "Cost Functions for a Service Firm with Variable Quality and Stochastic Demand: The Case of Hospitals." *Review of Economics and Statistics* 63, no. 4 (November 1981):620–24.

Hay, Joel W., and Michael J. Leahy. "Competition among Health Plans: Some Preliminary Evidence." *Southern Economic Journal* 50, no. 3 (January 1984):831–46.

Keppel, Bruce. "Recession, Costs Spur Changes in Health Benefits." *Los Angeles Times*, 21 February 1984, pp. 2, 9.

Leffler, Keith. *"Arizona v. Maricopa County Medical Society:* Maximum Price Agreements in Markets with Insured Buyers." *Supreme Court Economic Review*, 2 (1983):187–212.

Newhouse, Joseph P., and Charles E. Phelps. "Price and Income Elasticities for Medical Care Services." In Mark Perlman, ed., *The Economics of Health and Medical Care: Proceedings of a Conference Held by the International Economic Association at Tokyo*, pp. 139–61. New York: Wiley, 1973.

Newhouse, Joseph P.; Willard Manning, et al. "Some Interim Results from a Controlled Trial of Cost Sharing in Health Insurance." *New England Journal of Medicine* 305, no. 25 (December 17, 1981):1501–7.

Rorem, C. Rufus. *Affidavit of C. Rufus Rorem, Ph.D., C.P.A.* Presented to the U.S. District Court for the District of Maryland regarding *State of Maryland v. Blue Cross and Blue Shield Association*, et al., Civil Action No. HM 84-3839 (May 14, 1985).

Thompson, John Larkin. "Report Prepared for Presentation to the Advisory Council on Social Security." Boston: Blue Shield of Massachusetts, April 6, 1983.

9

PREMIUM REBATES FOR NO CLAIMS: THE WEST GERMAN EXPERIENCE

Peter Zweifel

INTRODUCTION

Recent debate about the pros and cons of cost-sharing in health insurance tends to be rather narrowly focused on two traditional instruments, the deductible and the coinsurance rate.[1] However, plans excluding full insurance coverage under all circumstances are likely to be unattractive to buyers, and for good reasons.[2] Therefore, the experience of private health insurers in West Germany who have been developing new, more flexible plans may be of some interest to U.S. readers.

German private health insurers have to compete with statutory health insurance (in particular, the substitute funds catering to the relatively well-to-do within the social insurance system) and among themselves.

Note: The author is grateful to Otto Waser for his expert computational assistance, and to the representatives of the two insurers involved for their cooperation.

1. M. S. Feldstein, "The Welfare Loss of Excess Health Insurance," *Journal of Political Economy* 81 (1973):251–80; J. P. Newhouse, "A Design for a Health Insurance Experiment," *Inquiry* 11 (1974):5–27; J. P. Newhouse, K. H. Marquis, and C. N. Morris, "Some Interim Results from a Controlled Trial of Cost Sharing in Health Insurance," *New England Journal of Medicine* 305 (1981):1501.

2. R. Zeckhauser, "Medical Insurance: A Case Study of the Tradeoff between Risk and Appropriate Incentives," *Journal of Economic Theory* 2 (1970):10–26.

Together they insure some 8 percent of the population.[3] Some of them, like "insurer A" (to be considered below), write traditional plans featuring deductibles and coinsurance. Others, like "insurer B," offer a no-claims rebate amounting to two to three months' worth of premiums. A third group of private health insurers operates a full experience-rated bonus system: The next year's premium is lower if the insured did not file a claim in the current year, and still lower if he also did not file a claim during the previous year(s). In this chapter, emphasis will be on the intermediate rebate offer, whereby the slate is wiped clean at the beginning of each year.

Such a plan offers three advantages to the buyer and two to the insurer. The buyer can always limit his out-of-pocket expenses under such a plan because there is no pro rata coinsurance when he decides to file the annual total as his claims. This first advantage is shared with a traditional deductible plan. But—and this is the second advantage—the pure rebate option relieves the insured from paying anything in the event of illness if he does not want to. This is important to people who are particularly risk averse when they are ill. These individuals will strongly dislike being faced with a loss in the guise of cost-sharing when they are in bad health. Under a rebate option, they do not have to face an outlay; rather, they forgo the extra rebate income—which is less of a burden to a risk-averse individual. To the extent that the same insureds are only slightly risk averse when they are well, the opportunity for gain offered by a rebate figures significantly, nearly compensating them for the premium-loading used to finance the rebate. Thus the rebate offer falls slightly short of an equivalent deductible plan in the event of good health, but is preferable by far in the event of illness. The third advantage applies only to individuals whose employer subsidizes part of the premium for their health insurance coverage, because such individuals hardly pay back the employer's share of any rebate they obtain. From the point of view of the insurance company, the rebate offer promises to relieve it of the processing of petty claims, thus saving administrative costs. More important, the rebate option also has the potential of limiting moral hazard (i.e., utilization of extra medical care because it is sub-

3. F. Beske, "Expenditures and Attempts of Cost Containment in the Statutory Health Insurance System of the Federal Republic of Germany," in Nuffield Provincial Hospitals Trust, ed., *The Public/Private Mix for Health: The Relevance and Effects of Change* (London: NPHT, 1982), pp. 233–63.

sidized by insurance) more effectively than do traditional methods of cost-sharing.

In this chapter we plan to test the hypothesis that rebate options are more effective in restraining utilization of medical care in minor episodes of sickness than are roughly comparable plans featuring deductibles and/or coinsurance. The test is based on the 1982 experience of insurer A (who wrote traditional plans) and insurer B (who wrote rebate plans) in the domain of ambulatory care. Hospital and dental care are disregarded for the time being. The traditional plans written by A are analyzed first, and some predictions relevant to those plans are tested in the following section. The third section will be devoted to a similar analysis of the rebate offer as introduced by insurer B in 1979, also supplemented by some empirical evidence.

The crucial step consists of juxtaposing the two families of plans and deriving a differential prediction about the impacts on utilization of medical care. The differential prediction can be shown to receive a good deal of empirical confirmation: Demand-increasing characteristics such as increasing age and female sex appear to be more strongly counteracted by the rebate offer than by traditional cost-sharing methods. Finally, some preliminary evidence points to an interesting phenomenon: While cost-sharing tends to have a stronger impact on the middle class than on the uppermost strata, the differential impact in favor of the rebate offer is preserved across income levels. This finding appears to commend new, more flexible cost-sharing provisions not only for private insurance, but also more generally for social health insurance, where problems of moral hazard loom as large.

INSTITUTIONAL BACKGROUND

Out of a population of about 62 million, some 90 percent of West Germans are enrolled in one of the not-for-profit statutory sickness funds, which number more than 1,250. About 2 percent are covered by public assistance, with the remaining 8 percent covered exclusively by private health insurance.[4] Of the enrollees in sickness funds, another 8 to 9 percent have bought supplementary private insurance, which provides coverage for a (semi)private ward in the hospital. But

---

4. Beske, "Expenditures and Attempts of Cost Containment"; J. M. Schulenburg, "Report from Germany: Current Conditions and Controversies in the Health Care System," *Journal of Health Politics, Policy and Law* 8, no. 2 (Summer 1983):320–51.

among dependent workers, only those earning a monthly income in excess of DM 3,900 in 1984 ($1,600) have the right to opt out of statutory insurance.[5] According to recent estimates, some 13 percent of enrollees could in fact opt out.[6]

Once the decision is made to leave statutory health insurance, however, there is no way back into the system. Even within private insurance, rate-setting according to age at entry keeps mobility low. Designed to guarantee a constant premium during an insured's lifetime, this type of rate-setting means that someone who changes insurance will lose the reserves accumulated while he was younger. Nevertheless, premiums are far from constant because of inflation in the health care sector. Premium rebates for no claims help to sweeten the pill for the insured.

Since the majority of private health insurers are mutuals,[7] they are legally obliged to redistribute profits to their members. Thus, loosely speaking, rebates have been common for a long time. But rebates for no claims are a much more recent phenomenon. Among the ten leading insurers (who account for 77 percent of all premium income),[8] two grant rebates for no claims (typically amounting to three months' worth of premiums—see insurer B below), while eight operate a full experience-rated system analogous to that used for automobile insurance (with a bonus typically amounting to a maximum of five months' worth of premiums). Before 1980, only one of these ten insurers offered a rebate for no claims, regardless of profits available for redistribution. These new options are thus spreading very rapidly. This development must await final assessment in terms of social welfare, however, because consumers who do not like rebate options have little choice but to change their insurer.

MODELING TRADITIONAL COST-SHARING: INSURER A

Insurer A is a private mutual company, catering mainly to independent businessmen, managers, and public officials. Insurance is written separately for ambulatory, hospital, and dental care. The emphasis

---

5. Bundesminister für Arbeit und Sozialordnung, *Sozialpolitische Informationen* (Bonn: Referat L6, 1985).

6. Gesamtverband der Deutschen Versicherungswirtschaft (GDV), *Marktentwicklung und Marktstruktur in der privaten Krankenversicherung* (Development and Structure of the Market for Private Health Insurance) (Cologne: Verlag Versicherungswirtschaft, 1984), p. 27.

7. Ibid., pp. 43ff.

8. Ibid., p. 36.

here will be on ambulatory care, because it is there that different cost-sharing provisions exist. There are two types of cost-sharing plans: one with deductibles varying from DM 250 to DM 1,500 per year ($80 to $500 at 1984 exchange rates), the other with coinsurance rates of 20, 30, and 40 percent and an upper limit of DM 2,400 ($800) gross billing.

Figure 9–1 illustrates the decision-making situation of two indi-

---

Figure 9–1. Propensity to Initiate an Ambulatory Care Episode, Insurer A.

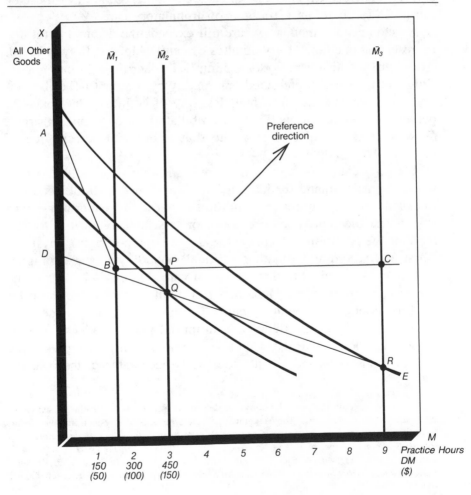

viduals who are thought to be identical in all but one respect. Alpha
has a plan with a deductible of DM 250 ($80), whereas Beta faces a
coinsurance rate of 20 percent. The two axes represent hours of ambulatory care received (M) and a composite of all other goods and
services (X). A physician hour is assumed to cost DM 150 ($50), all
included. Thus, a deductible of DM 250 means that Alpha has to pay
the first hour and forty minutes out of pocket. In other words, he has
to give up other goods and services in order to obtain medical care.

This trade-off is symbolized in Figure 9–1 by the falling segment
AB of the boundary ABC. The steepness of AB indicates that medical
care is relatively expensive, i.e., a lot of other goods (X) must be
sacrificed to obtain an extra hour of ambulatory care (M).

As soon as the ambulatory care bill exceeds the deductible (at $\bar{M}_1$,
representing one hour, forty minutes of care), Alpha is fully covered:
Additional medical care no longer implies a sacrifice of other goods.
This leveling off is represented graphically by segment BC of boundary ABC, which runs horizontal. By way of contrast, Beta pays 20
percent of every additional hour of ambulatory care, so his constraint
DE continues to fall, but at a rate that is only 20 percent that of
segment AB of Alpha.

The physician now enters the picture. Rather than fully conform
with patients' demand for his time, he is assumed to limit treatment
to exactly three hours for the condition in question.[9] Other physicians
might treat the same condition more or less intensively, but for the
moment the possibility of a patient searching out the "right" physician
is barred. Accordingly, another (vertical) boundary appears in Figure
9–1 at $\bar{M}_2$, equivalent to three hours of care. Figure 9–1 can now be
used to predict whether Alpha and Beta will take or leave the offer
of three hours of ambulatory care. To this end, a preference field
(common to Alpha and Beta by assumption) must be added. A preference field looks like the contours of a valuation hill, representing
combinations of M and X that are equally acceptable to the insured.

9. For evidence on the physician's role in determining intensity of treatment, see G. R.
Wilensky and L. F. Rossiter, "The Magnitude and Determinants of Physician-Initiated Visits
in the United States," in J. van der Gaag and M. Perlman, eds., *Health, Economics, and
Health Economics* (Amsterdam and New York: North-Holland, 1981), pp. 215–44; and P.
Zweifel, "Drugs, Physicians, and Hospitalization," in R. M. Scheffler and L. F. Rossiter,
eds., *Advances in Health Economics and Health Services Research*, vol. 5 (Greenwich, Conn.:
JAI Press, 1984).

Such an indifference curve is drawn at the three-hour limit of Alpha, passing through point P. Since the indifference curve hits the X axis below point A, point P (with $M = \bar{M}_2$ = three hours of care) must be of lower value to Alpha than point A (with zero hours of care). Alpha would therefore rather go without care than accept the treatment offer and pay the DM 250 deductible.

The same line of argument can be applied to Beta, but with the opposite result. Beta, operating on the DE boundary, reaches the indifference curve passing through point Q if he goes to see the physician. This indifference curve clearly hits the X axis at a higher level than point D (with zero hours of care). Beta would thus prefer to obtain the three hours of ambulatory care rather than save DM 90 (20 percent of DM 450). Casual inspection of Figure 9–1 reveals that a more limited treatment offer, such as $\bar{M}_1$ (one hour, forty minutes of care, worth DM 250 or \$85), would induce the same difference in behavior despite identical preferences: Alpha, having a plan with a minimal deductible, would decide against medical care, while Beta, having a plan with minimal coinsurance, would decide in favor of it.[10] This argument leads us to

> *Proposition A1:* For minor illnesses, plans with minimal deductibles, as well as plans with minimal coinsurance, will result in a smaller propensity to initiate an ambulatory care episode than plans without cost-sharing. The deductible's effect is stronger than the effect of coinsurance. These differences do not hold for major illnesses as judged by either the insured or the physician.

The last sentence of Proposition A1 becomes clear when one considers two cases. First, the insured may feel rather ill subjectively; highly valued combinations (M,X) will then contain more medical care than they do other goods and services. This implies rather steep indifference curves that would make the insured prefer point P ($\bar{M}_1$ hours of care) to point A (zero hours of care). Second, another physician may be willing to provide $\bar{M}_3$, owing, for example, to a more elaborate practice style. Under the deductible, the best point attainable is C; under coinsurance, it is R. The latter already lies on an indifference curve that is higher up the hill than any other point on either bound-

---

10. See also E. B. Keeler, J. P. Newhouse, and C. E. Phelps, "Deductibles and the Demand for Medical Care Services: The Theory of a Consumer Facing a Variable Price Schedule under Uncertainty," *Econometrica* 45 (1977):641–56.

ary. Thus, the patient will want to see the physician regardless of type of plan.

EMPIRICAL ESTIMATES ON TRADITIONAL COST-SHARING

This section contains estimation results based on a random sample of 10 percent of the population covered by insurer A in 1982 (see Appendix Table A9–1 for sample information). Since November 1981, the minimum deductible has been DM 250 ($85) and the next level, DM 450 ($150). Individuals facing these deductibles will usually not submit billings below these thresholds, so the probability of having positive outlays on ambulatory care cannot be studied. Instead, the analysis will focus on the probability that the annual bill will exceed the rather low thresholds of DM 250 and DM 450, which correspond to about one hour, forty minutes and three hours of medical care, respectively (Figure 9–1). The relevant findings, taken from Table A9–2 of the Appendix, are assembled in Table 9–1.

First of all, individuals insured under the leading plan with coinsurance (20 percent) are characterized by a smaller probability of

Table 9–1. Traditional Cost-Sharing and Utilization of Ambulatory Care, Insurer A (1982).

	Estimated Impact on Probability of Bill Exceeding . . .			
	DM 250 *($85)* *(N = 2,063)*	*DM 300* *($115)* *(N = 2,063)*	*DM 450* *($150)* *(N = 2,634)*	*DM 550* *($185)* *(N = 2,634)*
DM 250 ($85) deductible	−0.09	−0.06	[−0.06]	[−0.03]
DM 450 ($150) deductible	. . .	. . .	−0.12	−0.10
20 percent coinsurance	−0.09	−0.09	−0.09	−0.08
30 percent coinsurance	[−0.07]	[−0.09]	[−0.11]	[−0.11]
40 percent coinsurance	−0.21	[−0.16]	−0.20	−0.22

Note: Estimates in brackets are statistically not significant (differing from zero, at a confidence level of 0.05, two-tailed test). Some amounts were not tested for because they were irrelevant. Full details are given in Table A9–2.

exceeding the DM 250 threshold than are those without any cost-sharing, given the same age, sex, and risk class. The dampening effect of the minimal deductible (DM 250) assumes the same magnitude. At a threshold of DM 450, the DM 450 deductible turns out to be highly significant and more effective at reducing expenditures (12 percentage points, at a confidence level of 0.01) than 20 percent coinsurance (9 percentage points). But the DM 250 deductible does not seem to extend its impact very far beyond the DM 250 threshold; its coefficient (albeit negative, as predicted) fails to attain statistical significance, at a 0.05 confidence level, beyond the DM 300 ($100) level. On the other hand, the DM 450 deductible seems to reduce utilization at least up to DM 550 ($185). This discussion may thus be summed up in

Conclusion A1: The effects of traditional cost-sharing predicted by Proposition A1 are borne out to a considerable extent, with the dampening effect of the minimal deductible fading out rather quickly with increasing values of the annual bill for ambulatory care.

It is tempting to compare this conclusion with the findings of the Rand Health Insurance Study.[11] But in that case participants in the experiment were given financial incentives to submit all bills, irrespective of the deductible. It was therefore possible to test at the threshold of $0. The probability of expenditures on care (ambulatory or hospital) being positive was estimated to be about 19 points lower for insureds having a $150 deductible (in 1975 dollars).[12] At 1982 medical prices, the deductible amounts to $290, nearly twice as high as the $150 deductible entered in Table 9–1, the impact of which is some 12 points at that threshold. At the threshold of $150 rather than $0, the Rand estimate would have to be lower, coming closer to the figure presented here.

The Self-Selection Problem

Findings such as those reported here are frequently attributed to self-selection.[13] Some individuals may opt for plans with cost-sharing pro-

---

11. Newhouse, Marquis, and Morris, "A Controlled Trial of Cost Sharing."

12. N. Duan et al., *A Comparison of Alternative Models for the Demand for Medical Care*, R–2754–HHS (Santa Monica, Calif.: Rand, January 1982), pp. 9, 42.

13. C. E. Phelps, "Demand for Reimbursement Insurance," in R. N. Rosett, ed., *The Role of Health Insurance in the Health Services Sector* (New York: National Bureau of Economic Research, 1976), pp. 115–55.

visions because they know they are good health risks. Little wonder, then, if those having such plans stand out as having a favorable claims record; but these savings may stem from (unobservable) risk characteristics rather than from cost-sharing per se.

If the self-selection hypothesis is accurate, certain variables should emerge as powerful predictors of choice of plan. In particular, the propensity of an individual to select a cost-sharing option (either deductible or coinsurance) should depend on risk factors such as age and sex. Although true risk is unobserved, the risk class assigned by the insurer (on the basis of a medical examination) may serve as a rather good proxy; after all, assigned risk class is among the strongest predictors of utilization (see Appendix Tables 9A–2 and 9A–5). But in logistic regressions based on 1980, 1981, and 1982 data, risk class fails to significantly explain selection of options with cost-sharing provisions. Female sex is a significant explanatory variable (at a 0.05 confidence level) of plan selection only in 1980, while the probability of choosing a contract with cost-sharing provisions increases rather than decreases with age. Apparently, insurer A is rather successful at keeping bad risks out of full-coverage plans, perhaps by charging sufficiently high premium differentials. It may also be true that subjective (rather than objective) risk often determines the choice of contract. The age pattern noted above seems to reflect the fact that the generation that became active in the years of economic reconstruction after World War II is less risk averse than those born in the 1960s. Moreover, housewives shy away from contracts with cost-sharing provisions although they do not utilize ambulatory care services more than other groups when age and sex are taken into account (see Table A9–2 of the Appendix). This argument comes down to

> *Conclusion A2:* The effects of contract provisions put forth in Conclusion A1 cannot be attributed to self-selection of good risks, at least not within the population enrolled by insurer A.

The qualification stems from the fact that insurer A might still attract good risks from social health insurance or competitors in private health insurance. But these effects cannot be tested for in the context of the data available here.

REBATES FOR NO CLAIMS: INSURER B

Insurer B, although also a mutual, has some affinity with insurance companies. Along with independent craftsmen and professionals, merchants are overrepresented in the insured population. Insurance is written separately for ambulatory, hospital, and dental care, but these are taken into account jointly in the determination of the rebate. Thus, to be eligible for the rebate, an insured must have coverage under all three titles. In order to obtain the rebate, the insured must have no claims for one year under all three titles. The rebate offer applies to all plans issued by insurer B, precluding self-selection of risks within B according to the rebate offer. Rebates amount to three monthly premium payments; prior to 1980, they varied according to the operating results of the previous year.

The possibility of obtaining such a rebate complicates the analysis in at least two ways. First, the decision to file a claim after having received medical care gains importance. It introduces an additional element of censoring into the distribution of observed claims, one whose influence extends beyond the value of the deductible. Second, prior utilization of services affects the chance of receiving one's rebate and therefore the decision to see a physician and the choice of treatment intensity. On the other hand, this kind of rebate falls short of the full-blown experience-rated bonus system commonly found in European automobile insurance. Analysis of such a system would require multiperiod (and possibly dynamic) optimization methods.[14]

By way of contrast, the rebate will not even be discounted to present value in the simple two-goods models presented below. Nevertheless, a set of predictions can be derived bearing on the decision to initiate a treatment episode. Figure 9–2 can be used to illustrate how the rebate offer might affect the decision of Beta, whose plan does not contain any cost-sharing provisions. Beta now has a choice between two budget constraints: He can either foot the medical bill himself (resulting in the downward-sloping boundary FG) or file the claim (resulting in the horizontal boundary AC).

There exists, in principle, a medical bill that would equalize the two possibilities. It is drawn as $\bar{M}_1$ hours of care, where the two constraints FG and AC intersect (point P). At this point—DM 525 ($175), the assumed value of the rebate—filing the claim is financially equivalent to retaining it. The value of the rebate can also be read as the distance AF on the X axis. In the absence of a rebate offer, an individual with preferences as shown would prefer having $\bar{M}_1$ hours of

14. J. D. Hey, "No Claim Bonus?" *Geneva Papers on Risk and Insurance* 10 (1985): 209–28.

Figure 9–2.   Impact of Rebate Offer on Decision to Seek Care, Plan Without Cost-Sharing.

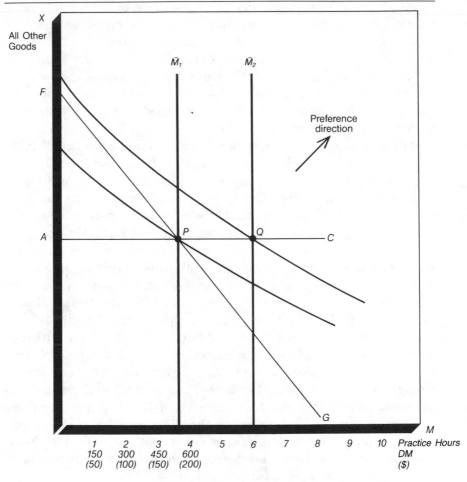

care to zero hours of care (compare points P and A). But with the rebate offer, Beta will rank point F (with zero hours of care) higher than point P (with $\bar{M}_1$ hours of care). As soon as the treatment offer increases to $\bar{M}_2$ hours of care, however, Beta will not want to forgo it, for point Q (where $\bar{M}_2$ = six hours of care) certainly ranks higher than point F (with zero hours of care). In general, the effect of "bonus hunger" should extend somewhat beyond the value of the bonus but fade away afterward.

The same line of argument can be applied to Alpha, who is covered by a plan with a deductible. In Figure 9–3, the rebate offer is attached to a plan with a DM 300 ($100) deductible, the leading option among deductibles offered by insurer B. Alpha, whose preferences are still assumed to be identical with those of Beta, faces the true cost of ambulatory care for the first two hours, whereas additional care is free (boundary *ABC*). If he saves his rebate, his available budget increases by *AF* in terms of other goods and services (*X*). This amount

Figure 9–3. Impact of Rebate Offer on Decision to Seek Care, Plan with Deductible.

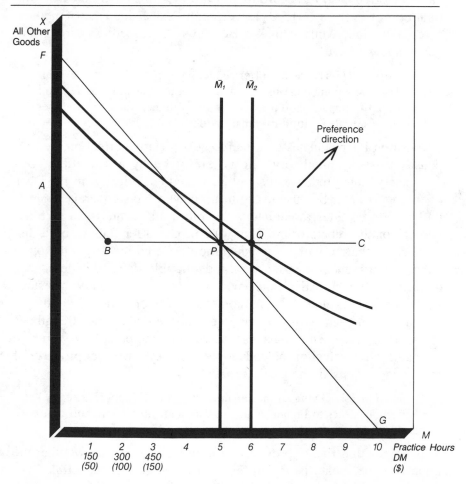

is smaller than *AF* in Figure 9–2 because the rebate amounts to one-fourth of the yearly premium, which is smaller for a plan with a deductible. Filing claims and paying them out of pocket are financially equivalent at a new point *P* (where $\bar{M}_1$ = five hours of care). With indifference curves drawn exactly as in Figure 9–2, Alpha ranks point *F* (zero hours of care and cashing in on the rebate) higher than point *P* ($\bar{M}_1$ hours of care). A similar prediction was derived from Figure 9–2, but in that case the treatment offer $\bar{M}_1$ contained fewer than four hours of care. If the treatment offer in Figure 9–3 is increased to $\bar{M}_2$ (six hours), Alpha would still prefer point *F* (zero hours of care) to point *Q*. In contrast, Beta, who is not subject to a deductible, would have preferred *Q* to *F*, according to Figure 9–2. Thus, increasing the treatment offer from $\bar{M}_1$ to $\bar{M}_2$ leaves Alpha's decision against medical care unaffected, while it makes Beta switch to medical care. More generally, we have

> *Proposition B1:* The rebate offer reduces the propensity to seek ambulatory care among both insureds with a deductible and those without. However, its impact should extend to even higher values of the medical bill if coupled with a minimal deductible.

Proposition B1 postulates that the rebate's negative effect on the propensity to seek ambulatory care is reinforced by a deductible. Unfortunately, this prediction cannot be tested empirically on the basis of insurer B data, because every insured who buys coverage from B under all three titles (ambulatory, hospital, and dental) can take advantage of the rebate offer. Thus, the rebate offer fails to be a distinguishing feature within the population covered by B. On the other hand, the presence or absence of a deductible does provide such a distinctive characteristic—one, moreover, that is shared with insurer A. In order to exploit this common feature, Proposition B1 must be cast into a different form. If it is true that the deductible strengthens the rebate effect, then it must also be true that the prospect of a rebate strengthens the effect of the deductible. This symmetrical property of interaction results in the easily testable

> *Proposition B2:* Owing to the rebate offer, the deductible extends its dampening effect to higher values of medical bills than could be expected otherwise.

This proposition finally provides a possibility for testing whether the impact of the rebate is any different from that of a deductible. We will be examining this possibility in the following section.

EMPIRICAL RESULTS ON REBATES FOR NO CLAIMS

As in the case of insurer A, the probability that the ambulatory care bill will exceed a series of thresholds is analyzed. In order to neutralize the filing decision, the analysis must start at a threshold of DM 300 ($100), the value of the minimum deductible. The impact of this deductible is estimated to amount to 8 percentage points (Table 9–2), with age, sex, and risk classification held constant. In other words, while about 71 percent of annual bills submitted by insureds having full coverage exceeded the limit of DM 300, only 63 percent of those submitted by comparable insureds having the minimum deductible exceeded it. This estimate corresponds quite well to those for insurer A, displayed in Table 9–1. In that case, the estimated impact was 9 percentage points measured at the slightly lower threshold of DM 250 ($85).

But from then on, it will be recalled, the effect of the deductible seemed to fade away rather quickly. In Table 9–2, however, the negative effect of the DM 300 deductible remains statistically significant at 10 to 12 percentage points up to a DM 700 ($235) threshold (significance judged at a 0.05 confidence level). By necessity, this result refers only to the subsample of individuals whose rebate is consumed by their dental bill, for only in those cases can one be sure that all those who incurred ambulatory care outlays submitted their bills. Maybe it bears repeating at this point that savings achieved through failure to submit the bill are of little interest from a social point of view because they amount to a mere shifting of costs from the insurer to the insured.

Table 9–2. Strengthening of the Deductible by the Rebate Option, Insurer B (1982).

	Estimated Impact on Probability of Bill Exceeding . . .					
	DM 300 ($100)	*DM 350 ($115)*	*DM 450 ($150)*	*DM 550 ($185)*	*DM 700 ($235)*	*Deductible + Rebate*
DM 300 deductible	−0.08	−0.10	−0.08	−0.11	−0.12	−0.06

Note: The sample includes 1,773 insureds whose rebate is consumed by the dental bill alone, except for the last column, where $N = 8,483$.

An alternative way of ensuring that all medical bills are reported is to put the threshold at the total of the deductible and the rebate. In fact, this total corresponds to point *P* in Figure 9–3. Point *P* allows five hours of care or DM 750, consisting of two hours' worth of deductible (DM 300) and three hours' worth of rebate (DM 450— the assumed yearly premium is thus DM 1,800 or $600). As soon as the bill for ambulatory care exceeds the sum of the deductible and rebate, the insured has every reason to submit the bill regardless of any dental outlays he may have incurred. These are rather high thresholds; nevertheless, efforts to save the rebate may still leave their traces, for the insured may realize only toward the end of the year that the rebate will be lost. In fact, these equivalence points are surpassed by a probability that is 6 percentage points lower if the insured has a plan with DM 300 ($100) deductible. In all, there is reason to formulate

Conclusion B1: The presence of the rebate option serves to strengthen the effect of the deductible on the propensity to consume an ambulatory treatment offer of given intensity up to rather high values, as stated in Proposition B2.

A similar effect was found by Knappe and Roppel, using different methods.[15] Unfortunately, it is not possible to directly compare the impacts of a deductible and a rebate offer of equal amount, since the rebate, being a fraction of the premium, differs from individual to individual. It is for this reason that its impact must be tested for indirectly, using (approximately) equal deductibles as a benchmark for comparison.

TRADITIONAL COST-SHARING VERSUS THE REBATE OFFER: THEORETICAL CONSIDERATIONS

The preceding sections have been devoted to the study of the impact of contract provisions, dealing with insurers A and B in isolation. Now the leading plans of insurers A and B will be directly juxtaposed in an attempt to derive a differential prediction. Moreover, the previous mode of analysis is generalized somewhat in that the insured is no longer confined to a take-it-or-leave-it situation but has the choice

---

15. E. Knappe and U. Roppel, *Zur Stärkung marktwirtschaftlicher Steuerungselemente im Gesundheitssystem: Probleme und Ansatzpunkte* (Increasing the Scope of Market Allocation in Health Care: Problems and Possibilities) (Cologne: Deutscher Institutsverlag, Beiträge No. 107/108, 1982), p. 69.

between two physicians, say, one having a more modest and the other an elaborate practice style. In Figure 9–4 these choices appear as two $(\bar{M}_0)$ and six $(\bar{M}_2)$ hours of ambulatory care. It is important that at least one of the choices remain below the reference billing, where submitting and not submitting the bill are equivalent financially (point U, equivalent to about three and a half hours of care). The boundary FG in Figure 9–4 is exactly the same as the boundary FG of Figure 9–2. There are three boundaries in Figure 9–4, beginning at the bottom.

Figure 9–4.   The Impact of Aging: Traditional versus Rebate Options.

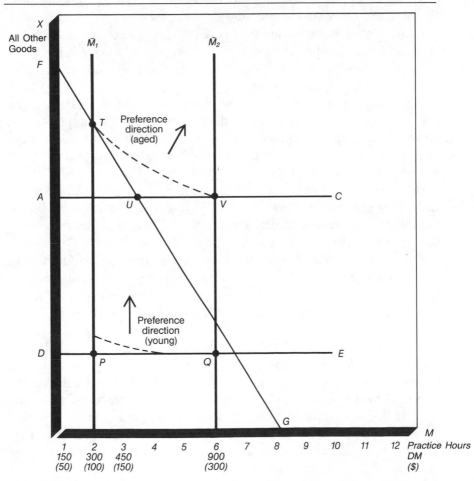

1. Boundary *DE*, symbolizing the full coverage plan as written by insurer A.
2. Boundary *AC*, symbolizing the full coverage plan as written by insurer B, if the insured files a claim (see Figure 9–2).
3. Boundary *FG*, symbolizing the full coverage plan as written by insurer B, if the insured receives the rebate (see Figure 9–2).

Care was taken to locate these constraints correctly on the graph. Insurer A does charge somewhat higher premiums for the two plans considered, with the result that point *D* on the *X* axis is relatively close to the origin. Thus, an individual with a given income has less to spend on other goods and services if insured by A than under a similar plan written by insurer B. However, it is also true that insurer B offers somewhat less comprehensive coverage of sundry items, such as hearing aids, than does insurer A. This point will be neglected in the line of thought that follows.

Imagine an individual becoming more and more interested, as he continues to age, in ambulatory medical care. The question then arises: How much aging does it take to make that individual switch from the modest to the more elaborate treatment offer under the different plans? To begin with, the typical young adult places little value on ambulatory care (*M*) compared to other goods and services (*X*). Graphically, his preference field is strongly oriented toward more *X*, as indicated by the almost vertical arrow. Accordingly, indifference curves must run flat, like the one passing through point *Q* on the *DE* boundary. But the diagram shows that even such a young individual would tend toward the elaborate treatment alternative with $\bar{M}_2$ hours of care (point *Q*) rather than make do with $\bar{M}_0$ hours of care (point *P*). All that is necessary is that he be covered by the no-cost sharing plan of insurer A.

Now suppose this individual is older. Graphically, this tilts his preference field toward the northeastern corner of Figure 9–4, and his indifference curves increasingly slope down. But under the rebate option of insurer B, a switch from the modest $\bar{M}_0$ care to the elaborate $\bar{M}_2$ care becomes attractive only if points *T* (on the *FG* boundary) and *V* (on the *AC* boundary) are subjectively equivalent. A glance at Figure 9–4 immediately reveals that the individual's preference field must be tilted rather strongly away from *X* and toward *M* to achieve indifference. Such a tilt would be the typical result of a good deal of aging. Clearly, a good deal of aging is necessary to put the insured on the brink of selecting more elaborate treatment when he is given the rebate option. Phrased somewhat more generally, this argument may be summed up by

> *Proposition D1:* Demand-increasing characteristics such as age (or female sex) should have less influence on the intensity of ambulatory care chosen when enrollees of insurer B are compared to those of insurer A. This statement is true only if the more modest treatment alternative costs less than the rebate, i.e., the maximum savings attainable.

The last proviso becomes clear from Figure 9–4. Under the rebate option, submitting and keeping the medical bill are equivalent financially where the boundaries AC and FG intersect. This intersection, marked as point U, corresponds to about three and a half hours of care (a rebate of DM 525 or \$175). If the choice between treatment offers had been between three and a half and six ($\bar{M}_2$) hours of care, a completely flat indifference curve would have sufficed to make the two offers equivalent. Thus, even a very young insured would tend to opt for the elaborate alternative if the modest one costs as much as the rebate itself.

TESTING FOR THE DIFFERENTIAL EFFECT OF THE REBATE OFFER

Proposition D1 can be tested rather easily by comparing the experience of insurers A and B in terms of the effects of age and female sex on the utilization of ambulatory care. For both samples, the age group below 44 years old serves as the benchmark. The first column of Table 9–3 indicates that, relative to the benchmark group, the probability of having positive ambulatory care outlays is 7 percentage points higher in the 45–54 age group of insurer A. For those above age 65, the estimated increment in probability amounts to 17 percentage points, but without attaining statistical significance. Therefore, if a young enrollee of insurer A has a 70 percent probability of making some outlay on ambulatory care, the probability might rise to about 87 percent in the high age group.

This increase in probability is much more moderate among the enrollees of insurer B, as predicted by Proposition D1. The third column of Table 9–3 shows that the age group above 65 has positive outlays with a probability that is but 5 percentage points higher than that of

Table 9–3.   Influence of Demand-Increasing Characteristics, Insurers A and B Compared.

| | *Impact on Probability of Ambulatory Care Bill Exceeding X (1982)* | | | |
| | *Insurer A (No Rebate Option) (N = 2,097)* | | *Insurer B (Rebate Option) (N = 1,726)* | |
	X = DM 0 ($0)	*X = DM 250 ($85)*	*X = DM 0 ($0)*	*X = 300 ($100)*
Age 45–54	0.07	0.11	0.08	0.14
Age 55–64	[0.11]	0.19	[0.02]	0.13
Age 65–99	[0.17]	0.23	[0.05]	[0.14]
Female	0.14	0.21	0.11	0.16

SOURCE: Tables A9–2, A9–5.

Note: Excluded from the sample are individuals with cost-sharing provisions (insurers A and B) and those whose dental bills remain below the rebate amount (insurer B). Bracketed values are statistically insignificant, at a confidence level of 0.05, two-tailed test.

the benchmark group. This is much less than the 17 points found for insurer A. Again, the hypothesis that these older enrollees have the same 70 percent probability of positive outlays as their younger counterparts cannot be rejected on statistical grounds, using the customary 0.05 level of confidence.

A very similar pattern emerges if the threshold is set at DM 250 (or DM 300—$100—for insurer B). As shown by the second column of Table 9–3, the probability of the medical bill exceeding the DM 250 threshold rises with age, becoming up to 23 percentage points higher than in the benchmark group of insurer A. Among the enrollees of insurer B, that probability remains just about the same from the age group 45–54 onward. Among the enrollees of more than 65 years of age, the estimated differential of 14 percentage points over and above the benchmark group fails even to attain statistical significance, judged at a 0.05 confidence level.

Table 9–3 contains another piece of evidence that supports the differential impact of the rebate offer. Enrollees of female sex have a higher probability of exceeding a given threshold with their ambulatory care outlays. This holds true for both insurers. However, the estimated probability of having positive outlays at all is 14 percentage points higher for female than for the male benchmark group of insurer

A, while it is only 11 points higher for insurer B (columns one and three).

The probability that the medical bill will be higher than DM 250/DM 300 is still higher for females than for males. But the differential amounts to 21 percentage points for insurer A and 16 points for insurer B (columns two and four). All these observations lend support to the view that the rebate offered by insurer B exerts a small but consistent dampening effect on the positive relationship between factors that increase demand (age, female sex) and utilization of ambulatory medical care. These considerations yield the very essential

> *Conclusion D1:* A comparison of age and sex differentials in medical bills for ambulatory care confirms Proposition D1. There is evidence to the effect that the rebate offer of insurer B dampens utilization of ambulatory medical care independently of traditional cost-sharing provisions.

This conclusion contains the strongest evidence in favor of the basic hypothesis stated in the introductory section: that rebate options are more effective in restraining utilization of medical care than are plans with only deductibles and/or coinsurance.

RELEVANCE TO SOCIAL INSURANCE

Owing to its data base, this study is limited to upper-income individuals. Nevertheless, an attempt can be made to extrapolate its findings to lower-income strata covered by social insurance schemes. Within the population segments covered by insurers A and B, as many insureds as possible have been assigned to uppermost, upper, or middle class. With only occupational status (but neither income nor wealth) known, such a classification necessarily involves a degree of judgment. Moreover, it can only be applied to men.

Preliminary statistical analysis suggested that the impact of increasing age on the utilization of ambulatory care was the same regardless of whether the insured belonged to the uppermost-, upper-, or middle-class group. However, there were some indications that assigned risk might have a specific effect on utilization according to strata. The crucial issue is, of course, whether cost-sharing provisions, traditional or of the rebate type, have a larger effect on the behavior of relatively lower income insured than on the members of higher strata.

The evidence turns out to be less clear-cut than expected (Table 9–4). For insurer A, the DM 450 threshold was selected because it allows us to test for the differential impacts of 20 percent coinsurance, the minimum DM 250 deductible, and the DM 450 deductible. Analyzed in isolation in each class, coinsurance does not seem to be statistically significant, but there is a weak hint that its negative effect on utilization may be most pronounced in the middle class. As in Table 9–1, the effect of the DM 250 deductible has faded to insignificance at the DM 450 threshold. Finally, the DM 450 deductible is estimated to have maximum impact among the upper class: It may lower the probability of the medical bill exceeding DM 450 by a full 15 percentage points. Statistically insignificant effects are found for the uppermost and middle strata.

This reversed ordering may well be of transitory nature, however, since insurer A increased the second-lowest deductible at the end of 1981, from DM 360 to DM 450 ($120 to $150). In 1981, the old deductible had a maximum effect of 21 percentage points (estimated at the DM 360 threshold) in the middle-class stratum and 8 points in the upper stratum. Its effect fell short of statistical significance in the top stratum. Thus, very high income individuals seem to react more quickly than others to changed financial incentives; in the long run, when the limited size of these incentives becomes clear, they can afford to neglect them.

Table 9–4.   Impact of Cost-Sharing, by Socioeconomic Class (1982).

	Estimated Impact on Probability of Ambulatory Care Bill Exceeding X		
Insurer A *X = DM 450 ($50)*	*Uppermost* *Class*	*Upper* *Class*	*Middle* *Class*
Coinsurance 20 percent	[−0.08]	[−0.06]	[−0.10]
Deductible			
DM 250 ($85)	[−0.05]	[−0.06]	[−0.04]
DM 450 ($150)	[−0.12]	−0.15	[−0.09]
Insurer B *X = DM 300 ($100)*			
Deductible			
DM 300 ($100)	[−0.03]	−0.10	−0.16

Note: Figures given are relative to enrollees of the upper socioeconomic class having plans without any cost-sharing provisions. Bracketed figures are not statistically significant, at a confidence level of 0.05, two-tailed test.

As regards male members of mutual insurer B belonging to the uppermost income group (lower half of Table 9–4), the DM 300 deductible fails to have a significant effect on the probability that the medical bill will exceed the threshold of DM 300. By way of contrast, the deductible is estimated to lower this probability by as much as 10 and 16 percentage points in the upper and middle strata, respectively.

In all, Table 9–4 contains sufficient evidence to support

> *Conclusion D2:* Whether reinforced by rebate offers or not, cost-sharing provisions tend to have a stronger impact on relatively lower income insured than on very high income individuals. Due allowance must be made in the short run, however, for a quicker reaction to such provisions by the well-to-do.

Although based on a high-income segment of the population, this conclusion is in full accordance with other studies focusing on the population covered by social insurance.[16] It even stands to reason that cost-sharing provisions will have an increasing impact the further one moves down the socioeconomic ladder. From the point of view of equal access, an important feature of any insurance scheme would therefore be that cost-sharing could be waived if necessary. Of course, a financial sanction would have to be attached to such a waiver. Rebate options of the type analyzed here may well provide the needed flexibility while limiting moral hazard at least as effectively as more traditional cost-sharing methods.

CONCLUSION

This chapter has examined the rebate offer for no claims recently introduced by West German private health insurers. Such an offer promises to have more appeal to buyers of insurance than do traditional cost-sharing arrangements. Moreover, theoretical analysis of leading variants of traditional and new plans suggests a dampening effect of the rebate offer on medical care costs over and above that afforded by traditional cost-sharing instruments.

These predictions were subjected to a series of empirical tests using individual data provided by two private insurers. For insurer A (selling traditional plans) it was found that coinsurance rates ranging from 20 to 40 percent restrained utilization of ambulatory medical care less

16. R. G. Beck, "The Effects of Co-payment on the Poor," *Journal of Human Resources* 9 (1974):129–42.

than did small deductibles (amounting to the equivalent of two to three practice hours), but the latter effect faded away rather quickly with increasing values of the bill. By way of contrast, a deductible and rebate of the same size appeared to retain its dampening effect for bills worth up to five practice hours.

Finally, older age and female sex increased the probability of a bill exceeding a given threshold, but these effects were found to be weaker among enrollees of insurer B than those of insurer A, as predicted. Since all cost-sharing arrangements seem to restrain utilization of ambulatory care most among middle-class enrollees and least among very high income earners, rebate offers could become an avenue for reintroducing cost-sharing in German social health insurance. Unlike traditional cost-sharing instruments, rebate offers allow the insured to reduce his out-of-pocket medical care costs to zero whenever he sees fit—at the fixed, calculable price of forgoing the premium rebate.

APPENDIX

Table A9–1. **Dependent and Explanatory Variables and Descriptive Statistics, Insurer A (1982).**

Variable	Explanation	Mean
DU250	= 1: Ambulatory care outlay exceeds DM 250	0.70
DU450	= 1: Ambulatory care outlay exceeds DM 450	0.59
A1924	= 1: Age 19–24	0.05
A3544	= 1: Age 35–44	0.28
A4554	= 1: Age 45–54	0.13
A5564	= 1: Age 55–64	0.09
A6574	= 1: Age 65–74	0.06
A7599	= 1: Age 75+	0.06
SEXF	= 1: Female	0.43
RISK	= 1–8: Risk class	1.23
SELF	= 1: Self-employed	0.43
HOUSEW	= 1: Housewife	0.08
COR40	= 1: Coinsurance rate 40 percent	0.01
COR30	= 1: Coinsurance rate 30 percent	0.02
COR20	= 1: Coinsurance rate 20 percent	0.17
DED450	= 1: Deductible DM 450	0.19
DED250	= 1: Deductible DM 250	0.12

Note: The sample includes all individuals with deductibles of DM 450 or less; it is used to calculate the third column of Table A9–2, bottom.

Table A9–2.   Probability of Having Ambulatory Care Expenditures in Excess of _X_, Insurer A (1982).

Variable	_X_ = DM0	_X = DM 250_ _($85)_	_X = DM 450_ _($150)_
No deductible (N = 1,686)			
A1924	−0.0533(−1.14)	−0.138**(−2.59)	−0.159*(−2.51)
A3544	0.0436(1.57)	0.0301(1.04)	0.0575(1.81)
A4554	0.129**(3.10)	0.138**(3.24)	0.183***(4.03)
A5564	0.137**(2.67)	0.160**(3.03)	0.230***(4.11)
A6574	0.301***(3.57)	0.340***(4.20)	0.430***(5.30)
A7599	0.398**(3.15)	0.340***(3.50)	0.465***(4.67)
SEXF	0.160***(5.75)	0.190***(6.96)	0.194***(6.83)
RISK	0.0328***(3.28)	0.0495***(4.97)	0.0539***(5.31)
SELF	−0.0818***(−3.45)	−0.0651**(−2.61)	−0.0467(−1.71)
HOUSEW	0.0119(0.04)	−0.0023(0.00)	−0.0315(−0.42)
COR20	−0.0787**(2.60)	−0.0776*(−2.44)	−0.0946**(−2.73)
COR30	−0.124(1.50)	−0.0582(−0.64)	−0.129(−1.39)
COR40	−0.272***(3.53)	−0.193*(−2.15)	−0.194*(−1.99)

	Chi2 = 157/df = 13 CONC = 0.709	Chi2 = 245/df = 13 CONC = 0.718	Chi2 = 292/df = 13 CONC = 0.721

Deductible = 0		≤ DM 250 (N = 2,063)	≤DM 250 or DM 450 (N = 2,634)
A1924		−0.140**(−2.79)	−0.186***(−3.54)
A3544		0.0442(1.66)	0.0391(1.54)
A4554		0.145***(3.76)	0.167***(4.68)
A5564		0.198***(3.91)	0.214***(4.51)
A6574		0.346***(4.52)	0.424***(5.56)
A7599		0.364***(3.63)	0.388***(4.34)
SEXF		0.208***(8.18)	0.232***(10.00)
RISK		0.0565***(5.77)	0.0644***(7.19)
SELF		−0.0769***(−3.33)	−0.0540*(−2.43)
HOUSEW		−0.0468(−0.68)	−0.116(−1.81)
COR20		−0.0869**(−2.65)	−0.0942**(−2.69)
COR30		−0.0678(−0.71)	−0.114(−1.19)
COR40		−0.212**(−2.26)	−0.198*(1.96)
DED250		−0.0871**(−3.09)	−0.0562(−1.78)
DED450		—	−0.124***(−4.49)

		Chi2 = 330/df = 14 CONC = 0.727	Chi2 = 483/df = 15 CONC = 0.730

Note: Intercepts are not shown. Coefficients (estimated impacts on probability) are derived from logistic regression coefficients through multiplication by $P (1 - P)$ where P = mean probability (see H. Theil, *Statistical Decomposition Analysis* [Amsterdam and New York: North-Holland, 1972], pp. 166–78, esp. 169). Asymptotic t − ratios are in parentheses.

*0.05 level of significance
**0.01 level of significance
***0.001 level of significance
CONC = share of concordant pairs

Table A9–3.   Dependent Variables and Sample Information, Insurer B (1982).

Variable	Explanation		Reference	Mean
DU0	= 1:	Ambulatory	Table A9–5 (top)	0.87
DU300	= 1:	care outlay	Table A9–5 (top)	0.71
DU300	= 1:	in excess	Table A9–5 (bottom)	0.71
DU bonus + deductible	= 1:	of X	Table A9–5 (bottom)	0.32

Table A9–4.   Explanatory Variables and Descriptive Statistics, Insurer B (1982).

Variable	Explanation	Mean
A1924	= 1: Age 19–24	0.02
A3544	= 1: Age 35–44	0.41
A4554	= 1: Age 45–54	0.18
A5564	= 1: Age 55–64	0.09
A6599	= 1: Age 65+	0.03
SEXF	= 1: Female	0.29
RISK	= Risk surcharge for coverage of ambulatory care (%)	4.55
SELF	= 1: Self-employed	0.48
HOUSEW	= 1: Housewife	0.08
DED300	= 1: Deductible DM 300	0.14

Note: The sample includes all individuals with deductibles of DM 300 or less; it is used to calculate the second column of Table A9–5, bottom.

Table A9–5.   Probability of Having Ambulatory Care Expenditures in Excess of X, Insurer B (1982).

	$X = DM0$	$X = DM\ 300$ ($100)	$X = Bonus +$ Deductible
No deductible (N = 1,726)			
A1924	−0.0634(−1.26)	0.0636(0.80)	
A3544	−0.0114(−0.58)	0.0220(0.85)	
A4554	0.0824**(2.66)	0.141***(3.83)	
A5564	0.0172(0.44)	0.129**(2.49)	
A6599	0.0541(0.88)	0.144(1.51)	
SEXF	0.109***(4.06)	0.158***(5.01)	
RISK	0.0099***(4.27)	0.0088***(4.97)	
SELF	−0.0579***(−3.28)	−0.0626**(−2.66)	
HOUSEW	−0.0558(−1.14)	−0.0936(−1.65)	
	Chi2 = 98/df = 9	Chi2 = 115/df = 9	
	CONC = 0.639	CONC = 0.620	
Deductible = 0		≤ DM 300 (N = 2,009)	≤ DM 300 (N = 8,483)
A1924		0.0622(0.84)	—
A3544		0.0350(1.41)	0.0710***(5.34)
A4554		0.162***(4.74)	0.152***(9.54)
A5564		0.138**(2.98)	0.217***(10.39)
A6599		0.127(1.62)	0.262***(9.41)
SEXF		0.145***(5.04)	0.0769***(5.97)
RISK		0.0080***(5.46)	0.0051***(11.18)
SELF		−0.0655**(−2.93)	−0.0540***(−4.79)
HOUSEW		−0.105*(−2.10)	−0.0599**(−2.67)
DED300		−0.0847**(−2.82)	−0.0630***(−3.98)
		Chi2 = 137/df = 10	Chi2 = 519/df = 9
		CONC = 0.624	CONC = 0.612

Note: The sample used in the first and second columns includes all individuals with dental care expenditures exceeding their bonuses. The sample used in the third column includes all individuals.

SELECTED BIBLIOGRAPHY

Beck, R. G. "The Effects of Co-payment on the Poor." *Journal of Human Resources* 9 (1974):129–42.

Beske, F. "Expenditures and Attempts of Cost Containment in the Statutory Health Insurance System of the Federal Republic of Germany." In Nuffield Provincial Hospitals Trust, ed., *The Public/Private Mix for Health: The Relevance and Effects of Change*, pp. 233–63. London: NPHT, 1982.

Duan, N.; W. G. Manning; C. N. Morris; and J. P. Newhouse. "A Comparison of Alternative Models for the Demand for Medical Care." R-2754-HHS. Santa Monica, Calif.: Rand, 1982.

Feldstein, M. S. "The Welfare Loss of Excess Health Insurance." *Journal of Political Economy* 81 (1973):251–80.

Hey, J. D. "No Claim Bonus?" *Geneva Papers on Risk and Insurance* 10 (1985):209–28.

Keeler, E. B.; J. P. Newhouse; and C. E. Phelps. "Deductibles and the Demand for Medical Care Services: The Theory of a Consumer Facing a Variable Price Schedule under Uncertainty." *Econometrica* 45 (1977): 641–56.

Newhouse, J. P. "A Design for a Health Insurance Experiment." *Inquiry* 11 (1974):5–27.

Newhouse, J. P.; Willard Manning, et al. "Some Interim Results from a Controlled Trial of Cost Sharing in Health Insurance." *New England Journal of Medicine* 305 (1981):1501–7.

Phelps, C. E. "Demand for Reimbursement Insurance." In R. N. Rosett, ed., *The Role of Health Insurance in the Health Services Sector*, pp. 115–55. New York: National Bureau of Economic Research, 1976.

Schulenburg, J. M. "Report from Germany: Current Conditions and Controversies in the Health Care System." In *Journal of Health Politics, Policy and Law* 8, no. 2 (Summer 1983):320–51.

Theil, H. *Statistical Decomposition Analysis*, pp. 166–78. Amsterdam and New York: North-Holland, 1972.

Wilensky, G. R., and L. F. Rossiter. "The Magnitude and Determinants of Physician-Initiated Visits in the United States." In J. van der Gaag and M. Perlman, eds., *Health, Economics, and Health Economics*, 215–44. Amsterdam and New York: North-Holland, 1981.

Zeckhauser, R. "Medical Insurance: A Case Study of the Tradeoff between Risk and Appropriate Incentives." *Journal of Economic Theory* 2 (1970): 10–26.

Zweifel, P. "Drugs, Physicians, and Hospitalization." In R. M. Scheffler and L. F. Rossiter, eds., *Advances in Health Economics and Health Services Research*, vol. 5, Greenwich, Conn.: JAI Press, 1984.

10

PREFERRED PROVIDER ORGANIZATIONS AND HEALTH CARE COMPETITION

H. E. Frech III

INTRODUCTION

The preferred provider organization (PPO) is the most dramatic and promising innovation in American health insurance since the early days of the health maintenance organization (HMO). PPOs are intended to reduce the costs of health care. They are so new that no official government or industry definitions or statistics for them exist. The limited literature available shows, however, that they are growing very rapidly, especially in the West.[1] In this chapter, I will examine the methods by which PPOs try to reduce health care costs and the potential effects of PPOs on costs and competition.

The PPO strategies for reducing health care costs can be boiled down to two: reduction of quantity and reduction of price. The former

1. For an informative review of the available literature, see Jon Gabel and Dan Ermann, "Preferred Provider Organizations: Performance, Problems, and Promise," *Health Affairs* 4, no. 1 (Spring 1985):24–40. For other new developments in health insurance, such as increasing copayment, see John Goodman, "The Changing Market for Health Insurance: Opting Out of the Cost-Plus System," Policy Report No. 118 (Dallas, Tex.: National Center for Policy Analysis, September 1985).

Note: Thanks are due to Richard Arnould, William Comanor, Alain Enthoven, Jon Gabel, Paul Ginsburg, William Lynk, Jack Meyers, Joel May, Joseph Newhouse, Mark Satterthwaite, and Jody Sindelar for excellent comments on an earlier draft.

is essentially identical to the quality control of the individual practice type of HMO. The latter is more interesting. It amounts to an attempt to improve the efficiency of competition in health care while retaining some of the consumer choice features of ordinary fee-for-service medicine. The major goal of this chapter is to analyze the competition-enhancing effect of PPOs. While they seem generally procompetitive, PPOs have some potential anticompetitive effects that bear watching.

WHAT IS A PPO?

A PPO provides a particular type of health insurance. It contracts with a limited number of providers—hospitals and/or physicians, to provide care for a particular group of consumers on preferential terms. The PPO stands between a specific, defined group of consumers and a specific, defined group of providers. Consumers are offered better terms (more complete insurance and possibly price discounts and/or utilization controls) if they patronize the preferred providers—hence the name. PPOs can be, and have been, organized by the providers, insurance companies, or employers. Union-organized PPOs cannot be far in the future. The PPO itself may not bear the risk; it may arrange for all or part of the risk to be assumed by others through reinsurance, or it may function as a contractual arm of an insurer. To make this concept more concrete, it will be useful to look at exactly what the consumers and the providers receive and relinquish in this contractual arrangement.

First, let us look at what the parties to the contract give up. The consumers relinquish free choice of provider—but only partially. The PPO contract provides certain insurance benefits for consumers who patronize the preferred providers, but it also provides some benefits for consumers who use other providers (often called out-of-plan utilization). This feature and the fee-for-service option distinguish the PPO from the HMO, which provides no benefits for out-of-plan use except for emergency care. The provider members of the PPO also give up some freedom, either pricing freedom and/or clinical freedom; that is, they either agree to provide care at a discount or at a fixed price, or they agree to be subject to the PPO's utilization controls, or both.

On the benefit side, PPO consumers are promised some savings in expected costs, based either on price reductions (through discounts and selection of low-priced providers) or utilization reductions. The providers receive more business in return. The procompetitive nature of the contract is evident here. Providers receive the promise of greater sales in return for the promise of lower costs and/or prices.

Relation to Other Forms of Health Insurance

For perspective, let us consider the whole spectrum of possible insurance arrangements. At one extreme is the currently typical third-party insurance. Under this sort of contract, the insurer simply reimburses the consumer for his expenses or pays the provider directly for the consumer's bills or costs. The insurer does not try either to establish prices in advance or to control utilization beyond some effort to eliminate very unusual or "unreasonable" utilization. Under this scheme, the consumer may use any doctor or hospital and receive the same insurance benefit, typically defined as some percentage of the cost. The insurer and the provider are, in principle, separate. At the other extreme is the group practice HMO. Here the insurer and the provider are integrated. The HMO is responsible for providing care to the insured, often with no out-of-pocket payment at all, if the insured goes to the HMO for care. If the insured purchases medical care from providers outside the HMO, he is entitled to no benefits whatsoever. Under this scheme, the HMO controls the price of the providers, since they are employees. It also controls utilization very easily, since it can simply limit the number of physicians and other personnel it hires and the number and type of hospital beds that its physicians are allowed to use. Somewhere in the middle of this spectrum between third-party insurance and HMO is the independent practice association (IPA) HMO, in which the HMO contracts with individual physicians and hospitals to provide care to its members. The physicians are paid by the HMO on a fee-for-service basis. Sometimes the fee is agreed upon in advance and set below the market fee. The hospitals and especially the physicians typically agree to be subject to some kind of (ordinarily loose) utilization control. IPAs are often, although not necessarily, organized by groups of physicians.

The economics of the fee-for-service PPO is closely related to that of the capitation HMO. From the consumer's viewpoint, the PPO may be thought of as a liberal version of the HMO, with one wrinkle: Consumers may still receive benefits, albeit reduced, if they use providers outside the PPO. Remember that HMOs provide zero benefits for out-of-plan utilization. It is this liberality that seems to make PPOs more attractive than traditional HMOs to many consumers.

Advantage over HMOs

Consumers who already have a valuable physician relationship outside the PPO can still benefit by using PPO hospitals and specialists, without giving up that relationship. Families can keep such relationships with some physicians for some family members and still gain from using PPO physicians for other members. In this respect, the PPO is like the Mexican or Chinese restaurant that includes hamburgers on its menu. It is thus patronized by families with one American-food lover who would otherwise have vetoed so exotic a cuisine. Individuals are not locked in to the PPO. At some reasonable cost, they can go outside the PPO if they are dissatisfied with a particular provider. This feature creates a form of market-based quality control, even if a particular medical specialty is represented by only one PPO member. Consumers need not tolerate a low level of quality or service by a preferred provider when they have this safety valve open to them.

Obviously, the option of paying for out-of-plan care offers advantages to consumers when compared to the harsher HMO policy. What is not so readily appreciated, however, is that properly designed coverage for out-of-plan care can save on PPO costs. The medical care thus purchased presumably costs somewhat more. If the PPO provides low enough benefits for such care, the PPO, on balance, profits from out-of-plan use. For example, suppose that out-of-plan medical care costs 10 percent more than in-plan use. If the PPO's benefits for out-of-plan care are reduced by more than 10 percent (say, by paying 75 percent of those costs compared to 90 percent of in-plan costs), the PPO gains. Also, non-PPO providers may respond to the PPO by behaving more competitively themselves, especially in competing for PPO members.

While it is closely related to the HMO economically, the PPO does not appear alien to consumers who are accustomed to the freedom of choice and procedures of traditional third-party insurance. From their viewpoint, they can still choose any physician or hospital. They still file their claims as usual, perhaps using the same claim forms as before. Aside from lower premiums, all that is new is that the benefits are better and the prices possibly lower if they use the PPO providers. This familiarity is a marketing advantage of the PPO, especially when compared to the HMO.

HISTORY OF PPOs

The history of the current PPO movement begins in the 1970s, but there have been important precursors. The earliest and most direct one is that of contract medicine as practiced around the turn of the century. Under this scheme, employers contracted with individual physicians for groups to provide medical care to their workers. Contract medicine was particularly popular in remote geographical areas. Much like the physicians of today, physicians who contracted with employers were content to accept lower prices in return for an assurance of more business. Not surprisingly, contract medicine was actively opposed by organized medicine.

HMOs can be traced more or less continuously to the early contract-medicine relationships. The most prominent HMO, Kaiser Foundation Health Plan, was originally established by Henry Kaiser for his California steel mill and shipyard employees. But HMOs evolved into a rigid system of benefits, whereby out-of-plan use was not reimbursed. Contract medicine and HMOs posed similar competitive threats to ordinary fee-for-service medicine, and both were actively opposed by organized medicine.[2]

In the early 1930s, the new Blue Cross hospital insurance began by contracting with a limited number of hospitals, which usually gave Blue Cross discounts. They can thus be regarded as early PPOs. Within a very few years, however, the Blue Cross plans began to contract with all or most area hospitals, and until recently they showed little interest—partly because most of them were controlled by the hospitals themselves—in reducing utilization, and thus evolved into models of conventional third-party insurance rather than into a form similar to modern PPOs.

It is likely that there have always been some small groups that contracted with selected providers in what would now be recognized as PPO arrangements. But the modern large-scale PPO movement

---

2. For an excellent summary of the early history of contract medicine and HMOs, and the opposition of organized medicine, see David M. Barton, "Alternative Institutional Arrangements for Medical Care Insurance" (Ph.D. Diss., University of Virginia, 1974).

dates back to the 1970s. The earliest pioneer seems to have been the Los Angeles firm Dual-Plus, which contracted with a panel of physicians on behalf of some insurance firms in 1970.[3] AdMar, also a Los Angeles company, was another early innovator. In its role as third-party administrator, it contracted with providers on a selective and preferential basis on behalf of employer and employee self-insured groups as early as 1978.[4] In 1980, the term *PPO* was apparently first used by Linda Ellwein of InterStudy, a respected Minneapolis consulting firm.

PPOs have been most successful in California. By 1985, that state accounted for 96 of the nations's 334 PPOs. Other states with many PPOs include Florida, with 27, and Ohio, with 26. California has 2.2 million PPO subscribers out of a national total estimated at 3.6 million. Part of the reason for California's leadership is due to the novel marketing strategy adopted by its Blue Cross plan. In areas where it had sufficient hospital and physician PPO contracts, Blue Cross simply put all of its individual subscribers into its PPO, called Prudent Buyer, and stopped writing traditional third-party individual health insurance. As of 1984, Prudent Buyer alone accounted for at least half a million PPO members.[5]

The organization and sponsorship of PPOs has varied widely. By 1985, providers had sponsored 52 percent of them and insurance carriers 16 percent. The remaining 32 percent were sponsored by investors, third-party administrators like AdMar, employees, or employers.[6] Of the PPOs whose ownership form was known in 1984, 52 percent were profit-seeking and 48 percent were nonprofit.[7]

Most of the provider- and insurer-based PPOs do not tailor their programs to the specific group being insured, while the consumer-based PPOs do. It is less expensive to administer a PPO contract that is not specifically tailored, but a generic contract can result in little or no cost savings. For example, suppose that the PPO contracts with

3. Undated sales materials, Dual-Plus (11 Golden Shore Drive, Long Beach, CA 90802).

4. This section relies heavily on Roger L. Arlen, "Preferred Provider Organizations: A History," University of California, Santa Barbara, February 1985. (Unpublished.)

5. Personal interview with Roger L. Arlen, University of California, Santa Barbara, February 1985.

6. "Industry Report on PPO Development," *Medical Benefits* 2, no. 13 (July 15, 1985): 8, 10, 11.

7. American Medical Care and Review Association, *Directory of Preferred Provider Organizations,* 3d ed., (Bethesda, Md.: AMCRA, 1984).

a hospital for a blanket charge of $800 per day, which is a 20 percent discount from the hospital's usual charge. If a particular group's past experience had been an average per diem cost of $750, perhaps because its members were very young, the PPO would actually be more costly than would the traditional plan. For this group, a customized PPO would be necessary to show real savings. This customizing requires data processing and statistical expertise, normally provided by a third-party administrator or consultant such as AdMar of Los Angeles or Affordable Health Concepts of Sacramento. It is likely that some insurers will start customizing their offerings for specific groups, especially large ones.

In California at least, legal changes have been important to PPO growth. Before 1982, health insurers were prohibited from selectively contracting with providers and from interfering with free choice of provider. Thus, early PPOs were organized by independent organizations, such as Dual-Plus or AdMar, on behalf of insurers or self-insured trusts. These firms avoided state insurance regulations. The passage of two important laws in 1982 changed all this. The first, AB 799, authorized MediCal (California's Medicaid) to contract selectively with hospitals. It became law in June 1982. The plan is considered a great success, having saved $230 million (13 percent) in its first year. Only a month later, California health insurance companies were given the same freedom by AB 3480, which allowed ordinary health insurers to compete with third-party administrators in offering PPO coverage of large groups, and to offer PPO coverage to individuals and small groups for the first time.

METHODS OF COST REDUCTION

Health care costs are equal to the price of care received times the quantity of care received. Cost-reduction strategies must operate on one or both factors. PPO cost-reduction strategies include utilization control, price discounts, provider selection for low price and low utilization, incentives for consumers to use PPO providers, and consumer copayments. PPOs share this last feature with traditional third-party insurance. Greater consumer copayments work primarily to reduce the quantity of care demanded, but they also have an important effect on reducing price by stimulating consumers to search for low price and by increasing providers' incentives to set a relatively low price.[8] PPOs differ widely in their use of consumer copayment. Some do not require any consumer copayment for in-plan care, while some require copayment as high as 20 percent.

PPOs' use of administrative utilization controls is very similar to that of independent practice–type HMOs and third-party insurers. Common examples include requirements for preadmission authorization for nonemergency hospitalization, second opinions for surgery, and concurrent review while the patient is hospitalized. Somewhat less common are programs of claims review that pinpoint physicians or hospitals with high utilization for given diagnoses. Some PPOs have no utilization controls at all; in some cases, these are new organizations that expect to institute controls in the future.

Naturally, PPOs expect that costs will be lower if consumers patronize the member providers. Most of the lower costs of using PPO providers probably comes from their lower prices, but if utilization controls have some effect, there would also be some savings in quantity of care. Thus, disincentives of various kinds and magnitudes are used to discourage out-of-plan use. Most commonly, the PPO raises the consumer copayment for out-of-plan use. Often the deductible is several hundred dollars per family higher for such use, and the copayment may be 20 percent for out-of-plan use but a small amount or nothing for in-plan use. Note that this consumer disincentive also has the salutary side effect of reducing costs, perhaps overall, but certainly to the PPO itself. On the other hand, there are some PPOs that do not penalize out-of-plan use; they try to channel their subscribers to the preferred providers by advertising the discount and other advantages. As the disincentives to out-of-plan use rise, PPOs become more like HMOs. The key feature of the PPO, however, is the idea of obtaining care at a lower price. It is this feature that makes the greatest difference for hospital and physician competition.

8. See H. E. Frech III and Paul B. Ginsburg, "Imposed Health Insurance in Monopolistic Markets," *Economic Inquiry* 13, no. 1 (March 1975):55–70, for theoretical analysis of how consumer copayment affects incentives for search and choice of low-priced providers. For empirical evidence, see Joseph P. Newhouse and Charles E. Phelps, "Price and Income Elasticities for Medical Care Services," in Mark Perlman, ed., *The Economics of Health and Medical Care: Proceedings of a Conference Held by the International Economics Association at Tokyo* (New York: Wiley, 1973), pp. 139–61; and Ronald Andersen and Odin W. Anderson, *A Decade of Health Services* (Chicago: University of Chicago Press, 1970), pp. 103–4.

Price Discounts, Provider Selection, and Competition

PPO contracts ordinarily establish a relatively low price for medical care. For example, the Ohio Health Choice Plan of Cleveland offers hospital discounts of 10 to 20 percent, and physician fees are reimbursed using a relative value conversion that amounts to discounts of 10 to 20 percent of average (not 90th percentile) physician charges.[9] The Met-Elect PPO, organized by the Metropolitan Insurance Company for Florida's Dade County School District, has negotiated hospital discounts of between 20 and 25 percent and physician discounts about 23 percent below "reasonable and customary fees," which are presumably the 90th percentile.[10] Many new plans that did not start with provider discounts have provisions for limiting price increases in the future. Note that many of these PPOs have very small market shares and therefore practically no monopsony power. Indeed, many PPOs obtain discounts from physicians and hospitals when they are still in the formation stage and have no membership.

Of course, individual consumers with no insurance or with conventional third-party insurance also would like to purchase care at such low prices. For the most part, PPOs can arrange lower contractual prices than are available to individual consumers. This is the real innovation of the PPO. To the extent that PPOs control utilization, they do nothing new. The question thus arises: How do PPOs, without market power, obtain discounts that individuals cannot?

Information and Incentives.   To answer this question, we must first consider the ordinary state of competition in medical markets in the absence of PPOs. One might think that physicians and hospitals would be very competitive, since there are hundreds of physicians and several hospitals in even a small city. However, two related factors hinder competition: poor consumer information and overly complete third-party health insurance, which removes much consumer incentive to reward competitive providers. Let us take up the information problem

---

9. See Department of Health and Human Services, *The Preferred Provider Organization Study*, Request for Proposal No. RFP–58–84–HHS–OS (Washington, D.C.: DHHS, July 11, 1984), p. C–27.
    10. Ibid., p. C–34.

first, concentrating on physicians. The situation is much the same for hospitals.

Consumers rely heavily on information from friends and relatives for physician referrals. Therefore, consumers do not know much about more than a handful of physicians. There may be excellent low-priced providers in the area, but most consumers simply do not know about them. Now consider the results of this consumer information problem for a physician considering a price cut. The physician has a problem in reaching consumers with the information about his price reduction. His ability to increase the volume of his business by cutting prices is thus limited. Further, since the price cuts will apply to all existing customers, they may not increase total revenue by very much. As a result, physicians must operate somewhat as isolated monopolists. The worse the information problem, the more economically isolated the physicians are from competition. Of course, the isolation is never complete. A great deal of economic evidence refutes the unlikely idea that there is absolutely no competition.[11]

Most third-party health insurance pays a certain percentage of expenditures. In some cases, especially for hospital care, it pays 100 percent. This sort of insurance gives scant incentive for consumers to change physician or hospital in response to a competitive price-cutting decision. For example, suppose that the insurance pays 80 percent of expenses. If so, an actual price difference of $300 means a difference of only $60 in the amount the consumer pays out of pocket. If the consumer prefers the more costly provider only a bit, perhaps because of convenience, he will not respond to the price difference. Of course, the situation is far worse for those with 100 percent insurance coverage. No price difference would induce them to change from a high-priced to a low-priced provider. They would always choose the one they favored—even if only slightly—over any other, regardless of price or cost differences. What is more, this kind of insurance reinforces the information problem. A consumer who cannot reduce his out-of-pocket payment much by careful choice of a competitive provider has little incentive to become informed about such providers. The result is imperfect competition. Providers act on the (correct) assumption that they are somewhat competitively isolated. Thus, even

11. See H. E. Frech III, "Competition in Medical Care: Research and Policy," *Advances in Health Economics and Health Services Research* 5 (1984):1–27.

where there are many providers, prices are set somewhat above the competitive level. This imperfect competition is a natural result of the information and incentive problems in the market and does not depend on collusion of any kind.[12]

The Effect of the PPO. The introduction of a PPO into the market improves both the information and the incentives available to consumers and providers. Consumers now know which providers offer lower prices—the PPO members. That greatly eases the information problem. Moreover, to the extent that the consumer's friends also use PPO providers, he gets better-quality information as well. What is more, the PPO offers built-in incentives for the consumer to use the low-priced PPO providers. In many cases, the coinsurance rate and the deductible—as well as the expected total price—are lower for PPO providers. These incentives are often very powerful. In fact, they can actually be stronger than the incentives to seek out a price-competitive provider in the absence of any insurance.

For example, suppose a PPO physician charges $90 for a procedure, while a non-PPO physician charges $100. Suppose also that the PPO requires no copayment for seeing member physicians, but a 20 percent copayment for out-of-plan physicians. In this case, the consumer's out-of-pocket payment would rise by $20 if he were to use the non-PPO physician rather than the member physician. A completely uninsured patient would save only the $10 difference in fees by choosing the lower-priced physician. One can see that a PPO can establish very strong incentives to use price-competitive providers without being perceived as overly harsh. As a result, both buyers and sellers in the market will become more price sensitive. Indeed, theoretical analysis by David Dranove, Mark Satterthwaite, and Jody Sindelar indicates that, at least for hospitals, price sensitivity may become so acute as to cause prices to become volatile.[13]

Discounting. For the provider, offering competitive discounts to a PPO can be very attractive. The discount information reaches the PPO

12. ibid. See also Mark V. Pauly and Mark A. Satterthwaite, "The Pricing of Primary Care Physicians' Services: A Test of the Role of Consumer Information," *Bell Journal of Economics* 12, no. 2 (Autumn 1981):488–506.

13. David Dranove, Mark Satterthwaite, and Jody Sindelar, "The 'New Competitiveness' in Health Care: Some Implications for Price and Capacity," (Department of Managerial Economics and Decision Sciences, Northwestern University, January 17, 1985). (Unpublished.)

subscribers very efficiently, as the provider is put on the PPO list. Moreover, the provider need not, and generally does not, reduce his prices to his other patients who have traditional third-party insurance. This in itself makes competitive price-cutting to a PPO more attractive than a general price cut. Also, the provider's low prices for PPO members are unlikely to be taken as a signal of low quality, while low prices in general might be.

The provider can often expect a large increase in volume from offering competitive prices to a PPO, because the consumer information problem is so effectively eased. But, even a case in which the PPO is small or includes so many providers that the potential volume increase is small does not constitute a serious drawback for the provider. Since the price reduction applies only to the PPO patients, the cost to the provider (in the form of lower, more competitive prices) is small when the gain (in the form of additional business) is small.[14] That explains why small PPOs with no monopsony power over physicians or hospitals nevertheless succeed in obtaining substantial discounts. In effect, by simultaneously improving incentives and information, PPOs make the market behave in a more competitive manner.

Provider Selection. Some PPOs do not obtain discounts from providers' normal prices. An example would be the Hewlett-Packard El Camino Hospital PPO in northern California. In that case, no discounts were negotiated. However, the hospital had already set prices 25 to 30 percent below the average for the area,[15] providing a price savings as a result of provider selection rather than discounting. Further, some of the price cuts reported as physician discounting are really a result of selection. When a PPO sends out a free list that is below average fees, there are already many physicians whose regular fees would be low enough to qualify, without discounting. Perhaps 20 percent of physicians ordinarily set fees that are 15 percent below

14. The "usual fee" requirements common to the Blue Shield plans are harmful to PPOs and to competition generally. These requirements, sometimes called "most favored nation" clauses, force the provider to give the Blue Shield plan the full benefit of any discounts made to another group, such as a PPO. Obviously, such a clause reduces the provider's incentive to offer selective price discounts. Luckily, it appears that these provisions are rarely enforced.

15. See Department of Health and Human Services, *Preferred Provider Organization Study,* p. C–15.

average. These low-priced physicians are, of course, especially likely to agree to the PPO terms, since they give up nothing at all. Thus, pure selection of low-priced providers is important, and this selection is beneficial to competition as well, even without the extra benefit of discounting.

Consider the provider who faces the choice of charging a high price or a low price for all patients. He is not considering offering a discount only to PPO subscribers. In the absence of the PPO, the low-price strategy for him is fraught with all the information problems discussed above. But if there is a PPO in the market, adoption of the low-price strategy means that the provider can be listed with the PPO. This improves the information flow to his consumers and leads to a larger increase in volume than would have been the case without the PPO. Not only is consumer information improved, but incentives to use the low-priced provider (through penalties for out-of-plan use) are also better than without the PPO. Thus, competitive pricing becomes a more attractive strategy to providers even if the PPO only selects low-priced providers, without attempting to obtain a discount.

Provider selection can affect the quantity of care received as well as the price. PPOs have good reason to select physicians who are less likely to use costly services and hospitalization. Even if a PPO does not purposefully select such conservative physicians, they are likely to be overrepresented on its provider lists. Physicians who practice in a conservative manner would be more comfortable practicing under strict utilization controls than would more aggressive physicians.

The Medicare Experience. The power of improved information to make the market more competitive can be seen in the experience of Medicare physician insurance. Medicare provides information, almost by accident, about which physicians are willing to provide care at competitive prices. Medicare was originally set up to pay physicians 80 percent of their normal market fees, with coinsurance paying the remaining 20 percent. After the program began, the incentives built into traditional third-party health insurance caused such enormous price and utilization increases that the government soon abandoned the idea of paying physicians their ordinary market fees. For the past several years, Medicare has limited physician fee reimbursement to a level about 25 or 30 percent below market fees. To prevent access problems for Medicare consumers, the government has permitted physicians to charge consumers for the difference between the Medicare allowance and the amount of the actual charge (to "balance-bill"). Physicians who choose not to balance-bill accept the Medicare allowance as payment in full for their services. In a confusing misnomer, this practice has come to be called accepting assignment. In effect, Medicare physician insurance has become an indemnity plan, with an allowance about 40 percent below market fees.

The informational advantage of this plan comes from the fact that Medicare is a well-known insurer; therefore, most of the elderly are likely to know exactly what it means to say that a physician usually accepts assignment. This phrase expresses concisely the idea that the physician offers substantial competitive discounts to Medicare patients. As if to underline the point, Medicare has recently started publishing lists of physicians who agree to accept assignment for all Medicare patients. Just as in the case of the PPO, the physician need not cut prices to other patients. As a result, physicians are often surprisingly willing to offer discounts to the elderly accepting assignment. Even though the average discount is about 25 to 30 percent, nationally, more than half of all physicians accept assignment. In Massachusetts, the figure is over 75 percent. Further, the percentage of physicians who discount to Medicare patients differs substantially within states. In general, assignment is much more common in the more competitive urban areas. For example, the assignment rate is 83 percent in Boston, but only 51 percent on rural Cape Cod,[16] which demonstrates not only the informational improvement due to the Medicare program, but also the lack of consumer information that keeps the market price high in areas with little Medicare, especially in cities. The last observation makes sense in light of research by Mark Pauly and Mark Satterthwaite that found that the consumer information problem is worse in larger cities.[17] The mere existence of a well-known scheme that pays less than market prices conveys information so well that competition is noticeably improved.

THE ANTICOMPETITIVE DANGERS

Because they might attain large market shares and because they must become intimately involved in the economics of medicine, PPOs pre-

16. See John Larkin Thompson, "Report Prepared for Presentation to the Advisory Council on Social Security," April 6, 1983.
17. See Pauly and Satterthwaite "The Pricing of Primary Care Physicians' Services."

sent some new dangers to competition, as well as the promise of improving it. There is a possibility that a large and independent PPO might attain monopsony power as a buyer. The opposite danger is that providers might use their own PPO to suppress competition among themselves. Thus, the PPO movement deserves close and continuing scrutiny by state and federal antitrust enforcement agencies.

Monopsony Power of the PPO

Some observers have suggested that the primary way that insurers can obtain discounts is by using their market purchasing power (i.e., their monopsony power) to exploit hospitals and physicians. For example, Mark Pauly notes that a provider is likely to accept a discount if the discounted price is still higher than the provider's marginal cost, and "if patients covered by this insurer represent a non-negligible share of [the provider's] business."[18] As Pauly observes, the only private insurers with a large enough market share to use their power to drive prices down are the Blue Cross hospital insurance and Blue Shield physician insurance plans that were founded by, and are generally controlled by, hospitals and physicians. In fact, there is evidence that the Blue Cross/Blue Shield plans do use their market power to depress prices below market level.[19] So far, the PPOs are far too small to do the same, so this market power explanation of how discounts are obtained must not apply. The only alternative explanation is the one discussed above. The PPO provides information and incentives so that price-cutting becomes a rational competitive strategy for individual providers.

Although not apparently an immediate problem, the danger of individual PPOs becoming so large that they have substantial market power is real. If that were to happen, the PPO that was largest would

18. See Mark V. Pauly, "Taxation, Health Insurance and Market Failure in the Medical Economy," *Journal of Economic Literature* 24, no. 2 (June 1986):629–75. Actually, the monopsonistic insurer can drive the price below the provider's marginal cost by threatening to withdraw a large amount of business.

19. For evidence that high Blue Shield market shares are associated with high physician discounts, see H. E. Frech III, "Monopoly in Health Insurance: The Economics of *Kartell v. Blue Shield of Massachusetts,*" chap. 8 of this volume. For analogous findings on Blue Cross and hospital discounts, see Killard W. Adamache and Frank A. Sloan, "Competition between Non-profit and For-profit Health Insurers," *Journal of Health Economics* 2 (1983):225–43; and Roger Feldman and Warren Greenberg, "The Relation between the Blue Cross Share and the Blue Cross 'Discount' on Hospital Charges," *Journal of Risk and Insurance* 48 (1981): 235–46.

be able to exploit providers the most. Its costs would be lower and it would obtain some cost advantages in the health insurance market. Its market buying power in the health care market would increase its market selling power in the health insurance market, which would in turn increase its monopsony power over providers. Note that, when measured in different health care markets, market *share* in the health insurance market provides the correct measure of market *power* in the health care market. The percentage of the buying market controlled by the insurer is the appropriate measure of its market power over physicians and hospitals. This monopsonistic exploitation analysis describes well what has happened in Massachusetts since physicians lost control of Blue Shield in the early 1970s. Blue Shield insures about 70 percent of the privately insured population and is thus able to extract a discount of about 30 percent from physicians.[20]

The monopsony power of a large PPO may lead to inefficiency as prices are depressed below the competitive level. That would tend to drive physicians out, artifically raising prices to the uninsured and those with other forms of insurance. Of course, such an outcome may be preferable to the status quo, in which physician prices exceed the competitive level. Also, the large PPO monopoly would become a virtual regulator of medical practice, with the ability to encourage or discourage innovations, high-quality practice, efficient geographical distribution, and almost all the details of medical care. Such a private regulatory system would be bad enough if the PPO monopsony regulator were a profit-seeking firm with no strongly held ideology of its own. However, if it were a nonprofit firm with a definite philosophy, it might impose its own narrow ideology on the health care system, with unpleasant and inefficient results. Further, a nonprofit firm is more likely to pursue its ideology because of the nonprofit legal constraint. A nonprofit firm cannot pay its profits directly to owners or controllers. Thus, nonprofit decision-makers will be willing to pursue nonpecuniary goals, including a particular vision of how the health care system should be structured.

The models for such powerful PPOs are the Blue Cross/Blue Shield plans that alone have a significant degree of market power.[21] The

20. See H. E. Frech III, "Monopoly in Health Insurance," this volume.

21. For a review of the evidence on the nonpecuniary goals that Blue Cross/Blue Shield nonprofit insurers have pursued, see H. E. Frech III, "Blue Cross, Blue Shield and Health Care Costs: A Review of the Economic Evidence," in Mark V. Pauly, ed., *National Health*

experience of Massachusetts shows that the preference of the Blue plans for low consumer copayment has led to a wasteful system with the highest overall medical care costs in the nation. Also, until recently, at least, Massachusetts Blue Shield discouraged office-based procedures. For the near future, the only serious danger of PPO monopoly power is the possibility that in some areas the large Blue Cross/ Blue Shield plans might move into the PPO market and dominate it. As in Massachusetts, the most likely ill effect would be their use of PPO discounts to subsidize overly complete insurance (with very small consumer copayment).

Monopoly of the Providers

A PPO signs complex contracts with many, perhaps most, of the providers in a local area. Further, to enforce these contracts, it must monitor the behavior of the providers. Therefore, a PPO under the control of providers is a natural vehicle for suppressing local provider competition, just as Blue Cross/Blue Shield, often under provider control, have done. The recent formation of the Stanislaus County PPO in central California is an especially clear illustration. Organized by the Stanislaus County Medical Society, the PPO quickly recruited 50 percent of the physicians in the city of Modesto and 90 percent of those in nearby Turlock. A key contractual provision of the PPO prohibited member physicians from joining any other PPOs. That made entry by competing PPOs difficult, as was surely the intention. After the Antitrust Division of the U.S. Department of Justice threatened a lawsuit, the Stanislaus PPO agreed to disband.[22] Here again, the most immediate danger is that Blue Cross/Blue Shield organizations that are already controlled by providers may form PPOs and quickly dominate their local markets.

Insurance: What Now, What Later, What Never? (Washington, D.C.: American Enterprise Institute, 1980), pp. 250–63. For empirical confirmation of the connection between large Blue Cross/Blue Shield market shares and high health care costs, see H. E. Frech III and Paul B. Ginsburg, "Competition among Health Insurers," in Warren Greenberg, ed., *Competition in the Health Care Sector: Past, Present and Future* (Germantown, Md.: Aspen Systems Corp./ Federal Trade Commission, 1978), pp. 210–37; and Joel W. Hay and Michael J. Leahy, "Competition among Health Plans: Some Preliminary Evidence," *Southern Economic Journal* 50, no. 3 (January 1985):831–46.

22. Gabel and Ermann, "Preferred Provider Organizations," p. 33.

CONCLUSION

PPOs offer an attractive compromise between the wide choice of provider inherent in the traditional third-party insurer and the cost savings of the HMO. They are successful because they improve consumer information about competing providers and thus make the health care industry more competitive and more efficient. The growth of PPOs does raise the long-run danger of individual or cooperating PPOs becoming too powerful, whether they are independent or controlled by providers. But these problems appear to be manageable. Overall, the emergence of PPOs is a very positive development. They promise greater efficiency, lower cost, and more competition in health care without compromising consumer choice.

SELECTED BIBLIOGRAPHY

Adamache, Killard W., and Frank A. Sloan. "Competition between Non-profit and For-profit Health Insurers." *Journal of Health Economics* 2 (1983):225–43.

American Medical Care and Review Association, *Directory of Preferred Provider Organizations,* 3d ed. Bethesda, Md.: AMCRA, 1984.

Arlen, Roger L. "Preferred Provider Organizations: A History." February 1985. (Unpublished, available from author, University of California, Santa Barbara.)

Barton, David M. "Alternative Institutional Arrangements for Medical Care Insurance." Ph.D. diss., University of Virginia, 1974.

Department of Health and Human Services. *The Preferred Provider Organization Study,* Request for Proposal No. RFP–58–84–HHS–OS. Washington, D.C.: DHHS, July 11, 1984.

Feldman, Roger, and Warren Greenberg. "The Relation between the Blue Cross Share and the Blue Cross 'Discount' on Hospital Charges." *Journal of Risk and Insurance* 48 (1981):235–46.

Frech, H. E. III. "Blue Cross, Blue Shield and Health Care Costs: A Review of the Economic Evidence." In Mark V. Pauly, ed., *National Health Insurance: What Now, What Later, What Never?* pp. 250–63. Washington, D.C.: American Enterprise Institute, 1980.

———. "Competition in Medical Care: Research and Policy." *Advances in Health Economics and Health Services Research* 5 (1984):1–27.

———. "Monopoly in Health Insurance: The Economics of *Kartell v. Blue Shield of Massachusetts.* Chap. 8 of this volume.

371

Frech, H. E. III, and Paul B. Ginsburg. "Imposed Health Insurance in Monopolistic Markets: A Theoretical Analysis." *Economic Inquiry* 13, no. 1 (March 1975):55–70.

Gabel, Jon, and Dan Ermann. "Preferred Provider Organizations: Performance, Problems, and Promise." *Health Affairs* 4, no. 1 (Spring 1985): 24–40.

Goodman, John. "The Changing Market for Health Insurance: Opting Out of the Cost-Plus System," Policy Report No. 118. Dallas, Tex.: National Center for Policy Analysis, September 1985.

Hay, Joel W., and Michael J. Leahy. "Competition among Health Plans: Some Preliminary Evidence." *Southern Economic Journal* 50, no. 3 (January 1985):831–46.

"Industry Report on PPO Development." *Medical Benefits,* 15 July 1985, pp. 8, 10, 11.

Milstein, Arnold, and Joan Trauner. *An Employer's Guide to Preferred Provider Organizations*. Sacramento: California Chamber of Commerce, 1984.

Newhouse, Joseph P., and Charles E. Phelps. "Price and Income Elasticities for Medical Care Services." In Mark Perlman, ed., *The Economics of Health and Medical Care: Proceedings of a Conference Held by the International Economics Association at Tokyo,* pp. 139–61. New York: Wiley, 1973.

Pauly, Mark V. "Taxation, Health Insurance and Market Failure in the Medical Economy." *Journal of Economic Literature* 24, no. 2 (June 1986): 629–75.

Pauly, Mark V., and Mark A. Satterthwaite. "The Pricing of Primary Care Physicians' Services: A Test of the Role of Consumer Information." *Bell Journal of Economics* 12, no. 2 (Autumn 1981):488–506.

Thompson, John Larkin. "Report Prepared for Presentation to the Advisory Council on Social Security." Boston: Blue Shield of Massachusetts, April 6, 1983.

Trauner, Joan B. *Preferred Provider Organizations: The California Experiment,* Institute for Health Policy Studies Monograph. San Francisco: University of California School of Medicine, August 1983.

INDEX

ABOUT THE EDITOR

H.E. Frech III is Professor of Economics at the University of California, Santa Barbara. He received his Ph.D. in economics from UCLA in 1974 and was awarded the U.S. Public Health Service Research Training Fellowship.

Professor Frech's expertise lies in health economics, industrial organization and antitrust economics. He is listed in the second edition of *Who's Who in Economics, Who's Who in the West, Contemporary Authors, Who's Who in California,* and *Who's Who in Western Finance.* In recent years, Professor Frech served as a Consultant to the American Medical Association, the Federal Trade Commission, the Department of Justice, and other organizations.

He has written numerous articles appearing in the *American Economic Review, The American Economist, Bell Journal of Economics, Journal of Economic Issues, Journal of Industrial Economics, Journal of Law and Economics,* and the *Journal of Political Economy.*

ABOUT THE AUTHORS

Paul B. Ginsburg is the Executive Director of the Physician Payment Review Commission, which was created in 1986 to advise the Congress on Medicare payment issues. His chapter herein was written prior to this appointment. Dr. Ginsburg's expertise lies in a wide variety of health care financing issues, including physician payment, hospital payment, health insurance, and alternative delivery systems. Dr. Ginsburg received his Ph.D. in economics from Harvard University in 1971.

From 1984 to 1986, Dr. Ginsburg was a Senior Economist at the Rand Corporation where he led projects on preferred provider organizations (PPOs), Medicare prospective payment of hospitals, physician payment, and cost containment in employment-based health plans. Prior to that, Dr. Ginsburg was Deputy Assistant Director for Income Security and Health at the Congressional Budget Office.

Dr. Ginsburg has authored *Containing Medical Care Costs Through Market Forces* and has co-authored several books including *A Private Health Plan Option Strategy for Medicare*. His numerous articles have appeared in *Economic Inquiry, Health Affairs, Health Care Financing Review, Journal of Health Economics, New England Journal of Medicine,* and *Research in Law and Economics.*

Clark C. Havighurst is William Neal Reynolds Professor of Law at Duke University. He received his J.D. from Northwestern University in 1958.

Professor Havighurst is a member of the Institute of Medicine of the National Academy of Sciences and an adjunct scholar of the American Enterprise Institute. He is currently serving as chairman of the executive and management committees of the *Journal of Health Politics, Policy and Law* and has also served as a consultant and advisor on health policy to the Federal Trade Commission.

Professor Havighurst's scholarly writings include articles on most phases of regulation in the health services industry, the role of competition in the financing and delivery of health care, medical malpractice, and a wide range of antitrust issues arising in the health care field. He is the author of *Deregulating the Health Care Industry* (1982) and *Health Care Law and Policy* (1988). His articles have appeared in major law reviews, *Bulletin of the New York Academy of Medicine*, *Encyclopedia of Bioethics*, *Health Affairs*, *Journal of Health Politics, Policy and Law*, and the *New England Journal of Medicine*.

Constance M. Horgan is currently a Senior Research Associate at Brandeis University, and formerly a Christopher Walker Fellow at the Center for Health Policy at Harvard University's Kennedy School of Government. Dr. Horgan received her Sc.D. in health policy and management from Johns Hopkins University School of Hygiene and Public Health in 1984.

Her research interests include alternative reimbursement mechanisms, differential HMO growth rates in urban markets, organizational changes in HMOs, enrollment of privately-insured populations, and inpatient-outpatient substitution in mental health care.

Dr. Horgan is coauthor of several publications in the area of reimbursement and financing of mental health.

Mark V. Pauly is Professor of Health Care Systems and Public Management at the Wharton School, and professor of economics in the School of Arts and Sciences at the University of Pennsylvania. He is also Executive Director of the Leonard Davis Institute of Health Economics and Robert D. Eilers Professor of Health Care Management and Economics. In 1967, he received his Ph.D. in economics from the University of Virginia.

Dr. Pauly has been elected an active member of the Institute of Medicine of the National Academy of Sciences and serves on the editorial boards of *Public Finance Quarterly, Health Services Research*, and the *Journal of Health Economics*, as well as Advisory Editor of the *Journal of Risk and Uncertainty*. He is also a board member of the Association for Health Services Research and the Hospital Research Foundation, a member of the Health Advisory Board, and a member of the Council on Research and Development of the American Hospital Association.

Dr. Pauly has written several books, among them *Medical Care at Public Expense*, and *Doctors and Their Workshops*, and he has coauthored *Controlling Medicaid Costs: Federalism, Competition and Choice*. His articles have appeared in the *American Economic Review, American Journal of Medicine, Bell Journal of Economics, Inquiry*, and the *Journal of Health Economics*.

Pamela Farley Short has been with the National Center for Health Services Research and Health Care Technology Assessment since 1980. She received her Ph.D. in economics from Yale University in 1984.

Dr. Short has focused her research in the area of health insurance, including gaps in public and private coverage, the connection between insurance and the use of health services, and the factors influencing insurance purchases. The results of her work have appeared in professional and scholarly publications such as *Advances in Health Economics and Health Services Research, Health Affairs, Inquiry*, and the *Journal of Health Economics*.

Jody L. Sindelar is Assistant Professor in the Department of Epidemiology and Public Health at the Yale School of Medicine. She has been appointed to the Institution for Social and Policy Studies at Yale University and is Adjunct Professor at Yale School of Management. She received her Ph.D. in economics from Stanford University in 1980.

Professor Sindelar currently serves on the Board of Directors of the Shirley Frank Foundation Alcoholic Treatment Center in New Haven, Connecticut, and is a Research Affiliate at the Center for Mental Health Services Research at the Yale Psychiatric Institute. She is cofounder and editor of *Medical Economics Group*, a Yale University Institution for Social and Policy Studies working paper series.

Her articles have appeared in *Economic Inquiry, Inquiry, Journal of Management Case Studies, Journal of Political Economy,* and the *Rutgers Law Journal.*

Frank Sloan is Chairman of the Department of Economics and Centennial Professor of Economics at Vanderbilt University. Professor Sloan received his Ph.D. in economics from Harvard University in 1969, and since 1976 has served as Director of the Health Policy Center at the Vanderbilt Institute for Public Policy Studies.

Dr. Sloan is currently studying malpractice reform and has published numerous articles on health care economics in, among others, the *American Economic Review, Bell Journal of Economics,* the *Journal of the American Medical Association,* and the *Quarterly Review of Economics and Business.*

He is coeditor of *Uncompensated Hospital Care: Rights and Responsibilities* and *Cost, Quality, and Equity in Health Care: Rights and Responsibilities.*

Amy K. Taylor is a Senior Economist at the National Center for Health Services Research of the U.S. Department of Health and Human Services. Dr. Taylor received her Ph.D. in economics from Harvard University in 1975, specializing in health economics, econometrics and public finance.

Support for Dr. Taylor's research has come from the National Science Foundation, the Carnegie Corporation and the Johnson Foundation. Her work in the areas of health economics, health policy and health services research has appeared in the *American Journal of Public Health, Econometrics, Industrial Relations, Journal of the American Statistical Association,* and *Public Health Reports.*

Peter Temin is Professor of Economics at the Massachusetts Institute of Technology and Research Associate at the National Bureau of Economic Research. He received his Ph.D. in economics from M.I.T. in 1964.

Professor Temin is the author of *Taking Your Medicine: Drug Regulation in the United States.* In addition, he has published numerous articles that have appeared in scholarly journals such as the *American Economic Review, Bell Journal of Economics, Drugs and Health:*

Economic Issues and Policy Objectives, Journal of Health Economics, Journal of Law and Economics, and the *Journal of Social History.*

Peter Zweifel has been Professor of Economics at the University of Zurich since 1983. He received his Ph.D. in economics from the University of Zurich in 1974 and later served as a research associate for the Center for Economic Research at the Swiss Institute of Technology.

Professor Zweifel specializes in consumer demand in Switzerland, economic models of physician behavior, and insurance in the Swiss health care sector. He is a member of the Federal Commission for Economic Stabilization, and serves on the Board of Editors of the *Journal of Health Economics.*

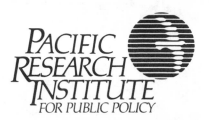

PACIFIC RESEARCH INSTITUTE FOR PUBLIC POLICY

The Pacific Research Institute produces studies that explore long-term solutions to difficult issues of public policy. The Institute seeks to facilitate a more active and enlightened discourse on these issues and to broaden understanding of market processes, government policy, and the rule of law. Through the publication of scholarly books and the sponsorship of conferences, the Institute serves as an established resource for ideas in the continuing public policy debate.

Institute books have been adopted for courses at colleges, universities, and graduate schools nationwide. More than 175 distinguished scholars have worked with the Institute to analyze the premises and consequences of existing public policy and to formulate possible solutions to seemingly intractable problems. Prestigious journals and major media regularly review and comment upon Institute work. In addition, the Board of Advisors consists of internationally recognized scholars, including two Nobel laureates.

The Pacific Research Institute is an independent, tax exempt, 501(c)(3) organization and as such is supported solely by the sale of its books and by the contributions from a wide variety of foundations, corporations, and individuals. This diverse funding base and the Institute's refusal to accept government funds enable it to remain independent.

OTHER STUDIES IN PUBLIC POLICY BY THE PACIFIC RESEARCH INSTITUTE

URBAN TRANSIT
The Private Challenge to Public Transportation
Edited by Charles A. Lave
Foreword by John Meyer

POLITICS, PRICES, AND PETROLEUM
The Political Economy of Energy
By David Glasner
Foreword by Paul W. MacAvoy

RIGHTS AND REGULATION
Ethical, Political, and Economic Issues
Edited by Tibor M. Machan and M. Bruce Johnson
Foreword by Aaron Wildavsky

FUGITIVE INDUSTRY
The Economics and Politics of Deindustrialization
By Richard B. McKenzie
Foreword by Finis Welch

MONEY IN CRISIS
The Federal Reserve, the Economy, and Monetary Reform
Edited by Barry N. Siegel
Foreword by Leland B. Yeager

NATURAL RESOURCES
Bureaucratic Myths and Environmental Management
By Richard Stroup and John Baden
Foreword by William Niskanen

FIREARMS AND VIOLENCE
Issues of Public Policy
Edited by Don B. Kates, Jr.
Foreword by John Kaplan

WATER RIGHTS
Scarce Resource Allocation, Bureaucracy, and the Environment
Edited by Terry L. Anderson
Foreword by Jack Hirshleifer

LOCKING UP THE RANGE
Federal Land Controls and Grazing
By Gary D. Libecap
Foreword by Jonathan R.T. Hughes

THE PUBLIC SCHOOL MONOPOLY
A Critical Analysis of Education and the State in American Society
Edited by Robert B. Everhart
Foreword by Clarence J. Karier

RESOLVING THE HOUSING CRISIS
Government Policy, Demand, Decontrol, and the Public Interest
Edited with an Introduction by M. Bruce Johnson

OFFSHORE LANDS
Oil and Gas Leasing and Conservation on the Outer Continental Shelf
By Walter J. Mead, et al.
Foreword by Stephen L. McDonald

For further information on the Pacific Research Institute's program and a catalog of publications, please contact:

PACIFIC RESEARCH INSTITUTE FOR PUBLIC POLICY
177 Post Street
San Francisco, CA 94108
(415) 989-0833